*Benzodiazepines Divided:*
*A Multidisciplinary Review*

# Benzodiazepines Divided

## A Multidisciplinary Review

edited by

MICHAEL R. TRIMBLE M.R.C.P., F.R.C.Psych.

*Department of Psychological Medicine,*
*National Hospital for Nervous Diseases,*
*Institute of Neurology,*
*Queen Square,*
*London*

A Beecham Symposium

*A Wiley Medical Publication*

JOHN WILEY & SONS

Chichester · New York · Brisbane · Toronto · Singapore

***British Library Cataloguing in Publication Data:***

Benzodiazepines Divided (A Wiley
medical publication)
1. Benzodiazepines — Congresses
I. Trimble, Michael R.
615′.7882 RM666.B42

ISBN 0-471-90199-7

Phototypeset by Dobbie Typesetting Service, Plymouth, Devon
Printed by Pitman Press, Bath, Avon

# List of Contributors


Professor A. Clare, *St. Bartholomew's Hospital, London.*

Dr. J. Cobb, *St. George's Hospital Medical School, Dept of Psychiatry, Jenner Wing, Cranmer Terrace, London.*

Dr. J. Cohn, *P.O. Box 7219, Newport Beach, California 92660, USA.*

Dr. Sandra E. File, *Dept of Pharmacology, The School of Pharmacy, 29/39 Brunswick Square, London.*

Dr. J. A. Gray, *University of Oxford, Dept of Experimental Psychology, South Parks Road, Oxford.*

Professor M. Hamilton, *University of Leeds, 30 Clarendon Road, Leeds.*

Dr. J. Herbert, *Department of Anatomy, University of Cambridge, Downing Street, Cambridge.*

Dr. L. L. Iversen, *MRC Neurochemical Pharmacology Unit, Medical Research Council Centre, Medical School, Hills Road, Cambridge.*

Dr. Susan D. Iversen, *University of Cambridge, Department of Experimental Psychology, Downing Street, Cambridge.*

Dr. D. A. W. Johnson, *Withington Hospital, West Didsbury, Manchester.*

Professor M. Lader, *Institute of Psychiatry, De Crespigny Park, Denmark Hill, London.*

Dr. P. Lascelles, *The National Hospitals for Nervous Diseases, Queen Square, London.*

Dr. M. Linnoila, *Room 48-239, Bldg.10, NIMH, 9000 Rockville Pike, Bethesda, Maryland 20205, USA.*

Professor I. Oswald, *University Department of Psychiatry, Royal Edinburgh Hospital, Morningside Park, Edinburgh.*

Professor A. Richens, *Welsh National School of Medicine, Heath Park, Cardiff, South Wales.*

Dr. A. J. Rose, *5 Sloane Avenue, London, SW3 3JD.*

Professor M. Sandler, *Queen Charlotte's Hospital, Goldhawk Road, London.*

Dr. M. Schmutz, *Ciba-Geigy AG, K-125.14.04, CH-4002 Basel, Switzerland.*

Dr. R. N. Straw, *CNS Diseases Research, The Upjohn Company, Kalamazoo, Michigan 49001, USA.*

Dr. M. Trimble, *The National Hospitals for Nervous Diseases, Queen Square, London.*

Dr. P. Tyrer, *Mapperley Hospital, Porchester Road, Nottingham.*

# Preface

D. H. Tuke (1882), in the closing pages of his *Chapters in the History of the Insane in the British Isles*, commented on the statement of Paracelsus that 'what avails in mania except opening a vein? Then the patient will recover. This is the arcanum. Not camphor, not sage, and marjoram, not clysters, not this, not that, but phlebotomy' by stating: '. . . this treatment of 1841 has been supplanted by the more rational therapies which we witness in 1882.'

Since Tuke's day, various 'modern' rational therapies have been brought into treatment in psychiatry, each with its supporters and opponents. The introduction of insulin coma therapy, convulsive seizures, chlorpromazine and other major tranquillizers, and the antidepressants, have each in their turn been acclaimed as a turning point in treatment, as indeed they were. The same was also true for the benzodiazepines. First marketed in 1960, they seemingly heralded a breakthrough in tranquillizer treatment. Less addictive than the barbiturates, safer in overdose than most psychotropic drugs, and apparently without side effects, their popularity was immense, with both patients and doctors.

One hundred years on from Tuke's comments finds us in almost perpetual debate regarding the efficiency, dangers, and necessity of psychotropic drugs in general, and benzodiazepines in particular. So widely used have these drugs become, that, as some authors in this book point out, few of us escape taking a dose of one of them in the course of a year. As with other remedies however, their widespread acclaim has been met in the fullness of time by disquieting reports about their abuse, our addiction, or our doctor's seduction to 'easy treatment' for the ills of all mankind.

It seems therefore appropriate now, to try to reappraise their use and value —especially in the light of knowledge recently gained at the more fundamental experimental level regarding their mode of action. The discovery of the benzodiazepine receptor, followed by the possibility that the brain itself manufactures an 'endogenous benzodiazepine', and the development of benzodiazepine antagonists, have all led to much renewed research activity with this class of drugs, and leads us further down the path towards a biological understanding of anxiety and the neuroses.

In this book, based on a symposium held in Harrow Weald, London, in late 1982, experts from several disciplines have been brought together to discuss the benzodiazepines from as many different angles as possible. Included are the views of general practitioners and consultant psychiatrists on their clinical use (chapters 5, 6, 16, and 17); the latest data with regard to the side effects and withdrawal symptoms (chapters 2, 22); biochemical and animal data from researchers working both at the level of receptor technology, and with models of anxiety (chapters 7–13); and information on the pharmacology and laboratory measurement of the benzodiazepines (chapters 14, 15).

An attempt has been made to set the social problems of these drugs alongside those of alcohol and nicotine (chapter 1), and non-drug treatments of anxiety are also discussed (chapter 4). Finally, several specific clinical topics are included, reviewing the measurement of anxiety (chapter 3), and the value of benzodiazepines in sleep disorders, depression, epilepsy and alcoholism (chapters 18–21).

The approach has been multidisciplinary, and it has been the editor's intention to bring together workers from different fields, to pool their information, teach each other, and hopefully recognize new challenges that arise from areas of interest adjacent to their own.

> Use three physicians still: first Dr. Quiet
> Next Dr. Merryman: and then Dr. Diet (Salerni *c.* 1484)

This book is about the first of these three.

## Reference

Tuke, D. H. (1882). *Chapters in the History of the Insane in the British Isles*, Kegan, Paul, Trench & Co., London.

# Acknowledgements

Sincere thanks go to those who have most helped coordinate the meeting upon which this book was based. The staff from Beecham Research Laboratories and Marge Zietsman are especially acknowledged for their expert secretarial help and assistance with planning and coordination. Also the Palantype Organization, who worked so industriously throughout the meeting to record all the participants' comments, are to be thanked for providing accurate typescripts of the discussions.

Finally, I am personally grateful to all those who took part in the meeting, and provided chapters for this volume. It is hoped that they will find in it a true reflection of their ideas which were put forward and discussed at the symposium, and that its contents will provide a stimulus for further work in this field.

# Conversion Factors to Molar Units for Benzodiazepines and some Anticonvulsants*

| Drug | Conversion factor |
|---|---|
| Bromazepam | 3.16 |
| Carbamazepine | 4.23 |
| Chlordiazepoxide | 3.34 |
| Clobazam | 3.32 |
| Clonazepam | 3.17 |
| Desmethyl diazepam | 3.69 |
| Diazepam | 3.51 |
| Ethosuccimide | 7.08 |
| Flunitrazepam | 3.19 |
| Flurazepam | 2.58 |
| Ketazolam | 2.71 |
| Lorazepam | 3.11 |
| Nitrazepam | 3.55 |
| Oxazepam | 3.49 |
| Phenobarbitone | 4.31 |
| Phenytoin | 3.96 |
| Primidone | 4.58 |
| Valproic acid | 6.94 |

*Supplied by Dr. Goldberg, Department of Chemical Pathology, Institute of Neurology, London.

# Contents

Benzodiazepines Divided
Edited by M. R. Trimble


# 1

# Benzodiazepines, Alcohol or Nicotine?

ANTHONY W. CLARE

## INTRODUCTION

It is customary these days, at the beginning of a book devoted to such matters as this text, for one of the contributors to utter some comments, ritualistic yet fresh, pungent yet balanced, pointed yet sanguine concerning the use of mind-altering substances in our society. Depending as much upon the author's temperament as on the state of our knowledge, such remarks can take the form of a dire warning that our society is hell-bent on drugging itself into a state of terminal euphoria and malaise, or a reassuring reminder that there has not been a society on this earth since life began which has not experimented with psychotropic substances. The example of alcohol is often held up for our consideration with its history of misuse and use, illustrating the pendular swing between these two positions from prohibitionism and temperance on the one hand to widespread drunkenness and insobriety on the other, a swing which various societies over the centuries have manifested.

Doctors, understandably, see their role as that of detached professionals providing information, psychological, biological and social, concerning such drugs. Yet, very easily, almost imperceptibly, we can slip into the role of moralizer and priest. We possess our fair share of that quality which is the hallmark of many a professional moralizer, namely the ability sturdily to refuse to practise what we preach. If you doubt that, consider for a moment the medical profession's reputation vis-à-vis alcohol abuse (Murray, 1975, 1976) while, simultaneously, we render ourselves vulnerable to the charge that we actually fuel the anxiety that psychotropic substances are used to relieve (Comfort, 1968). In short, if we are not to aggravate matters which many of us may believe to be fairly serious as it is, then we must avoid as far as is possible contaminating our clinical and scientific knowledge with our morality.

The title of this chapter ends with a question mark. The implication is of a weary acceptance that psychotropics will always be with us, so which poison appears to be the most acceptable? Of course, this begs the question whether we need the psychotropics at all. But the choice, if there is to be a choice, is which is it to be—a cigarette, a drink, or a Valium? (Of course, many take all three.) Making it requires a balancing of the indicators of benefit against those of harm.

## TOBACCO

In the light of the long-standing discussion concerning smoking and ill-health, the persistent and increasingly successful campaign against the habit, and the growing public restrictions and private disapproval, it would now appear that the use of tobacco is circumvented by more disadvantages than benefits. It is estimated that in any one year there are 50,000 deaths directly or indirectly associated with its use, the death rate for adults being 250 per 100,000 per year. A leading cancer expert, commenting on the history of the debate concerning smoking and cancer, recently observed that 'in retrospect, it is almost as if Western societies had set out to conduct a vast and fairly well controlled experiment in carcinogenesis bringing about several million deaths and using their own people as the experimental animals' (Cairns, 1978). To continue to smoke now it is insufficient to plead ignorance. As Mishan (1972) remarked:

> If smoking tobacco causes 20,000 deaths a year, no subtracting from the benefits, on account of this risk, need be entered in a cost-benefit analysis of the tobacco industry in as much as smokers are already aware that the tobacco habit is unhealthy . . . the economist has no choice but to assume that they consider themselves better off despite the risks.

At the present time, 42% of males and 37% of females aged 16 and over appear to consider themselves 'better off despite the risks' for they continue to smoke (DHSS, 1982). Doctors might counter by pointing out that some people smoke because they cannot give it up—they are addicted—but that cannot be the whole answer and certainly does not explain the thousands who take up the habit each year. There must be other 'benefits' which, in some people's judgement, outweigh the losses. What might these be?

One explanation may be linked with the fact that it tends to be the richer and better educated section of society who are smoking less than they used to. In contrast the smoking patterns of the less well off have changed relatively little. It has been suggested (Cairns, 1978) that the better-off recognize the advantages that can accrue from extending life into the sixth and seventh decades; after all, it can be a time of maturing dividends and life insurance policies. For the poor, giving up the immediate pleasures of nicotine inhalation for the dubious benefit of extending their lives by 5 or 10 years exercises less of an appeal, particularly in the light of the fact that the personal and social circumstances of the aged poor, even in Britain's welfare state, are far from attractive. The prosperous elderly own their own homes and live on index-linked pensions—the poor can be found congregating in the less salubrious parts of our inner cities and what passes as community facilities for the elderly but which are often little more than geriatric bins.

The influence of age in this discussion is important. Whereas the great majority of smokers begin the habit in their late teens or early twenties, the peak incidence of lung cancer occurs between 50 and 75. The majority of those affected do not pay the price of their youthful indulgence until they have successfully negotiated young adult and middle age, have reared families, carried out careers and virtually completed their working lives. The impact of lung cancer, while serious, wasteful and avoidable, is not as shattering, as antisocial and as personally disruptive as disorders of a chronic and potentially fatal kind which affect individuals earlier in life—such as chronic alcohol abuse.

Another barrier to the elimination of lung cancer, and indeed of the smoking that causes it, is economic. Nicotine is known to cause death not only from chronic bronchitis and heart disease (cigarette smoking doubles the mortality from coronary heart disease (Reid *et al.*, 1976)), and the relationship between smoking and ill-health in general is well accepted. It is possible to estimate fairly accurately what the economic consequences would be if any given percentage of the population stopped smoking. In 1972, the Department of Health and Social Security published a report which included just such a calculation (DHSS, 1972). Not unexpectedly, it showed that a reduction in smoking would increase the gross national product (partly by reducing absence from work and partly by saving lives and therefore increasing the population) and would decrease the amount of chronic respiratory disease and therefore the costs of health care. But, from the government's viewpoint, such gains are only temporary. Leaving aside any consideration of revenue from the tax on tobacco, the gains would be wiped out after about 20 years by the resulting increase in the population who are past retirement age and who, therefore, require social security and more than the average amount of health care but do not generate much income for the state. From that time, the losses will always be greater than the gains. The calculated savings on social security payments and health care that the cigarette apparently brings because it diminishes the number of old people 'is enough to pay many times over for all government sponsored medical research' (Cairns, 1978). In addition, the revenue from the tobacco tax is almost enough to pay for all the salaries and running costs for all the hospitals in the country. Faced with such economic considerations, most governments do not seem benevolent enough to forego revenue in order to support preventive medicine. Rather they have preferred to plough large sums of money into research into the cure of cancer and to encourage the design of a cigarette that is safer but still addictive, and still contains some unique taxable ingredient.

## ALCOHOL

A recent publication by the Office of Health Economics, entitled *Alcohol: Reducing the Harm* (Taylor, 1981), points out that the scale of ethyl alcohol consumption in Britain can be seen to be enormous if compared to, for instance, that of medically legitimated drugs and medicines. The most frequently prescribed group of psychotropics, namely the benzodiazepine tranquillizers, accounted for some 30 million scripts filled in 1979. The cost to the NHS was a little over £30 million. 'In the same year', the OHE report continues, 'the British population drank 40 million proof gallons of spirits, 1500 million gallons of beer and 100 million gallons of wine. This is equivalent to over 17 pints of absolute (pure) alcohol for every individual aged over 15 in the country. The cost to the public was almost £9000 million.'

Table 1 UK consumption of alcohol

| Year | Beer* | Spirits† | Wine‡ | Annual per capita aged 15 + litres of absolute alcohol |
|---|---|---|---|---|
| 1950 | 26 | 10 | 13 | 5.2 |
| 1955 | 25 | 12 | 18 | 5.3 |
| 1960 | 27 | 15 | 27 | 5.8 |
| 1965 | 30 | 18 | 36 | 6.5 |
| 1970 | 34 | 20 | 46 | 7.3 |
| 1974 | 39 | 33 | 83 | 8.9 |
| 1976 | 41 | 36 | 81 | 9.7 |

*Million bulk barrels; †million proof gallons; ‡million gallons.
*Source: Alcohol and Alcoholism*, p.94, Royal College of Psychiatrists, 1979. Reproduced by permission of the Royal College of Psychiatrists.

Between 1950 and 1976, the annual per capita consumption of alcohol rose from 5.2 litres to 9.7 litres per head (Table 1). Such a trend has been accompanied by equally dramatic increases in alcohol-related conditions and problems. Between 1950 and 1977 the numbers of offences for drunkenness rose from 47,717 (14 per 1000) to 108,871 (27.9 per 1000) (Table 2). Cirrhosis deaths per million rose from 23 to 37 between 1950 and 1975 (Table 3), drinking and driving prosecutions over the ten years 1966–1976 from just over 10,000 cases to approximately 60,000 (Figure 1), while the number of premature deaths associated with alcohol use is somewhere in the order of between 5000 and 10,000 per annum (Taylor, 1981). In March 1982 values, the

Table 2 Offences for drunkenness

| Year | No. of offences | No. per 1000 pop. |
|---|---|---|
| 1950 | 47,717 | 14.0 |
| 1955 | 54,210 | 15.8 |
| 1960 | 68,109 | 19.3 |
| 1965 | 72,980 | 19.8 |
| 1970 | 82,374 | 21.6 |
| 1975 | 104,452 | 27.0 |
| 1977 | 108,871 | 27.9 |

*Source:* Annual Home Office Reports, and *Offences of Drunkenness, 1970*, London, HMSO.

Table 3 Cirrhosis deaths

| Year | Total | Death rates per million |
|---|---|---|
| 1950 | 1016 | 23 |
| 1955 | 1159 | 25 |
| 1960 | 1272 | 28 |
| 1965 | 1384 | 29 |
| 1970 | 1387 | 28 |
| 1975 | 1835 | 37 |

*Source:* Registrar General's *Annual Statistical Reviews*, London, HMSO.

total social and health costs of alcoholism to Britain have been estimated as lying somewhere between £698 million and £1064 million (Maynard and Kennan, 1981) but, as an editorial in the *British Journal of Addiction* recently pointed out, 'the costs in suffering which lie behind these figures defy any easy reckoning' (Editorial, 1982).

The problem of arriving at a somewhat more precise estimate of the social and health costs of alcohol abuse is in part due to the wide discrepancies concerning that most basic of statistics, namely the national prevalence of alcohol abuse. In one study, involving England and Wales, the number of problem drinkers, including alcoholics, was estimated by age, social class and country of origin, using information on incidence from Wilkins' (1974) study of alcoholism in a general practice population, and population figures from the 1971 Census (Holtermann and Burchell, 1981). This approach yielded a total of 360,000 problem drinkers. However, given the nature of Wilkins' survey, this was considered to be an underestimate and an alternative upper estimate of 600,000 based upon an alternative approach (quoted in Taylor, 1981) has been advanced. Holtmann and Burchell estimate the annual resource costs of lost output attributable to alcohol misuse to be between £330 and

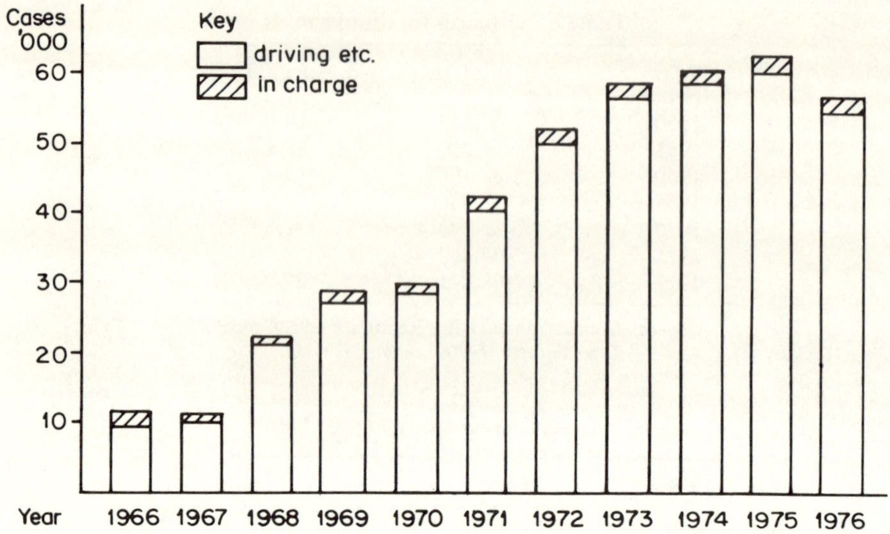


Figure 1 Drinking and driving prosecutions (England and Wales): *Source:* adapted from a figure in the Report of the Departmental Committee on Drinking and Driving (1976) (Blennerhassett Committee) with additional information obtained by personal communication with the DHSS

£540 million at 1977–8 prices and the resource costs incurred by the health and social services to be between £38 and £52 million. The cost to society of road traffic accidents has been extensively studied by the Department of Transport and it has estimated that the cost of such accidents attributable to alcohol misuse was approximately £85 million at 1977–8 prices while the cost of law enforcement was £11 million (Weeden and Burchell, 1982). The total cost, aggregating across cost components and eliminating double-counting because the cost of road traffic accidents includes an allowance for lost output, has been estimated to be between £430 and £650 million at 1977–8 prices depending upon prevalence assumptions (Weeden and Burchell, 1982).

Road traffic accidents are but one measure of the price paid by individuals and society for alcohol misuse and abuse. The other consequences, related to physical health and functioning, marital and family life, work and public order are no less important. Approximately 6–10% of alcoholics commit suicide while Kessel and Granville-Grossman (1961) found the suicide rate of ex-Maudsley inpatient alcoholics to be 75 times that expected. Mortality studies have consistently revealed increased death rates in samples of alcoholics and other heavy drinkers (Bruun *et al.*, 1975) while non-specific gastritis, pancreatitis, peptic ulceration and upper alimentary bleeding are all most commonly seen in those who drink excessively (Cogbill and Song, 1970). The central nervous system bears a particularly heavy brunt with such consequences of long-term heavy drinking as peripheral neuropathy, Wernicke's encephalopathy, Korsakoff's psychosis, epilepsy and dementia (Victor *et al.*, 1971; Ron, 1977). The grim dismal picture of the cost of our failure to drink moderately and in a controlled fashion is systematically documented in the Royal College of Psychiatrists' brief review of the subject (Royal College of Psychiatrists, 1979).

There is considerable controversy concerning the precise relationship, but little disagreement that there is a relationship, between per capita consumption and alcohol-related harm (Bruun *et al.*, 1975; Schmidt, 1977). This has turned attention towards social and political responses to the problem of misuse in addition to clinical approaches. One argument concerns increasing the price of alcohol through taxation, an argument which derives some force from the fact that the relative price of alcohol has actually fallen since the second world war. However, such a suggestion immediately brings medical and social policies into collision with political and economic ones. The Department of Health and Social Security, in a policy statement entitled 'Drinking Sensibly', had this to say on the central question whether taxation is to be used to control the liquor supply:

> Taking account of the economic as well as the health and social considerations, and bearing in mind the practical difficulties involved, the Government cannot accept recommendations that have been made for the systematic use of tax rates as a means of regulating consumption.

There then follows a passage which a *British Journal of Addiction* editorial termed 'so Janus-faced that surely even the wolf must blush' (Editorial, 1982):

> Health and social implications are, however, clearly of great importance and the Government intends within the context of its overall economic strategy to continue to take these into account when changes of duty and wider taxations are considered.
>
> (DHSS, 1981)

What this all amounts to is that while the Government is concerned that alcohol misuse may be costing in excess of £1000 million, it is not that concerned for the very good reason that the estimated figures for consumer expenditure on beer in 1981 are £6361 million and on wine and spirits for the same year, £4983 million. The net tax accruing from that £11,344 million is in the region of £4000 million. Add to the benefits the 70,000 jobs provided by the brewing, distilling and alcohol sales business, and the £1000 million earned in exports, and you may begin to see why the well-founded medical and social arguments in favour of curbing the growth of alcohol consumption do not

Table 4 Real resource costs (estimated 1982 costs)

| | £ million |
|---|---|
| Road accidents | 140 |
| Direct health care costs | 85 |
| Law enforcement | 18 |
| Lower industrial production | 820 |
| Total | 1063 |

Economic benefits (estimated 1981)

| | £ million |
|---|---|
| Taxation | 4000 |
| Exports | 1000 |
| Total | 5000 |

Information derived from Weeden and Burchell (1982) and from Taylor (1981).

quite cut as much ice with our political masters as one might have anticipated (Table 4).

However, whereas alcohol and nicotine are psychotropic drugs readily available to those who wish to use and abuse them, there are psychotropic drugs which can only be obtained on prescription. The abuse and misuse of these drugs are, therefore, much more the responsiblity of doctors than the abuse of alcohol and nicotine ever can be.

## TRANQUILLIZERS

As Paul Williams has pointed out, the last two decades have seen large increases in the number of psychotropic drugs that are prescribed and dispensed each year (Williams, 1981). The scale of the increases are well known and are merely summarized here. In England and Wales, between 1965 and 1970, there was a 19% increase in the prescribing of psychotropic drugs (Parish, 1971). Prescribing of non-barbiturate hypnotics increased by 145%, tranquillizers by 59% and antidepressant prescribing by 83%. The prescribing of barbiturate hypnotics fell by 24% and stimulants and appetite suppressants by 36%. Williams (1981) examined the position for the period 1970–5 and found that, taken as a whole, psychotropic drug prescribing had increased by 8% over the study years, a slower rate of increase than in the previous five years and less than the increase, 15%, in the prescribing of non-psychotropic drugs over the same period. There was a 45% decrease in the prescription of barbiturate hypnotics and a 47% increase in the prescription of non-barbiturate hypnotics. The trends for tranquillizer and antidepressant prescribing were very similar to each other with increases of 28% and 32% respectively. In view of the remarkable fall in barbiturate, appetite suppressant and stimulant prescribing as well as the more publicized rise in non-barbiturate psychotropic drug prescribing, there may well be substance in Fry's claim that 'drug therapy has changed remarkably in content but less remarkably in volume', and that in respect of the total volume of prescriptions for psychotropic drugs in the NHS over the past 30 years 'there has been no great change' (Fry, 1982).

At the present time, it is estimated that about 10% of adults in the UK consume a psychotropic drug during any one year and that about 15% of all prescriptions written by GPs are for psychotropic substances. Similar figures have been obtained from surveys in the United States. The US National Survey of Psychotherapeutic Drug Use reported that about 14% of women and 7.5% of men had used a medically prescribed antianxiety agent one or more times during the year prior to the interview (Mellinger and Balter, 1981). It is important to put these usage figures into a context of social psychotropic use. Approximately 75% of the adult population drink alcohol regularly while 40% are regular smokers. There is some evidence, too, that psychotropic drug use, or more particularly use of tranquillizers, may be falling—certainly the US survey, quoted above, and conducted in 1979, found no evidence of an increase and some signs of the beginning of a fall in the rate of prescribing of these drugs compared with an earlier survey undertaken in 1971.

The use of tranquillizers has been criticized on at least three grounds (Williams and Clare, 1979). First, such prescribing is criticized on clinical grounds. General practitioners, who are the main prescribers, are criticized for prescribing unnecessarily (Dunlop, 1970; Trethowan, 1975), and for using antidepressants and tranquillizers interchangeably (Weissman, 1981). Attention has recently been drawn to the manner in which patients become long-term users of tranquillizers (Mellinger and Balter, 1981) and a study in press revealed that some 20% of patients prescribed a psychotropic for the first time for 3 months were still taking the drugs twelve months later (Murray *et al.*, personal communication). Second, such prescribing is criticized on moral grounds; in the view of one critic, if 'man takes tranquillisers in order to withdraw from universal difficulties which man is born to cope with, this undermines social character' (Parry *et al.*, 1973). Others regard psychotropic drug prescribing as a form of social exploitation (Stoessel, 1973; Waldron, 1977). Third, psychotropic drug use is criticized on financial grounds, attention being drawn to the cost of these drugs, with the implication that the money spent on tranquillizers and related drugs could and would be better spent elsewhere (Tyrer, 1978).

Taking these criticisms in reverse order, financial criticisms seem weak. Williams (1981), in a thoughtful analysis, showed that the total tranquillizer bill for the period 1972–7 was £68.17 million. In 1977, just one of those years, the British spent over £6500 million on beer, wine and spirits. Mellinger and his colleagues have wondered whether patients with psychological distress turn to alcohol when denied psychotropics (Mellinger *et al.*, 1978), a query which led *The Lancet* to wonder about the wisdom of exhortations concerning the reduction of such prescribing given the fact that 'the problems of alcohol abuse are far greater than the mild degree of dependence that may result from abusing the alternatives' (Editorial, 1978). Not all of us are quite so certain that we are concerned with a 'mild degree of dependence' but from the financial perspective at least it is difficult to contest William's view that psychotropic drugs account for a very small proportion of total health expenditure. It is equally difficult to see how the many treatments suggested to replace psychotropic drugs could be provided as cheaply.

The moral objections are more difficult to meet, being based, in part at any rate, on the view that the anxieties and stresses for which many people seek pharmacological relief are more appropriately faced with stoicism and overcome by drawing on personal coping skills and resources and on non-medical supports.

The clinical objections would appear the most substantial. One of the reasons for the popularity of the modern non-barbiturate tranquillizers was the fact that they appeared to be non-addictive and they seemed extremely safe. In contrast with antidepressants, for example, it is quite difficult for patients to kill themselves by taking large doses of benzodiazepine tranquillizers. However, there is growing evidence that benzodiazepine tranquillizers are capable of inducing dependence, and can do so in normal dosages (see chapter 2). While it is difficult to document such a phenomenon save in somewhat atypical groups, for example patients who have been taking such drugs for many years and who are well motivated to stop, the evidence from epidemiological surveys indicating quite substantial numbers of patients taking such drugs in normal and often quite low doses for lengthy periods of time does add support to the argument that the proportion of patients who are dependent may actually be quite high.

Does it matter that patients are regularly consuming such drugs if there is no evidence of escalation of drugs or serious sequelae? At the moment we cannot be sure of the actual and the long-term consequences of such use. Much interest is currently focused on the possible impact of such long-term use on levels of psychomotor performance and efficiency, and a number of researchers have examined the possible role of tranquillizers in road traffic accidents. While it is widely recognized that alcohol is an important factor in such accidents, the role of other psychotropic substances is much less clear. Yet such drugs could be related to road accidents as a result of their effects on driving skills, interaction with other substances, such as alcohol, or their effect on psychiatric ill-health (the latter could of course contribute to a reduction of road accidents). Williams, in a detailed literature review (Williams, unpubl.), found only one controlled study, in which a series of 74 consecutive injured motor vehicle drivers admitted to an Oslo hospital were compared with 204 non-accident drivers attending for routine medical check-ups (Bo *et al.*, 1975). The two groups were compared in terms of blood alcohol and plasma diazepam concentrations. Of the control group 4 (2%) and 3 (1.5%) had detectable levels of diazepam and alcohol respectively. None had detectable levels of both. In contrast, 7 (9.5%) and 31 (42%) of the accident drivers had detectable diazepam and alcohol in the blood, and 8 (10.8%) had both. Of the 7 accident drivers with diazepam only, the plasma concentration exceeded the upper limit of the therapeutic range in 4. The authors concluded that diazepam consumption represented a significant, but in relation to alcohol, a minor causative factor in road accidents.

Skegg and his Oxford colleagues (1979) compared the drugs prescribed for 57 people injured or killed while driving cars, motorcycles or bicycles with those prescribed for 1425 age- and sex-matched controls. They found that 6 (10.5%) of the accident and 36 (2.5%) of the control group had been prescribed sedatives and tranquillizers, yielding a relative risk for accidents while taking these drugs of 5.2. When the analysis was performed for minor tranquillizers only, the relative risk was 4.9. These results suggest that a person taking such drugs is five times more likely to have an accident than one who is not.

But what does this association mean? Whitlock (1979) commented on the cases who were on minor tranquillizers and who had an accident: one was a 52-year-old man who died in a head-on collision with a lorry; Whitlock suggested that he may have been committing suicide. Another was a 37-year-old man who had a long history of heavy drinking but who denied drinking before the accident. However, no blood alcohol estimations were done and alcohol cannot be outruled. A third case was a 58-year-old woman taking Equagesic who was knocked off her bicycle when a car door was opened in front of her—it is quite possible that the state of the man opening the door was more relevant. The fourth case was that of a 50-year-old female diabetic on insulin and a variety of psychotropics who fell off her bicycle. This could have been a transient episode of hypoglycaemia.

Thus, while an association has been demonstrated, it is not possible to say with certainty that there is any causal connection. Summarizing over 20 years of research, Williams (personal communication) regards the return as 'poor' and concludes that 'we are certainly not yet in a position to disentangle the effects of psychotropic drugs on driving from the effects of any underlying illness, psychiatric or physical, for which they may be prescribed'.

However, the fact that, according to a recent longitudinal study of psychotropic drug prescribing published by researchers at the General Practice Research Unit, about one in five patients who begin a new course of psychotropic drug use are still receiving the drugs 6 months later, suggests that we must not be too sanguine concerning the problem (Williams *et al.*, 1982). Certain variables were found to be associated with long-term use, most notably age, a positive history of previous use of such drugs and, for women, the coexistence of marital social difficulties. The results also suggested that long-term use is, not surprisingly, more likely in those with severe psychological symptoms.

## SUMMARY

No psychotropic drug is without its undesirable consequences. Nicotine, or at least tobacco, is currently the most condemned although it is arguable that its social impact is anything like as severe as the currently more tolerated (and abused) alcohol. Alcohol exacts a formidable price in terms of physical and psychological morbidity, social disintegration and economic distortion—its role in the appalling epidemic of road fatalities and mutilations is itself sufficient for us to give pause and consider again the responsibility of the medical profession regarding the raising of the level of public awareness. Tranquillizers are more within the profession's power but if the profession is to influence public attitudes towards such drugs it does need to put their use into perspective. It may well be that simple guidelines concerning their use in acute crises, their dangers when used chronically, the relationship between duration of use and the development of dependence, the clinical indications favouring the prescribing of antidepressants rather than anxiolytics and consideration of practical alternatives to drugs in the management of psychologically distressed patients, would be of more help in reducing inappropriate prescribing and indiscriminate use than fussing about their cost, moralizing over their effects or demanding their prohibition.

## REFERENCES

Bø, O., Haffner, J. F. W., Langald, Ø., Trumpy, J. H., Bredesen, J. E. and Lunde, P. K. M. (1975). Ethanol and diazepam as causative agents in road traffic accidents. In: *Alcohol, Drugs and Traffic Safety*, pp.439–448 (Eds. Israelstam, S. and Lambert, S.), Addiction Research Foundation, Toronto.

Bruun, K., Edwards, G., Lumio, M., Makela, K. *et al.* (1975). *Alcohol Control Policies in Public Health Perspective*, Finnish Foundation for Alcohol Studies, Helsinki.

Cairns, J. (1978). *Cancer, Science and Society*, Freeman & Co., Reading, England.

Cogbill, C. L. and Song, K. T. (1970). Acute pancreatitis. *Arch. Surg.*, **100**, 673–676.

Comfort, A. (1968). *The Anxiety Makers*, Penguin, London.

Dept. of Health and Social Security (1972). *Smoking and Health: A study of the effects of a reduction in cigarette smoking on mortality and morbidity rates, on health care and social security expenditure and on productive potential*, HMSO, London.

Dept. of Health and Social Security (1981). *Prevention and Health: Drinking Sensibly*, HMSO, London.

Dept. of Health and Social Security (1982). *On the State of the Public Health for the year 1980*, HMSO, London.

Dunlop, D. (1970). The use and abuse of psychotropic drugs. *Proc. R. Soc. Med.*, **63**, 1279–1282.

Editorial (1978). Stress, distress and drug treatment. *Lancet*, **ii**, 1347–1348.

Editorial (1982). Cirrhosis as a growth investment opportunity. *Brit. J. Addict.*, **77**, 113–122.

Fry, J. (1982). Psychiatric illness in general practice. In: *Psychiatry and General Practice*, pp.43–47 (Eds. A. W. Clare and M. Lader), Academic Press, London.

Holtermann, S. and Burchell, A. (1981). *The Costs of Alcohol Misuse*, Government Economic Service Working Paper, No. 37, DHSS, London.

Kessel, W. I. N. and Granville-Grossman, K. (1961). Suicide in alcoholics. *Brit. med. J.*, **2**, 1265–1270.

Maynard, A. and Kennan, P. (1981). The economics of alcohol abuse. *Brit. J. Addict.*, **76**, 339–345.

Mellinger, G. D. and Balter, M. B. (1981). Prevalence and patterns of use of psychotherapeutic drugs: results from a 1979 national survey of American adults. In: *Epidemiological Impact of Psychotropic Drugs*, pp.117–135 (Eds. G. Tognoni, C. Bellantuono and M. Lader), Elsevier/North Holland, Amsterdam.

Mellinger, G. D., Balter, M. B., Manheimer, D. I., Cisin, I. H. and Parry, H. J. (1978). Psychic distress, life crisis and use of psychotherapeutic medications. National Drug Survey data. *Arch. gen. Psych.*, **35**, 1045–1052.

Mishan, E. J. (1972). *Cost Benefit Analysis: An Informal Introduction*, Allen and Unwin, London.

Murray, R. M. (1975). Alcoholism and employment. *J. Alcoholism*, **10**, 23–26.

Murray, R. M. (1976). The characteristics and prognosis of alcoholic doctors. *Brit. med. J.*, **2**, 1537–1539.

Parish, P. A. (1971). The prescribing of psychotropic drugs in general practice. *J. R. Coll. gen. Pract.*, **21**, Suppl. 4, 1–77.

Parry, H. J., Balter, M. B., Mellinger, G. D., Sisin, I. H., and Manheimer, D. I. (1973). National patterns of psychotherapeutic drug use. *Arch. gen. Psych.*, **28**, 769–783.

Reid, D. D., Hamilton, P. J. S., McCartney, P., Rose, G., Jarrett, R. J. and Keen, H. (1976). Smoking and other risk factors for coronary heart disease in British civil servants. *Lancet*, **ii**, 979–984.

Ron, M. (1977). Brain damage in chronic alcoholism: a neuropathological, neuroradiological and psychological review. *Psychol. Med.*, **7**, 103–112.

Royal College of Psychiatrists (1979) *Alcohol and Alcoholism*, Tavistock, London.

Schmidt, W. (1977). Cirrhosis and alcohol consumption: an epidemiological perspective. In: *Alcoholism: New Knowledge and New Responses*, pp.15–47 (Eds. G. Edwards and M. Grant), Croom Helm, London.

Skegg, D. C. G., Richards, S. M., and Doll, R. (1979). Minor tranquillisers and road accidents. *Brit. med. J.*, **1**, 917–919.

Stoessell, J. (1973). *Psychopharmaka: die verordnete Anpassung*. Piper & Co., Munchen.

Taylor, D. (1981). *Alcohol: Reducing the Harm*, Office of Health Economics, London.

Trethowan, W. H. (1975). Pills for personal problems. *Brit. med. J.*, **3**, 749–751.

Tyrer, P. (1978). Drug treatment of psychiatric patients in general practice. *Brit. med. J.*, **2**, 1008–1010.

Victor, M., Adams, R. D. and Collins, G. M. (1971). *The Wernicke-Korsckoff Syndrome*, Blackwell, Oxford.

Waldron, I. (1977). Increased prescribing of Valium, Librium and other drugs. *Int. J. Health Serv.*, **1**, 37–62.

Weeden, R. and Burchell, A. (1982). Alcohol and disease: economic aspects. *Brit. med. Bull.*, **38**, 1, 9–11.

Weissman, M. M. (1981). Depression and its treatment in an U.S. urban community. *Arch. gen. Psych.*, **38**, 417–421.

Whitlock, F. A. (1979). Minor tranquillisers and road accidents. *Brit. med. J.*, **2**, 670.

Wilkins, R. W. (1974). *The Hidden Alcoholic in General Practice*, Elite Science, London.

Williams, P. (1981). Trends in the prescribing of psychotropic drugs. In: *The Misuse of Psychotropic Drugs* (Eds. Murray, R., Ghodse, H., Harris, C., Williams, D. and Williams, P.), Gaskell Publications, Royal College of Psychiatrists, London.

Williams, P. and Clare, A. (1979). Management of psychological disorder in general practice. In: *Psychosocial Disorders in General Practice*, pp.133–134 (Eds. P. Williams and A. Clare), Academic Press, London.

Williams, P., Murray, J., and Clare, A. W. (1982). A longitudinal study of psychotropic drug recipients. *Psychol. Med.*, **12**, 201–206.

## DISCUSSION

## CHAIRMAN: DR SUSAN IVERSEN

DR. P. LASCELLES: I am tempted to try to link the benzodiazepines and alcohol through the action, perhaps at the receptor, of the beta-carbolines?

PROFESSOR M. SANDLER: I do not know.

DR. L. L. IVERSEN: I do not know the answer, either. There are bits of evidence that suggest that the end result of benzodiazepine receptor activation and the effects of alcohol, at least as far as inhibitory systems in brain are concerned, may be similar. There are now good neurophysiological data that seem to show that ethanol can prolong the effectiveness of the main inhibitory transmitter substance, GABA, which is also thought to be the final common pathway through which benzodiazepines exert many of their actions. There is no direct interaction between ethanol and benzodiazepine receptors. Nobody has identified an ethanol receptor, if such a thing exists.

DR. P. LASCELLES: But are the beta-carbolines active at the benzodiazepine receptor?

DR. L. L. IVERSEN: Beta-carbolines more directly relate to the benzodiazepine receptor, although even that is not a simple story.

DR. M. TRIMBLE: Are the people who become addicted to alcohol the same ones who become addicted to benzodiazepines? I suppose I am chasing a biochemical link with the addictive link. Do we know anything about the relative addiction of these compounds, and the people that actually take them? That is epidemiological work which I should have thought would have been rather important.

DR. A. CLARE: One of the first papers I ever wrote was of a woman at the Bethlem Royal Hospital who had become dependent on diazepam. She was taking vast quantities of it—around 300 mg or 400 mg a day, and she had previously been dependent on alcohol. Certainly for our purposes we succeeded in showing that the symptoms that she had of withdrawal were, indeed, due to the diazepam. She was a cross-abuser of the most remarkable kind. But she had been helped to abuse by doctors. Indeed the only substance that she abused that doctors had not given her was alcohol. She had had barbiturates and indeed doctors put her on diazepam for anxiety, and she became very dependent on it.

The literature on dependence to diazepam is greatly confused by the issue of cross-dependence. There is certainly a large number of people in whom dependence on diazepam seems to be very well established, but there is the problem that many also have a history of abusing alcohol.

With regard to the numbers, you asked what proportion of people who abuse alcohol abuse diazepam. I do not know. However, it will partly be affected by the medical treatment of alcoholics, which in some places relies very heavily on the use of psychotropics, while in others does not involve them at all.

THE CHAIRMAN: With regard to driving, there have been a number of published studies within the last twelve months indicating that in volunteer subjects benzodiazepines do impair skilled performance in simulated driving tests.

DR. A. CLARE: But the problem with those is that the people who take tranquillizers may be taking them for therapeutic and medical reasons, whereas volunteers are just healthy subjects taking diazepam. You could argue that actually there is a case to be made that diazepam actually reduces road traffic accidents because some of the people in high states of arousal released on the roads without it might be as much of a menace. It is difficult to test this in that kind of experimental situation.

DR. J. COBB: Dr Clare was saying that, whether we like it or not, people are going to take mind-altering drugs, and they are going to take tranquillizers. Therefore, what we need to do in the future is to develop a safe, palatable tranquillizer, perhaps some sort of benzodiazepine that could be sold in liquid form over the bar, which would have a built-in indicator to tell people when they had had too much. I really wanted to ask if that is, in fact, a fair representation of his views.

DR. A. CLARE: Yes, I suppose it is. If you take the three substances, tobacco has turned out to be a disaster, and it is a disaster that apparently we show some general political, social and medical will to correct. If the trends that are being slowly established in the United States and elsewhere continue, then perhaps by the turn of the century that particular epidemic will be under much greater control. Most of my colleagues and I accept that alcohol is inevitably part and parcel of our culture. No one I know would willingly release a substance like alcohol on to the market freely now if we knew what we now know about it.

That, then, leaves us with the psychotropics. I am not for a minute suggesting that they be dispensed like aspirin in a chemist's, although no doubt some might argue that. What I am suggesting is that, given the nature of these drugs, and given what we increasingly know about their side effects, I would suggest that, by paying attention to one or two very simple things, we can do a great deal to modify the undesirable impact of benzodiazepines while accepting some of their obvious benefits.

There are two very simple things that I would suggest. One is that doctors, general practitioners, for example, who prescribe the great bulk of these, are given much clearer instructions concerning their use and abuse. The second is that if patients are going to use these drugs they should be encouraged to use them over the short term and not the long. One of the simplest things you can advise a general practitioner is that if someone, for whom he has prescribed a benzodiazepine to tide them over a crisis, has failed to respond after 2 or 3 weeks, that is not an indication for maintaining the patient on a benzodiazepine. That is an indication for reviewing the situation, and looking then to some of the other treatments which may, indeed, be more costly than benzodiazepines but which offer much less in the way of undesirable side effects.

PROFESSOR M. LADER: I have two very brief points: the first is that tobacco is a disaster; we do not know whether nicotine is. Nicotine in some pure form, like a nasal spray, might be useful.

Second, I agree that, if faced with a choice between continuing alcoholism and long-term benzodiazepine use, it is definitely preferable, on present knowledge, to change that alcoholic into a potential long-term benzodiazepine user.

PROFESSOR M. SANDLER: Some people have been busy dismantling the model of alcoholism based on the concept of a small number who abuse it, trying to rule out the possibility of pharmacogenetic variation or, if you like, individual susceptibility to alcohol as a factor. I do not think it is right to do so. The evidence is pointing the opposite way. If we look, for instance, at the first article in this week's *Lancet* by Peters and his colleagues, they demonstrate a deficit in acetaldehyde dehydrogenase, thus providing a possible basis for some people being more susceptible to the dire effects of ethanol intoxication than others. We ourselves are still working on another aspect of this problem, the possible generator of addictive metabolites. It is well known also that the geographical distribution of alcoholics throughout the world is discontinuous. There is substantial variation: very high in Scotland; very high in Hungary; rather low in certain warmer countries. These are all facts that have to be explained somehow. I would suggest indeed that it may eventually be practicable to pick out the susceptible individual as a public health measure, and warn him that he may be susceptible; this is one possible ploy that we should not neglect.

Benzodiazepines Divided
Edited by M. R. Trimble


# 2

# Benzodiazepine Withdrawal States

MALCOLM LADER

## INTRODUCTION AND DEFINITIONS

Operationally defined terms are the most relevant to the clinical situation and provide a useful basis for the theoretical formulations. The prescribing doctor is concerned with the two major types of drug dependence:

1. *Psychological dependence* is an inference from the drug-seeking behaviour of the patient that the patient makes careful provision to ensure his supply.
2. *Physical dependence* is an inference from the development of a clinically definable syndrome which supervenes on discontinuation of chronic medication.
3. The specific *withdrawal syndrome* is the emergence of a well-defined syndrome with predictable onset, duration, and offset of action containing psychological and bodily symptoms *not previously complained of by the patients*. It can be suppressed by reinstitution of the discontinued medication. Identification of a specific withdrawal syndrome is of crucial importance in establishing the dependence-inducing propensities of a drug.
4. *Tolerance* is an inference from a state in which repetition of the same dose of a drug has progressively less effect, or in which the dose has to be progressively increased to maintain the original pharmacological effect.

## BENZODIAZEPINES

The benzodiazepines are among the most widely used of all prescribed drugs. The benzodiazepines have largely replaced the barbiturates because:

1. they are more effective in alleviating anxiety and stress responses;
2. they have fewer and less severe side effects;
3. they are much safer in overdosage;

4. they induce liver enzymes much less and so do not interact with other drugs; and finally,
5. they are believed to be less liable to induce dependence with subsequent withdrawal states.

However, the abuse potential of the bromides, paraldehyde, chloral, barbiturates and meprobamate was belatedly recognized. Escalation of dosage was noted, tell-tale signs of drug-seeking behaviour were detected, and a characteristic withdrawal syndrome described. The current situation with the benzodiazepines is now reviewed with particular emphasis on withdrawal states.

## Dependence-inducing properties

### *Animal studies*

One method is to implant an indwelling catheter into a vein so that when the animal presses a bar, a bolus of drug-containing solution is injected into the blood stream. Rats will bar-press at a very high rate in order to maintain an input of a powerful dependence-inducing agent such as heroin but less rapidly for barbiturates. The benzodiazepines show low activity in this model.

A definite withdrawal syndrome can be recognized on discontinuation of benzodiazepines and they can also be cross-substituted in animals previously rendered dependent on other drugs (Deneau and Weiss, 1968).

### *Human studies*

Hundreds of papers have reported cases of dependence on the benzodiazepines. This literature has been comprehensively reviewed by Marks (1978), and by Greenblatt and Shader (1978), Palmer (1978), Jepsen and Haastrup (1979), and Petursson and Lader (1981a); Maletzky and Klotter (1976) have reviewed the literature on the dependence potential of diazepam. Marks (1978) estimated that just over a hundred of these publications contained authenticated cases of physical dependence with a definite withdrawal syndrome or carefully documented cases of psychological dependence. The cases collected by Marks fell into two categories:

1. those within the context of the 'drug scene' with evidence of multiple drug abuse or alcoholism;
2. those occurring in a therapeutic situation.

### *Multiple drug abuse with high doses*

Marks collected 151 case worldwide of benzodiazepine dependence within the framework of multiple drug abuse or alcoholism, plus 250 less definite cases.

In most cases excessive doses of benzodiazepines were used. A few individuals stayed within the therapeutically recommended doses for several years. The duration of use varied from a few months to a few years.

*Clinical dependence*

Cases of benzodiazepine dependence reported to have arisen solely within the therapeutic situation, and in which other forms of drug dependence played no major contributory role, comprise only a few of the cases reported in the literature.

*High doses.* Several reports indicate that in patients on 2–5 times therapeutic doses, physical dependence can develop within 2–3 weeks (Woody *et al.*, 1975), and certainly within 4 months (Hayashki *et al.*, 1974). In most cases, however, the drugs have been taken for much longer, usually a few years.

In one study (Hollister *et al.*, 1961), psychiatric inpatients were given chlordiazepoxide, 100–600 mg daily for 1–7 months. Eleven patients were changed abruptly to placebo. Ten of the 11 patients reported new symptoms or developed new signs. Psychoses were aggravated in five patients, insomnia and agitation supervened in five, and four lost their appetite. Two patients had major epileptiform convulsions on the seventh and eighth days following discontinuation.

*Therapeutic doses.* Studies of benzodiazepine withdrawal following ingestion of therapeutic doses have been few. Covi and his associates (1969, 1973) abruptly stopped chlordiazepoxide treatment, 45 mg daily for 20 weeks, and described a mild abstinence syndrome, consisting mainly of subjective feelings of anxiety and tension as well as minor symptoms, such as trembling, poor appetite, and faintness or dizziness.

Further confirmation of normal dose dependence comes from a recent study by Tyrer *et al.* (1981). Forty patients who had taken lorazepam or diazepam alone in regular dosage for a mean period of 3.6 years had their benzodiazepines replaced by propranolol or placebo for 2 weeks under double-blind conditions. Depending on the criteria for the definition of an abstinence syndrome, 27–45% of the patients had withdrawal symptoms during the study. Propranolol did not affect the incidence of withdrawal symptoms but reduced their severity. The rate of fall in plasma drug levels was significantly greater in those patients who experienced withdrawal symptoms.

Khan *et al.* (1980) studied eight cases of benzodiazepine withdrawal syndromes in a general psychiatric hospital. All the patients had been taking therapeutic doses for periods ranging from 4 weeks to 10 years. The patients, two men and six women, were all keen to stop the drugs and some had previously attempted withdrawal unsuccessfully on their own.

Several case have been described recently of withdrawal symptoms, including seizures, from short-term and long-term lorazepam treatment. Haselrud and Heskestad (1981) have reported withdrawal reactions to therapeutically administered flunitrazepam in four patients, two of whom experienced psychotic episodes.

## Personal studies

### *Pilot study*

In our first study (Hallstrom and Lader, 1981), we compared the findings associated with the gradual discontinuation of medication in patients who had taken high doses of benzodiazepines with those in patients on a normal dose. The ten patients studied had asked for help in stopping their benzodiazepine medication and gave informed consent to clinical and electrophysiological studies. During an initial period of at least 10 days' observation and acclimatization to the ward for the inpatients or three outpatient sessions at weekly intervals for the two outpatients, benzodiazepines were administered in the dosages which the patients claimed they were taking. Following this period the medication was gradually reduced over a period of 10 days to 7 weeks, as the clinical condition permitted. The patients were tested at predetermined intervals corresponding to full dose of benzodiazepines, and then 75%, 50%, 25% of the initial dose and immediately on termination. They were then studied at approximately 5, 10, 15, and 30 days after stopping medication and at follow-up when they had resumed their normal life. On each occasion, the subjects were evaluated on a battery of tests in the morning, 12 hours after the last dose of drug. Random urine specimens were taken to exclude the taking of other drugs by the patients.

The high dose group ($n = 4$) took an average dose of 135 mg diazepam (or diazepam equivalent) per day (range 80–200 mg). The low dose group ($n = 6$) took an average of 20 mg per day (range 8–30 mg). The peak plasma concentration for the high dose group was 4126 ng/ml diazepam equivalents, (s.d. 3138 ng/ml) and the mean for the low dose group was 778 ng/ml (s.d. 351 ng/ml). Ten days after stopping medication both groups still had detectable amounts of drugs in their plasma.

The Hamilton Anxiety Ratings of symptoms were low before reduction of the drug but increased markedly after the drug was stopped. The pattern of the curves was similar in both groups but the low dose group had a higher and later peak in symptoms than the high dose group. The exacerbation resolved slowly over 2–4 weeks. However, other symptoms not typical of anxiety were also reported and are listed in Table 1.

The main implication of the study was that the subjective and objective changes on discontinuing benzodiazepine medication were much the same in

Table 1 Main symptoms and numbers of patients experiencing them (pilot study)

| Symptom | No. of patients |
|---|---|
| Anxiety | 9 |
| Sleep disturbance | 7 |
| Intolerance to bright light and loud noise | 6 |
| Unsteady gait | 5 |
| Numb feelings/tingling feelings | 4 |
| Muscle pains | 4 |
| Loss of appetite/nausea | 4 |
| Pressure on face | 3 |
| Aggressive feelings | 3 |
| Depression | 3 |
| Weakness | 3 |
| Sore eyes | 2 |
| Hallucinations, illusions, paranoid ideas | 2 |
| Fits | 1 |

quality and quantity in high and low dose subjects. As some of these symptoms were not typical of a recrudescence of anxiety and tended to remit in time, they must be considered as a possible true withdrawal syndrome. To look at this in more detail, we mounted a double-blind study of withdrawal (for preliminary data, see Petursson and Lader, 1981b). Twenty-two patients were studied, their psychiatric diagnoses being anxiety neurosis, depression or

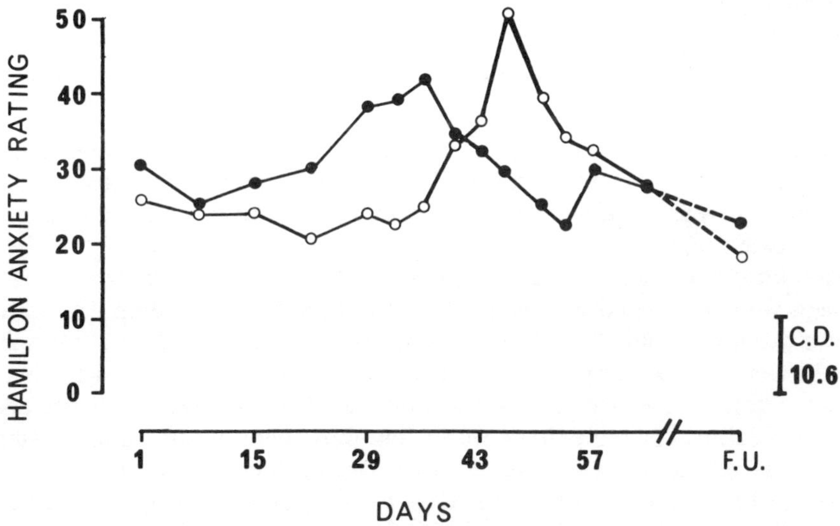


Figure 1 Mean Hamilton Anxiety Ratings in group A patients (●—●) and group B patients (○—○). C.D. represents the 0.05 critical difference: means further apart than this statistic are significantly different at the 0.05 probability level or beyond. F.U. = follow-up

Table 2 Withdrawal symptoms and numbers of patients ($n = 22$) experiencing them 0–2; 2–4 weeks post-withdrawal and at follow-up

| Symptoms | 0–2 weeks | 2–4 weeks | Follow-up |
|---|---|---|---|
| Anxiety, tension | 22 | 11 | 5 |
| Agitation, restlessness | 9 | 5 | 0 |
| Irritability | 9 | 2 | 0 |
| Lack of energy | 7 | 0 | 1 |
| Impaired memory and concentration | 7 | 1 | 0 |
| Depression | 5 | 7 | 1 |
| Depersonalization, derealization | 5 | 1 | 0 |
| Sleep disturbance | 20 | 7 | 2 |
| Loss of appetite | 15 | 3 | 0 |
| Headache | 12 | 2 | 0 |
| Muscle pains, aches, twitchings | 11 | 2 | 1 |
| Nausea, dry retching | 10 | 1 | 1 |
| Tremor, shakiness | 10 | 1 | 0 |
| Perspiration | 9 | 1 | 0 |
| Other bodily symptoms | 8 | 1 | 0 |
| Metallic taste, hyperosmia | 14 | 2 | 0 |
| Paraesthesia | 14 | 4 | 0 |
| Sore eyes, photophobia | 13 | 5 | 0 |
| Incoordination, vertigo | 11 | 4 | 0 |
| Hyperacusis | 9 | 2 | 0 |
| 'Flu-like' illness | 9 | 0 | 1 |
| Hypersensitivity to touch, pain | 4 | 1 | 0 |
| Paranoid reaction | 3 | 1 | 0 |
| Visual hallucinations | 1 | 0 | 0 |

personality disorder with anxiety, and none was alcoholic or took other drugs. They had all received benzodiazepines in therapeutic doses for at least one year (range: 1–16 years). Seventeen were on diazepam (mean daily dose 17 mg, range: 10–30 mg).

The withdrawal was gradual, double-blind and placebo-controlled. The patients were recruited over a period of one year, and were randomly allocated to two groups (A and B). Both groups continued with their drugs, full dose, for the first 2 weeks; group A was then reduced to half dose for a further 2 weeks, before the medication was discontinued. Group B received the full dose of their medication for the first 4 weeks, but were then withdrawn in the same manner as group A, i.e., 2 weeks later. During these phases placebo was substituted for the active drugs, and after withdrawal of the drugs both groups continued on placebo only for 4 and 2 weeks respectively, followed by 2 weeks without any tablets or capsules. In the course of the study period which lasted 10 weeks, patients were assessed at regular intervals of 3, 4 or 7 days on a battery of clinical, physiological, and psychological variables.

Plasma concentrations of benzodiazepines fell steadily in both groups with a 2-week delay in group B. Concentrations were undetectable by 3–4 weeks after final discontinuation.

All the patients experienced some form of withdrawal reaction which was most pronounced 3–7 days after stopping the medication. Anxiety rose sharply during the withdrawal, and to a point of panic in several patients, but usually subsided to prewithdrawal levels over the next 2–4 weeks.

Figure 1 depicts the Hamilton Anxiety Ratings. Anxiety symptoms were mild before dosage reduction but rose to a peak 3–7 days after stopping the medication ($F_{9,12}$ = 8.51; $P<0.001$). These high anxiety levels gradually resolved over the next 2–4 weeks. Self-ratings showed a pattern of withdrawal effects in each case with symptoms of anxiety, agitation, shaking, trembling, palpitations, nausea or sickness, and muscular tension. Table 2 lists the main symptoms elicited at interview and the number of patients complaining of them 0–2 and 2–4 weeks postwithdrawal, and at follow-up 12 weeks later. The symptoms have been assigned to three categories—psychological symptoms of anxiety, somatic symptoms of anxiety, and perceptual changes. The last are untypical of anxiety, and, together with the time course of the other symptoms, suggest that a true withdrawal syndrome is experienced and not merely a return of the original anxiety.

Fast-wave (13.5–26 Hz) activity in the EEG is characteristically increased by benzodiazepines. Control data were available for this and other physiological

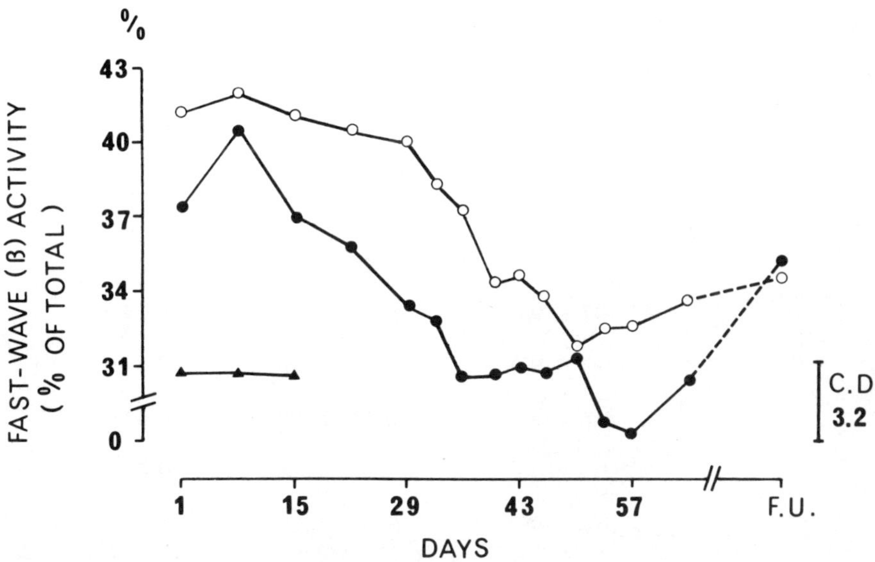


Figure 2 Mean fast-wave (13.5–26 Hz) EEG activity (expressed as a percentage of total) in control subjects (▲—▲), group A (●—●) and group B (○—○) patients. C.D., critical difference; F.U., follow-up

measures from a group of 14 drug-free healthy individuals (mean age 35) tested on three successive weekly occasions. Fast-wave activity is initially markedly above normal (Figure 2), and on withdrawal, a marked decrease occurs from mean values of over 40% (fast-wave activity as a percentage of total EEG activity) to almost 30%. Similar drug withdrawal effects were seen in the 4–7.5 Hz waveband of the EEG, some components of the averaged auditory-evoked response of the EEG, and skin conductance level and fluctuations. Indeed, some evidence for a 'rebound' effect is apparent in some of these variables (e.g. Figure 2).

### *Biochemical measures*

Biochemical measures were taken in a subgroup of seven patients (four males, three females) withdrawing from benzodiazepines in the manner described earlier. Six 24-hour urine samples were collected for each of the patients and assayed for the following by Dr. P. A. Bond and Dr. B. Smith:

1. MOPEG glucuronide and sulphate (Bond and Howlett, 1974). This is a glycol metabolite of noradrenaline.

Table 3 MOPEG levels in 24-hour urines during chronic benzodiazepine treatment and withdrawal (means + s.e.m.). Data in parenthesis express results in percentages of the control values

| Day | ng/ml | mg/24-h | mg/g creatinine |
|---|---|---|---|
| | | Controls ($n$ = 5) | |
| 1 | 1058 ± 228 | 1.28 ± 0.24 | 0.87 ± 0.15 |
| 8 | 1320 ± 361 | 1.64 ± 0.31 | 1.09 ± 0.14 |
| 15 | 1628 ± 587 | 1.62 ± 0.36 | 1.09 ± 0.25 |
| Mean ± s.e.m. | 1336 ± 249 | 1.51 ± 0.18 | 1.02 ± 0.11 |
| (%) | (100) | (100) | (100) |
| | | Patients ($n$ = 7) | |
| 7 | 447 ± 95† | 0.68 ± 0.15† | 0.54 ± 0.14* |
| | (33) | (46) | (53) |
| 14 | 395 ± 93† | 0.66 ± 0.16† | 0.51 ± 0.11† |
| | (30) | (44) | (50) |
| 28 | 486 ± 193* | 0.73 ± 0.25* | 0.42 ± 0.11† |
| | (36) | (49) | (41) |
| 31 | 365 ± 89‘ | 0.58 ± 0.14‡ | 0.41 ± 0.09‡ |
| | (27) | (39) | (40) |
| 35 | 514 ± 109† | (0.98 ± 0.25) | 0.60 ± 0.16* |
| | (38) | (66) | (59) |
| 49 | 614 ± 121* | 1.05 ± 0.25 | 0.65 ± 0.16 |
| | (46) | (71) | (64) |

Differences from controls: *$P$0.05; †$P$0.01; ‡$P$0.001.

2. 5-HIAA. This is the main metabolite of 5-HT (serotonin).
3. free cortisol concentrations.

In addition, five healthy drug-free subjects acted as controls.

*Results.* Urine volume and creatinine content remained fairly constant over the withdrawal period, although patients' urine volumes were above normal. MOPEG excretion was greatly reduced below normal prior to benzodiazepine withdrawal, with levels gradually rising after the drug discontinuation. When expressed as ng/ml, MOPEG concentrations never exceeded 50% of control values (Table 3). However, expressed as ng MOPEG/24 hours, values on days 35 and 49 are not significantly different from normal.

5-HIAA, free cortisol and cortisol/creatinine ratio were not different from normal at any time. The rise in MOPEG levels was not due to the general stress of withdrawal as initially they were abnormally low and cortisol levels were never high.

## TOLERANCE

Tolerance is a complex phenomenon generally seen as a waning of drug effect over time or as an increment in dosage to maintain the drug effect. It can be pharmacokinetic with alterations in drug metabolism or pharmacodynamic with tissue tolerance at the effector site such as the receptor complex. In a previous study (Lader *et al.*, 1980), tolerance to some effects of clorazepate was demonstrated in normal subjects after 2 weeks of once-daily administration. Also tolerance is seen clinically, anxious patients commencing benzodiazepines reporting that the initial drowsiness wanes over a few days. Tolerance on long-term use has not been much studied so we investigated it using a 'probe' injection of diazepam.

In this study, eight male patients withdrawing from benzodiazepines were compared with eight healthy male controls. The patients were tested:

1. during the first 2 weeks while on their full dose of benzodiazepine;
2. 4 days after complete benzodiazepine withdrawal;
3. 21 days after withdrawal.

Controls were tested once.

Following an overnight fast the subject attended the laboratory and some physiological variables were continuously monitored. An intravenous cannula was inserted and an hour later 10 mg of diazepam/75 kg body weight was injected over 5 minutes. Recordings were carried out and blood samples taken over the next two hours.

Plasma benzodiazepine receptor binding activity in the two groups is shown in Figure 3. On the first occasion, plasma drug levels were significantly higher

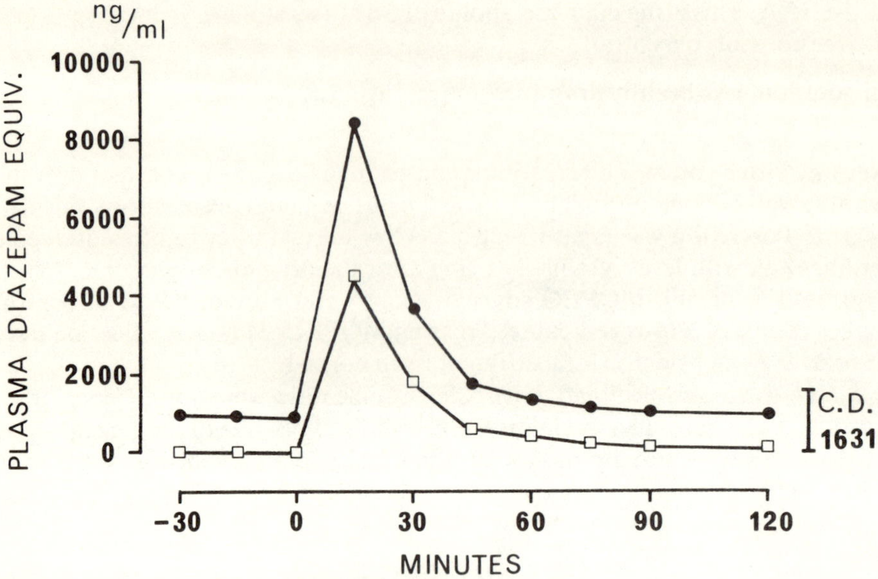


Figure 3 Mean plasma benzodiazepine concentrations in patients on long-term benzodiazepines (●—●) and drug-free controls (□—□) before, during and after an intravenous injection of diazepam. C.D., critical difference

in the patients, 15 minutes after the injection. By 21 days after withdrawal, the peak post-injection level in the patients had approximated to normal values. The enhanced levels in patients while on their benzodiazepine presumably reflects the saturation of a tissue compartment with the drug, hindering the passage out of the plasma.

EEG fast-wave activity was significantly higher in the patients on drugs than in control subjects (Figure 4). After withdrawal, fast-wave activity decreased but had still not reached normal values 21 days after drug cessation (Figure 5). A clear 'ceiling effect' is apparent in response to the diazepam challenge: the EEG fast-wave activity increases to the same point after the injection but this represents a major restoration of activity after withdrawal as the baseline drops.

Subjective tolerance was also found. Both patients and controls experienced a mild and brief episode of euphoria within 5 minutes of the diazepam injection. Thereafter, the controls felt drowsy and sedated whereas the patients, although prior to the injection somewhat less alert, showed no such change (Figure 6). After withdrawal, the patients showed a significant increase in sedation after the injection.

Diazepam is known to produce a release of growth hormone into the plasma and this was very evident in our control subjects (Figure 7). By contrast, the

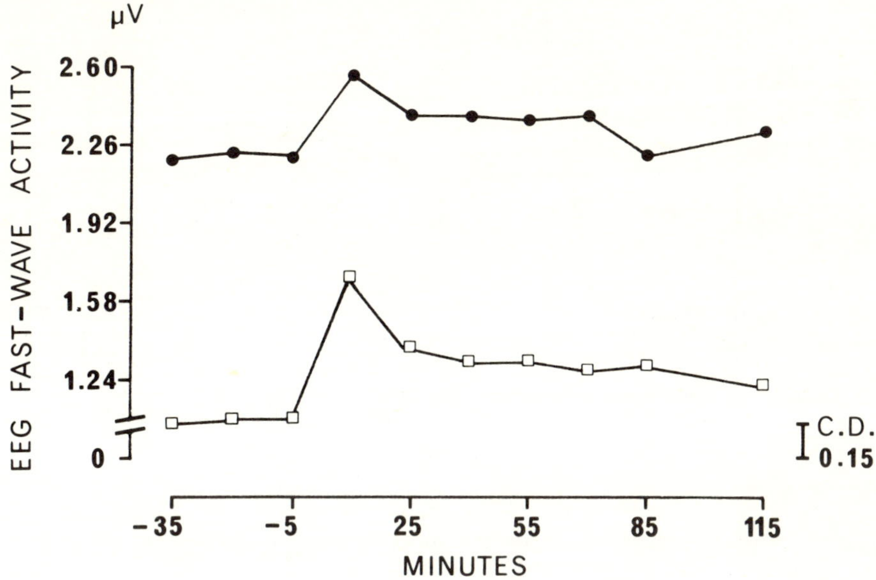


Figure 4 Mean EEG fast-wave activity (μV) in patients and controls. Symbols as in Figure 3

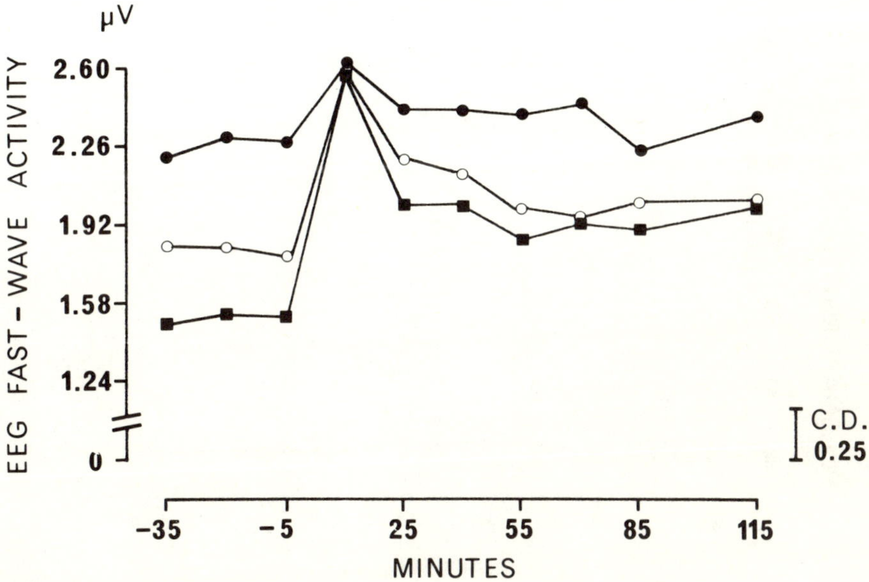


Figure 5 Mean EEG fast-wave activity (μV) in patients prior to withdrawal (●—●), 4 days (○—○) and 21 days (■—■) after discontinuation of long-term benzodiazepines. C.D., critical difference

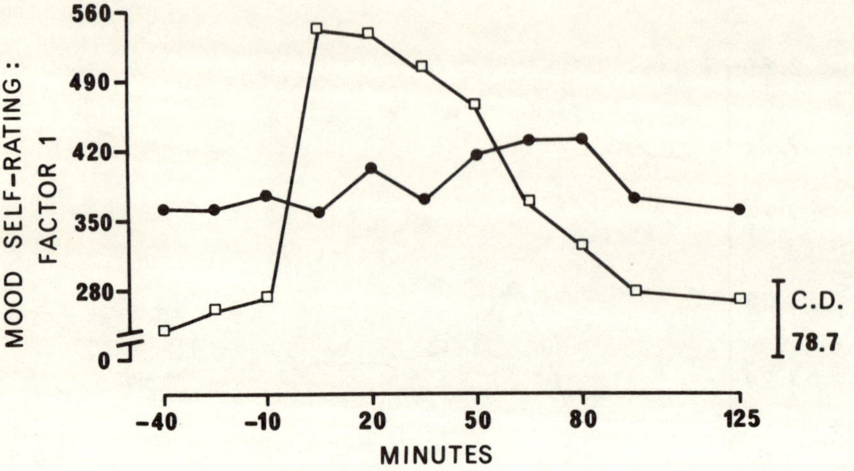


Figure 6 Mean self-ratings of mood (factor 1: alertness–drowsiness) in patients and controls. Symbols as in Figure 3

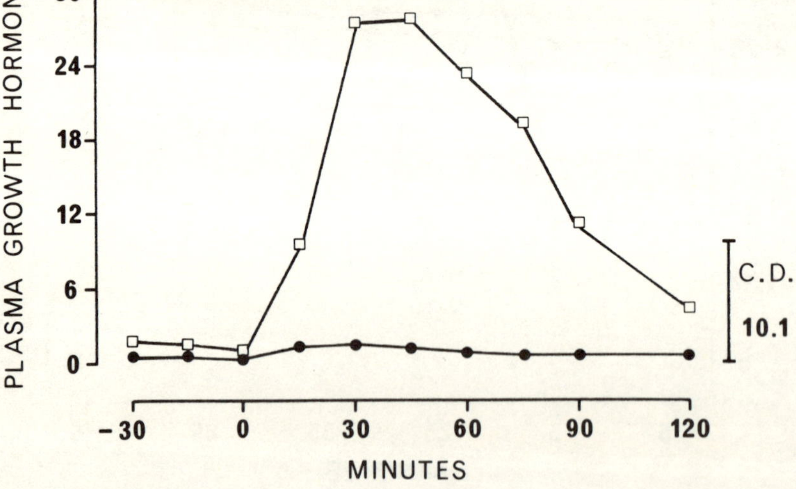


Figure 7 Mean plasma growth hormone concentrations in patients and controls. Symbols as in Figure 3

patients on benzodiazepines showed almost total tolerance. After withdrawal, growth hormones reappeared. Prolactin levels showed no clear patterns.

## Comment

Our definitions of withdrawal syndromes need refinement. Three components must be separated. Many psychotropic drugs have autonomic side effects and withdrawal is followed by a peripheral rebound. Similar effects are seen with many other classes of drugs, for example, the $\beta$-adrenoceptor antagonists. A second rebound is seen with central effects. Both stimulant and depressant drugs on withdrawal are associated with phenomena which are the reverse of the therapeutic action; oversedation follows stimulant withdrawal, anxiety and insomnia follow sedative withdrawal. But with some psychotropic drugs, especially the sedative/hypnotic/tranquillizers including alcohol, the barbiturates and the benzodiazepines, specific symptoms are seen on withdrawal which cannot be interpreted as either rebound peripheral or rebound central phenomena nor as a recrudescence of the original symptoms for which the depressant drug was initially prescribed. In particular, perceptual symptoms supervene in every modality. This constitutes a drug-specific withdrawal syndrome.

A second point concerns the relationship between tolerance and dependence. It has been implied if not overtly stated that tolerance is a prerequisite of dependence. Almost all theories of dependence rely on mechanisms of tolerance whether this is hypothesized to involve intracellular mechanisms, cell membranes, receptors, neurotransmitter synthesis, storage or release. Our demonstration of widespread normal dose dependence without evidence of clinical tolerance suggests that two types of physical dependence should be distinguished—high dose dependence with tolerance and low dose dependence supervening on chronic usage. Even so, the clinical situation is far from settled: our tolerance data shows a complex pattern with some variables showing tolerance, others continuing to be responsive to the test dose of diazepam.

The liability to benzodiazepine dependence is greater than hitherto suspected. For example, Kemper *et al.* (1980) analysed the case notes of all inpatients at the Psychiatric Clinic, Göttingen, for a 3-year period (1977–80). This showed that for this short period alone, many more patients had been admitted to their clinic because of benzodiazepine dependence than Marks (1978) found that for the years 1960–77 for the whole of the Federal Republic of Germany. While in previous years secondary benzodiazepine dependence ('switchers from bottle to pill') was most frequent, among the admissions in recent years a growing number of patients had never before taken addictive agents other than benzodiazepines (primary dependence).

The second implication arising directly from our work, and that of Tyrer, is that normal dose dependence can and does occur frequently, especially in patients taking benzodiazepines for several months or more. Non-escalation of dosage is no longer an indication that dependence has not occurred. The only marker we have left is the onset of the specific withdrawal syndrome on discontinuation of the drug. A rough estimate from Tyrer's figures and from the known usage of tranquillizers (Balter *et al.*, 1974) would be that 200,000 people in the UK would experience withdrawal symptoms if they tried to stop their benzodiazepines. In some these symptoms would be major and/or persistent.

## REFERENCES

Balter, M. B., Levine, J. and Manheimer, D. I. (1974). Cross-national study of the extent of anti-anxiety/sedative drug use. *New Engl. J. Med.*, **290**, 769–774.

Bond, P. A. and Howlett, D. R. (1974). Measurement of the two conjugates of 3-methoxy-4-hydroxyphenylglycol in urine. *Biochem. Med.*, **10**, 219–228.

Covi, L., Lipman, R. S., Pattison, J. H., Derogatis, L. R. and Uhlenhuth, E. H. (1973). Length of treatment with anxiolytic sedatives and response to their sudden withdrawal. *Acta psychiat. scand.*, **49**, 51–64.

Covi, L., Park, L. C., Lipman, R. S., Uhlenhuth, E. H. and Rickels, K. (1969). Factors affecting withdrawal response to certain minor tranquillizers. In *Drug abuse: Social and Psychopharmacological Aspects*, pp.93–108 (Eds. Cole, J. O., and Wittenborn, J. R.), pp.93–108, Thomas, Springfield, Illinois.

Deneau, G. A. and Weiss, S. (1968). A substitution technique for determining barbiturate-like physiological dependence capacity in the dog. *Pharmacopsychiatrie, Neuro-psychopharmakologie*, **1**, 270–275.

Greenblatt, D. J. and Shader, R. I. (1978). Dependence, tolerance and addiction to benzodiazepines: clinical and pharmacokinetic considerations. *Drug Met. Rev.*, **8**, 13–28.

Hallstrom, C. and Lader, M. H. (1981). Benzodiazepine withdrawal phenomena. *Int. Pharmacopsychiatry*, **16**, 235–244.

Haselrud, J. and Heskestad, S. (1981). Abstinens og forvirringsreaksjoner etter Rohypnol-bruk. *Tidsskrift for den Norske Laegeforening*, **101**, 112.

Hayashki, T., Higashki, T. and Kadota, K. (1974). Three cases of chronic chlordiazepoxide intoxication and their withdrawal symptoms. *Clin. Psychiat.*, **16**, 77–83.

Hollister, L. E., Motzenbecker, F. P. and Degan, R. O. (1961). Withdrawal reactions from chlordiazepoxide ('Librium'). *Psychopharmacologia*, **2**, 63–68.

Jepsen, P. W. and Haastrup, S. (1979). Abstinensreaktioner efter benzodiazepines. *Ugeskrift for Laeger*, **141**, 1121–1125.

Kemper, N., Poser, W. and Poser, S. (1980). Benzodiazepin-Abhängigkeit. *Deutsche Medizinische Wochenschrift*, **105**, 1707–1712.

Khan, A., Joyce, P. and Jones, A. V. (1980). Benzodiazepine withdrawal syndromes. *N.Z. med. J.*, **92**, 94–96.

Lader, M. H., Curry, S. and Baker, W. J. (1980). Physiological and psychological effects of clorazepate in man. *Brit. J. clin. Pharmac.*, **9**, 83–90.

Maletzky, B. M. and Klotter, J. (1976). Addiction to diazepam. *Int. J. Addict.*, **II**, 95–115.

Marks, J. (1978). *The Benzodiazepines. Use, overuse, misuse, abuse*, MTP Press, Lancaster.

Palmer, G. C. (1978). Use, overuse, misuse and abuse of benzodiazepines. *Alabama J. med. Sci.*, **15**, 383–392.

Petursson, H. and Lader, M. H. (1981a). Benzodiazepine dependence. *Brit. J. Addict.*, **76**, 133–145.

Petursson, H. and Lader, M. H. (1981b). Withdrawal from long-term benzodiazepine treatment. *Brit. med. J.*, **283**, 643–645.

Tyrer, P., Rutherford, D. and Huggett, T. (1981). Benzodiazepine withdrawal symptoms and propranolol. *Lancet*, **i**, 520–522.

Woody, G. E., O'Brien, C. P. and Greenstein, R. (1975). Misuse and abuse of diazepam: an increasingly common medical problem. *Int. J. Addict.*, **10**, 843–848.

## DISCUSSION

## CHAIRMAN: DR SUSAN IVERSEN

PROFESSOR I. OSWALD: In defence of the benzodiazepines, while I agree that the withdrawal syndrome has all the characteristics associated with the barbiturate withdrawal syndrome, in practical clinical life one does not often come up against things like seizures in the way that one used to in the barbiturate days. The relative rarity may be something to do with the benzodiazepines, or it may be due to the fact that many of them in the past have had a long half-life. You cannot abruptly withdraw something like flurazepam beacuse its active metabolites are going to take a couple of weeks to be got rid of.

PROFESSOR M. SCHMUTZ: We have some new animal evidence that the shorter the presence of benzodiazepine on the receptor sites, the greater the chance that withdrawal fits occur. We have done experiments on monkeys, with alumina hydroxide induced epileptic seizures. This is a chronic seizure state, and the monkeys usually have focal seizures. You can antagonize these seizures with benzodiazepines, yet only for a limited time because of the occurrence of tolerance. When you stop the treatment abruptly you get rebound seizures, that is, from simple focal seizures you either get generalized seizures, more frequently occurring simple focal seizures or focal seizures with loss of consciousness. When you add, at the time the benzodiazepines are withdrawn, a benzodiazepine antagonist such as CGS/8216 then this rebound phenomenon is made worse. We think that this is due to the fact that by adding the antagonist, the benzodiazepine is displaced much more rapidly from the receptor sites than without adding the antagonist during the withdrawal period.

PROFESSOR M. HAMILTON: From the clinician's point of view, is it worthwhile slowing down the withdrawal, and if so, for how long?

PROFESSOR LADER: Tyrer suggests that if withdrawal is slow enough symptoms are few. That is not our experience however. Also, when you go very slowly, the person's life revolves around their withdrawal schedules and experiences for months on end. On balance it is probably optimal to withdraw over about 4 and 8 weeks.

DR. M. TRIMBLE: Dr. Iversen, can you help us about changes in receptors with these drugs in relation to dependence?

DR. L. L. IVERSEN: I do not think one can predict the nature of the withdrawal syndrome, e.g. whether it will be an unpleasant experience. You might have a 'withdrawal syndrome' which simply was a readaptation of your brain receptors to not having the drug around, but it need not be unpleasant.

This adaptation process cannot, I am afraid, be related simply to changes in receptor number. In the case of the opiates, where you have classical withdrawal syndrome which is heavily dose-related, there are no changes in opiate receptor numbers that one can easily measure. In this case, we do not understand the mechanism at all.

I do not think there is any evidence for changes in benzodiazepine receptor numbers after chronic treatment.

PROFESSOR M. LADER: There is much imprecision about withdrawal syndromes. To establish physical dependence one must establish the emergence of symptoms previously not present in that individual. That is why I emphasize the perceptual symptoms, because they are untypical of anxiety.

Benzodiazepines Divided
Edited by M. R. Trimble


# 3

# The Assessment of Anxiety

MAX HAMILTON

## INTRODUCTION

It is convenient to regard all mental disorders as being constituted of disturbances of three components: subjective well-being (symptoms), interpersonal relationships and social adjustment. It is clear that from this viewpoint the patient is regarded as a whole. Although it is customary to think of general medicine as being concerned with the effects of malfunction of organs, this is a very one-sided view: the physician is concerned with the treatment of a patient. Although symptoms are the focus of attention, when it comes to the management of the patient, the other aspects of disease can be critical for the outcome. Much of current criticism of 'orthodox' medicine is based on the dissatisfaction of the public which feels that doctors are far too much preoccupied with aetiology and biochemical and physiological disturbances, and not enough with the disturbance of life and the suffering of the patient.

The criticism is exaggerated, even if not wholly untrue. Physicians have recognized for over half a century that the management of diabetes is not purely an exercise in metabolism. Orthopaedic surgeons have long been aware that the morale of the patient is basic to the outcome of treatment of fractures. Current debates on the treatment of breast cancer are not so much concerned with subsequent mortality as with the 'quality of life'. These are just a few examples but there are plenty of others. Nevertheless, it can be said that criticisms of current medical practice have led to greater attention being paid to the personal and social problems of patients.

In psychiatry, treatment is not based on aetiology (with a few exceptions) because not enough is known of the causes of mental illness to provide a treatment based thereon. Treatment is concerned with the manifestations of illness, and therefore on its three aspects. As this symposium is concerned with drug treatments, which affect mainly symptoms, this will be the major concern here, although the other aspects will be mentioned below.

## ASSESSMENT OF SYMPTOMS

It is an empirical fact that the more severely ill patients have more symptoms than the milder cases. In consequence, a count of the number of symptoms experienced by a patient gives a crude measure of the severity of illness. This is the basis of the 'check list' of symptoms. Surprisingly, this apparently crude measure is quite successful in practice, and has a high correlation with 'global' assessments made by the physician or even by the patient. How symptoms are defined and demarcated cannot be considered here.

A simple check list suffers from two deficiencies: each symptom contributes one point to the total, regardless of its severity or its nature. Obviously a severe symptom is more disabling than a mild one and undoubtedly some symptoms are more disabling than others, e.g. fainting attacks are more disturbing than dizziness.

Both of these deficiencies can be remedied, with improvement in the assessment, by giving a greater weight to disabling symptoms and to greater severity. Thus trivial, mild, moderate, and severe levels of a symptom can be given 1, 2, 3, and 4 points, as is the usual custom, or 1, 2, 4, and 8 points, as was used in one of the pioneer scales (Moore, 1929). The use of graded levels changes the check list to a rating scale.

The greater disability of a particular symptom can be dealt with either by giving it a greater weight, i.e. the score on that symptom is multiplied by an appropriate factor, so that it contributes more to the total score than minor symptoms, or by increasing the number of items related to that symptom. For example, the symptom 'agoraphobia' can be given greater weight by providing a separate item for each situation in which it occurs, such as street, buses, shops, and so on. This is the basis of the construction of current scales.

To the outsider, the simple basis of rating scales begs all sorts of questions. In the first place, how is it possible to add scores on different symptoms? Surely there can be no meaning to a sum of scores derived from assessment of loss of weight, headaches, and palpitations. This is quite true when we are concerned with the specific items and the changes that occur in them. When interest is directed to the difference between treatments and the way they affect various symptoms, e.g. when comparing a $\beta$-blocker with an anxiolytic, then indeed the individual symptoms have to be considered separately. It is only when severity is being considered as a whole that the scores on different symptoms are summed. The justification for this is that every extra symptom is a source of additional disability or suffering and so contributes its share to the total.

From the psychometric point of view, when two items are positively correlated, they have a common variance and each can be regarded as a sort of measure of the other. When all the items in a scale are positively correlated, then all of them have a common variance, and it is this common variance which is measured by a total score.

To the statistician, it is the arbitrary nature of the weights which is disturbing. Giving the grades of severity of a symptom the weights of 1–4 implies that a grade of 'severe' is four times greater than 'trivial'. The numbers 1–4 here are ordinal measures, signifying no more than the order in which the grades lie. The methods of customary (parametric) statistical analysis are inappropriate to ordinal measures, and results obtained with them are meaningless. From the theoretical point of view, this is quite true. There are indeed methods by which the weights (scores for the grades and even for the symptoms) can be assigned with such values that summation becomes legitimate. However, it has been shown empirically that the difference between the 'correct' method and the customary crude one comes to very little. Furthermore, the more items there are in a scale, the smaller is the difference. For the scales of 10 or more items, the difference is less than the errors of measurement. That is to say, if the assessment is made by two different judges at the same time, or the same judge makes a second assessment within a short time of the first, the two scores will differ by more than the difference between 'true' and crude weighting.

There is much misunderstanding about the nature of measurement in physiology and biochemistry. Many measurements have the appearance of being quite straightforward; technically, they are 'ratio' measurements, but functionally they are not. A pulse rate of 80/min is four times greater than one of 20/min but functionally there is a world of difference. A blood glucose of 70 mg/dl is seven times greater than one of 10 mg/dl, but in the latter case, the patient is dead.

Another point that is often raised concerns the possibility that two patients may have the same total score and yet have completely different symptoms. Even though their scores are identical they are obviously not comparable. Assuming that this is the case, then unless these two individuals are unique in this respect, we must accept that there is a group of patients who score on one set of symptoms and another group which scores on the second set. We have here an either–or situation. The patients have either one set of symptoms or the other. The implication of this is that the disorder we are measuring with the scale is not a unitary condition and that we are dealing with two different types of patients. It is easy to detect this situation.

When the intercorrelations of the items are calculated, it will be seen that the items fall into two sets: within each set the intercorrelations are positive, but between them they are negative. This indicates that it is illegitimate to sum the scores of all the items to produce a grand total. The two sets of items should be summed separately, and the scale used to give two scores for subsequent analysis.

A complete separation is not likely to occur because the two groups would have been recognized as being different long before any attempt would have been made to construct a scale. However, partial separation (or partial overlap) does occur (Hamilton *et al.*, 1960).

The argument can be extended to more than two groups. Many scales are designed to give a set of scores which are intended to be handled separately.

It goes without saying that any instrument for making measurements should be used properly by one who knows how to do so. The practical value of the scores obtained from a rating scale depends on the skill and judgement of the rater. Raters should know how to recognize the symptoms when they are present and should be able to grade their severity appropriately. They should also know how to use the scale and how to avoid common errors and biases. A good scale should be backed by definitions of the items and their grades. With such a background, rating scales stand up well when compared with ordinary instrumental methods such as are used in physiology and clinical biochemistry. When two raters use a scale at the same interview, e.g. for depression, it is my experience that they will not often differ by more than 10% for a total score.

It is still regarded as a serious deficiency of rating scales that they are based on subjective judgement. Oddly enough, nobody complains about subjectivity when it comes to evaluating wines, mixing varieties of tea, or even awarding medals in Olympic Games ice skating championships. What matters about a measurement is not whether it is subjective or objective, but whether it measures what it is supposed to measure (validity) and does so with sufficient freedom from error (reliability). When we are considering complex patterns of behaviour, there is no way of assessing them except by the exercise of human judgement. Human judgement is extraordinarily sensitive. Anybody can tell the difference between paintings by Rembrandt and Van Gogh, but an expert can look at a Rembrandt and tell when it was painted. When a patient feels ill, he is making a subjective judgement, and another when he says he feels better. Observers can make judgements which correspond closely with that of the patients.

Of the other methods available for the assessment of symptoms, the only one in common use is the 'analogue' scale. At the two ends of a line drawn on a sheet of paper, the two extremes of a symptom are recorded, e.g. for anxiety, 'completely calm' and 'panic fear'. Alternatively: 'quite calm' and 'the most anxious I have ever been'. The patient is asked to make a mark along the line to indicate what he feels at the moment. Despite the vagueness of the directions and the apparent lack of a good basis for making a judgement, it has been found that patients are quite capable of producing meaningful assessments. The score on an analogue scale is the distance of the mark from one end of the line. A deficiency of analogue scales is that they are subject to 'contrast effects', i.e. when the patient's condition changes, the change is apt to be exaggerated.

Similar methods can be applied to the rating of interpersonal relationships and social adjustment. Such scales are now being introduced but they have not been used extensively. Whereas the description and demarcation of symptoms have a long history and have now reached a stage of great refinement, there are still many difficulties with these other two kinds of scales. Social adjustment presents special problems, because its characteristics differ between the sexes and among classes and cultures.

## ASSESSMENT OF ANXIETY

It has always been known that anxiety and fear are accompanied by bodily changes, and these obviously provide an alternative method for measuring anxiety. Of course, the need to confine measurement to the use of non-invasive techniques is a considerable limitation. There are more important difficulties. There is ample evidence that the physiological and biochemical changes associated with anxiety vary considerably among individuals (Lacey and VanLehn, 1952). Even within one system, e.g. cardiovascular, in a particular individual, different measurements (pulse rate, pulse pressure, blood pressure) can give very different results. Some subjects show a fixed pattern of responses to different anxiety-producing stresses and others give a variety of responses (Lacey *et al.*, 1953). In consequence, the correlations among physiological measures are low and, what is worse, the correlations with clinical state are equally low (Greer *et al.*, 1973). As anxiety is a psychological state (at least patients think it is) it is therefore difficult to establish the validity of physiological measurements. Much the same applies to the various behavioural characteristics of animals that are supposed to correspond to anxiety in humans.

The word 'anxiety' has three different meanings in psychiatry. It is used to signify the normal reaction of an individual who is in a stressful situation, e.g. making a speech in public; an abnormal state occurring as a symptom in many psychiatric disorders; and a syndrome 'anxiety neurosis' or 'anxiety state'. Many individuals have a low threshold for anxiety when exposed to stress, however mild. In common speech they have an anxious disposition. In the language of psychology they show marked traits of anxiety. It is important to distinguish characteristics of personality from anxiety neurosis, which is an abnormal state, occurring in individuals who do not necessarily have an anxious disposition. In the early days of clinical research on anxiolytic drugs, many investigators did not appreciate the importance of this distinction and used in their trials various scales which had been designed for assessment of personality. Some still do. Two of such scales are the Manifest Anxiety Scale (Taylor, 1953) and the Eysenck Personality Inventory (Eysenck and Eysenck, 1964).

## EVALUATION OF TREATMENT

Compared with other mental disorders, anxiety states (neurosis) have comparatively little effect on interpersonal relationships and social adjustment. In consequence, in the overwhelming majority, published trials of treatments confine themselves to evaluating improvement in symptoms. Except in the rare extremely severe cases, patients retain their insight and can give good account of themselves. For this reason, self-rating scales are most commonly used.

In the evaluation of treatments, interest is directed specifically towards the symptom of anxiety (anxious mood) or more generally towards all the symptoms of anxiety neurosis. For the former, the simplest method is to use the visual analogue method. Although it has minor disadvantages, it has the supreme merit that it can be used repeatedly as often as is required. For the latter purpose there are available many self-rating scales. Only a few will be considered here.

The Hopkins Symptom Check List (Parloff *et al.*, 1954) has been much used in the USA. It contains 64 items, covering both psychological and somatic symptoms and has been shown to be sensitive to the effects of treatment with drugs (Rickels *et al.*, 1972). The Lipman Scale (Lipman *et al.*, 1969) is an abbreviated version and appears to be equally effective.

The Symptom Rating Test (Kellner *et al.*, 1968) contains 39 items, 21 of which are concerned with psychological symptoms and 18 with somatic ones. Although it is described as a check list, the items can be rated on a four-point scale. They can be grouped into subscales for anxiety, depression, somatic symptoms, and 'inadequacy'. It has been found to be fully sensitive to treatment effects in drug trials.

Scales can be designed for the measurement of duration, frequency or intensity of symptoms. Sheffield and Kellner (1970) showed that measurement of the duration of symptoms did not differentiate between neurotics and normals, though frequency of symptoms did. Neither was sensitive to changes in clinical state. Only scales measuring intensity differentiated between neurotics and normals and also reflected changes in clinical state. Perhaps this is why the Self-rating Anxiety Scale of Zung (1971), which concentrates on the duration of symptoms, is now little used.

In contrast with the great number of self-rating scales for anxiety states which has been published, it would appear that there are only three observer-rating scales. The first one was that of Buss *et al.* (1955) but apparently it has not been used in clinical trials. Zung (1971) designed an Anxiety Status Inventory which consisted of the same 20 items as in his SAS, but the symptoms are graded for severity.

Only one observer scale is in regular current use and that is the one designed for measurement of severity of illness of anxiety neurosis (Hamilton, 1959). It consists of 13 items, scored 0–4, covering symptoms and also behaviour at

A

**ASSESSMENT OF ANXIETY**

Case No. . . . . . . .

Dept. No. . . . . . . . . . Date. . . . . . . . . . . . . . Name . . . . . . . . . . . . . . . . . . . . . . . . . . . . . . . .
Age . . . . . . Sex . . . . . . N.S.W.D. . . . . . . Reln. to Treatment . . . . . . . . . . . . . . . . . . . .

| Item No. | Score Range | Symptom | Comments |
|---|---|---|---|
| 1 | 0–4 | Anxious Mood | |
| 2 | 0–4 | Tension | |
| 3 | 0–4 | Fears | |
| 4 | 0–4 | Insomnia | |
| 5 | 0–4 | Intellectual | |
| 6 | 0–4 | Depressed Mood | |
| 7 | 0–4 | Gen. Som. Muscular | |
| 8 | 0–4 | Gen. Som. Sensory | |
| 9 | 0–4 | Cardiovascular | |
| 10 | 0–4 | Respiratory | |
| 11 | 0–4 | Gastrointestinal | |
| 12 | 0–4 | Genitourinary | |
| 13 | 0–4 | Autonomic | |
| 14 | 0–4 | Behaviour at Interview | |
| | | TOTAL | Further Notes |

0 = Absent  1 = Mild or trivial  2 = Moderate  3 = Severe  4 = Very severe to grossly disabling

Figure 1 The Hamilton Anxiety Rating Scale

interview (see Figure 1). Inter-rater reliability for the total score was found to be 0.89, but others have obtained higher figures, e.g. 0.94 (Lader *et al.*, 1974). Robinson *et al.* (1965) found that for individual items, two raters did not differ by more than one point in 66–93% of ratings. The items can be divided into two groups, dealing with 'psychic' and 'somatic' symptoms. The two groups are effectively independent, e.g. the above authors found that the correlation between them was −0.02. Scores on the one subscale therefore bear no relation to those on the other. This brings out clearly the problems which arise from measurement of physiological changes. The scale has been found to be more discriminating between drug and placebo responses than any other (Kellner *et al.*, 1968).

In his invaluable reviews, Kellner (1971, 1972) came to the conclusion that the Lipman and Kellner self-rating scales were the best and were about as good as the Hamilton scale. He also considered that in trials comparing active drugs against placebo, the 'physician's guess' about medication was an adequately sensitive method.

## SUMMARY

The best method of assessment of complex patterns of behaviour, as in mental disorders, is by means of subjective judgement, properly standardized. The empirical basis for rating scales is described and some of their problems considered briefly. Despite their apparent crudity, it can be shown that rating scales have adequate reliability and validity for the purposes for which they are used. Some of the most useful scales are briefly described.

## REFERENCES

Buss, A. H., Wiener, M., Durkee, A. and Baer, M. (1955). The measurement of anxiety in clinical situations. *J. cons. Psychol.*, **19**, 125–129.

Eysenck, H. J. and Eysenck, S. B. G. (1964). *Manual of the Eysenck Personality Inventory*, University of London Press, London.

Greer, S., Ramsay, I. and Bagley, C. (1973). Neurotic and thyrotoxic anxiety: clinical, psychological and physical measurements. *Brit. J. Psychiat.*, **122**, 549–554.

Hamilton, M. (1959). The assessment of anxiety states by rating. *Brit. J. med. Psychol.*, **32**, 50–55.

Hamilton, M., Smith, A. L. G., Lapidus, H. E. and Cadogan, E. P. (1960). Controlled clinical trial of thiopropazate, chlorpromazine and occupational therapy in chronic schizophrenics. *J. ment. Sci.*, **106**, 40–55.

Kellner, R. (1971). Improvement criteria in drug trials with neurotic patients I. *Psychol. Med.*, **1**, 416–425.

Kellner, R. (1972). Improvement criteria in drug trials with neurotic patients II. *Psychol. Med.*, **2**, 73–80.

Kellner, R., Kelly, A. V. and Sheffield, B. E. (1968). The assessment of changes in anxiety in a drug trial: a comparison of methods. *Brit. J. Psychiat.*, **114**, 863–869.

Lacey, J. J., Bateman, D. E. and VanLehn, R. (1953). Autonomic response specificity. *Psychosom. Med.*, **15**, 8–21.

Lacey, J. J. and VanLehn, R. (1952). Differential emphasis in somatic response to stress. *Psychosom. Med.*, **14**, 71–81.

Lader, M. H., Bond, A. J. and James, D. C. (1974). Clinical comparison of anxiolytic drug therapy. *Psychol. Med.*, **4**, 381–387.

Lipman, R. S., Rickels, K., Covi, L., Derogatis, L. R. and Uhlenhuth, E. H. (1969). Factors of symptom distress. *Arch. gen. Psychiat.*, **21**, 328–338.

Moore, T. V. (1929). The empirical determination of certain syndromes underlying praecox and manic-depressive psychoses. *Am. J. Psychiat.*, **9**, 719–738.

Parloff, M. B., Kelman, H. C. and Frank, J. D. (1954). Comfort, effectiveness and self-awareness as criteria of improvement in psychotherapy. *Am. J. Psychiat.*, **111**, 345–351.

Rickels, K., Lipman, R. S., Garcia, C. and Fisher, E. (1972). Evaluating clinical

improvement in anxious outpatients: A comparison of normal and treated neurotic patients. *Am. J. Psychiat.*, **128**, 1005–1009.
Robinson, J. T., Davies, L. S., Kreitman, N. and Knowles, J. B. (1965). A double-blind trial of oxypertine for anxiety neurosis. *Brit. J. Psychiat.*, **111**, 527–529.
Sheffield, B. E. and Kellner, R. (1970). The temporal stability of self-ratings of neurotic symptoms. *Brit. J. soc. clin. Psychol.*, **9**, 46–53.
Taylor, J. A. (1953). A personality scale of manifest anxiety. *J. abnorm. soc. Psychol.*, **48**, 285–290.
Zung, W. W. K. (1971). A rating instrument for anxiety disorders. *Psychosomatics*, **2**, 371–379.

## DISCUSSION

## CHAIRMAN: DR MICHAEL TRIMBLE

DR. JOHNSON: Rating scales are very useful, and many of the criticisms arise, I think, from the way in which they are used rather than the scales themselves. Certainly two very common fallacies and mistakes, in my opinion, are that when you see drug A compared to drug B the results are expressed as a statistical difference between two scores. Obviously the number which you need to achieve a statistical difference depends partly upon the severity of symptoms or the number you start with. I have even seen in one study—this was on lithium, looking at memory—changes which were deemed to be statistically significant below the normal cut-off score for a depressed and non-depressed person. Clearly to have a meaningful clinical change, a patient has to have a change of a certain score which varies with the severity of illness he is suffering from. I think that is a very major error in the way many results are expressed.

Another, separate point, which I think is a problem with individual items as well as with the total score, is that the score can sometimes come from sources other than the illness being tested. For instance, I think it is true to say that one cannot really score depression in the setting of schizophrenia in the same way that one can score depression in the setting of a normal personality.

If we are looking at the side effects of a drug, we always take a zero score of the side effects before the person starts treatment. Or I suggest that we should. I think this is also true, perhaps, in terms of the score that a treatment might produce in terms of changes. Certainly with the antidepressants, and the ones with anticholinergic effects and the ones that do not have anticholinergic effects, this is relevant to looking at patients. If you try to divide them according to the constellation of symptoms which they present you with and try to look at the symptom response or try to pick up the patients who respond. Since certain somatic symptoms are affected by the drugs, you can get differences which I would suggest are false in terms of treatment, but reflect the difference in side effects of the two drugs being treated.

I am making a plea for a more sophisticated use.

PROFESSOR HAMILTON: I agree with your plea. Clinicians who are evaluating treatments should use their clinical judgement in doing so. If they use a rating scale, they should recognize that the scale is only a particular way of recording their judgement.

If the person doing a trial has no sense and does not know what he is up to, he can obviously produce anything. Clearly, as you say, a trial has to be carried out and scales used with clinical understanding.

The point you make that you can get statistical significance by having a sufficiently large number of cases is perfectly true, which means that when you read a clinical trial report one of the first things you have to ask yourself is: these patients differ significantly from a statistical point of view but how significant is it from a clinical point of view? Remember what Karl Pearson said once. 'The trouble is not that figures lie but that liars figure.'

PROFESSOR SANDLER: It was lying that I wanted to bring up! The patient would not necessarily want to admit to being frightened by anything or that he was worried about sexual prowess. There must be tremendous error, perhaps from the personality of the observer and the interaction with the patient.

PROFESSOR HAMILTON: I was once involved in organizing a trial in which just these points were taken into account, and surprisingly enough they made very little difference indeed. But I would accept that in principle there is something to it, and that is, of course, the main criticism of self-rating scales as opposed to observer scales. If I ask a patient, 'Have you ever got so low that you have wished you were dead or thought of killing yourself?' and the patient first of all gulps, goes pale, hesitates a bit and then says, 'No, of course not,' I write him down as suicidal. This is where one has to use clinical judgement in evaluating a patient's symptoms. I do not ask a patient, for example, questions about suicide, nor do I ask him questions about libido, until I have talked to him and he has talked to me sufficiently long to make me feel that I am likely to get an honest answer. I have a saying about psychiatric interviewing: never ask a question today if you can put it off till tomorrow. Do not rush the patients. Do not put them into a corner and say, 'Deliver or else.' You must take it leisurely, and try to recognize that they are sick people and must be treated gently. That is what they come for.

This, of course, is the great advantage of the observer scale. You can take these difficulties into account, and others as well.

PROFESSOR LADER: I strongly believe that the use of rating scales on their own in a clinical trial is a retrograde step. I recently reviewed all placebo control trials of benzodiazepines between 1977 and 1982. The Hamilton rating scale for anxiety is used almost routinely, and I could pool the data from many of these trials. Despite difficulties, the means for 1000 patients on benzodiazepines, 1000 patients on a test benzodiazepine, and 1000 on placebo were obtained. I could then establish the mean changes on the rating scale. But having gone through these papers carefully I had no idea whether the benzodiazepines were of any use clinically. By using the rating scale, triallists had dropped the old 1950's way of counting heads and saying 'patient recovered' or 'patient did not recover'. As far as the practising clinician is concerned, he is not concerned whether he has a mean drop of six, eight or ten points on a rating scale. He wants to know, at the end of his 4 weeks' course of treatment, whether that patient is better: will the patient continue on that medication because it is showing some evidence of effectiveness, or is the patient going to be changed from the medication? The plea I make, is that rating scales should be used in conjunction with head-counting to carefully defined operational criteria.

DR. R. ANCILL: Some of our current clinical projects involve a comparison of doctor-derived observer ratings, clinical judgements and computer-derived patient self-ratings in anxiety as well as depression. The patients appear to be falling into two groups: a majority group where the correlation between the observer and the patient is, during initial assessment and follow-up, very high—in excess of 0.8. However there is consistently a much smaller group of patients where, although there is initial agreement, over the treatment period of several weeks the doctor rates and judges the patient as progressively improving, but the patient rates himself as not changing. This is difficult to explain in terms of loss of insight, because the conditions are not those usually associated with loss of insight, and in any case, loss of insight usually implies that the patient sees himself as not ill rather than not well. If it is a genuine disagreement between the doctor and the patient, who is right, and why?

PROFESSOR HAMILTON: Without looking into the details of how these observations were made, especially how the observer ratings were carried out, it is not possible to say. However, I can make a general statement: self-ratings and observer ratings do measure something different. If you want to be comprehensive, use both.

Benzodiazepines Divided
Edited by M. R. Trimble


# 4

# Psychological Methods of Treating Anxiety

JOHN COBB

Psychological advice concerning ways of coping with anxiety has a long history and does not stem solely from specialist therapists. A hundred years ago, W. S. Gilbert suggested:

> when you're lying awake with a dismal headache, and repose is taboo'd by anxiety,
> I conceive you may use any language you choose to indulge in, without impropriety.
>
> *Iolanthe*, 1.

What has happened in the last 20 years is that 'commonsense' methods have been labelled and systematically studied. Gilbert's method might be classified as 'ventilation'! Most of this work has been done on volunteer, analogue populations. Empirical results have generated new suggestions concerning the mechanism of anxiety and this has, in turn, led to the development of therapeutic 'packages' that are just starting to be tested on clinical populations, in controlled studies. New terms such as 'anxiety management training' and 'cognitive behaviour therapy' have appeared in the literature. Before discussing these critically, it is necessary to look at the conceptual framework from which therapists develop their work.

## CONCEPTUAL ISSUES

Factor analytic studies (Hamilton, 1959) confirmed the long recognized assumption that anxiety could be divided into psychic and somatic components. Lang (1971), while conducting psychophysiological studies

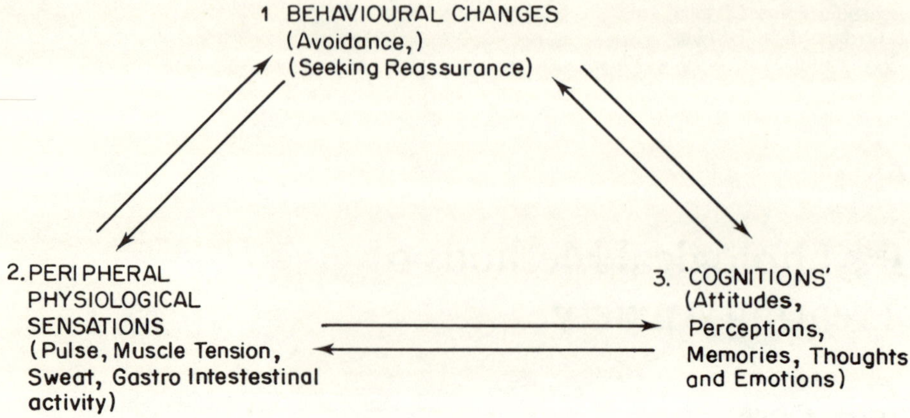


Figure 1 Pragmatic clinical model of anxiety—slightly modified from Lang (1971)

related to the clinical work of Wolpe, relabelled these components 'cognitive' and 'physiological' and added a third, 'behavioural'. In the James Lange/ Cannon Bard tradition, debate has continued concerning the direction of causality between these three factors. However, to most therapists this argument is irrelevant since the relationship between the three aspects of anxiety is seen as being a circular one (Figure 1)—a view which has considerable pragmatic merit when it comes to treatment.

Psychological methods of treatment may be aimed, with some degree of specificity, at any of these three levels. In theory, changes in one should lead to changes in the other two. However, anxiety is not a diffuse, undifferentiated internal state, but rather reflects a set of specific psychobiological variables, and the physiological, cognitive and behavioural patterns are not highly correlated (Hodgson and Rachman, 1974). Thus in clinical practice the relationship is not always as simple as Figure 1 suggests. The case of the socially phobic man, who learns to take part in social situations who thinks very differently about himself and the way that others see him, but whose dry mouth and sweatiness is as bad as ever when talking to other people, illustrates the way in which elements in the model can at times operate independently. Similarly in a study comparing frontalis EMG feedback training with progressive relaxation (Leboeuf and Lodge, 1980), it was shown that though the EMG training was superior in reducing muscle tension, both methods were equally effective in reducing scores on the State-Trait Anxiety Inventory and Taylor Manifest Anxiety Scale.

## PSYCHOPATHOLOGICAL ISSUES

Differing viewpoints concerning the psychopathology of anxiety often reflect no more than the training of the individual concerned. Neurophysiologists emphasize the importance of the ascending reticular formation and the limbic system. Psychobiologically trained psychiatrists stress the importance of inherited and developmental factors and psychoanalysts concentrate on internal psychic conflict. Therapists using psychological methods of treatment described in this review are no exception and pay great attention to whether or not contingencies can be identified when a particular patient is being assessed. Conventional diagnostic categories can be loosely arranged along a dimension according to the degree of specificity of external stimuli which precipitates the anxiety (Figure 2).

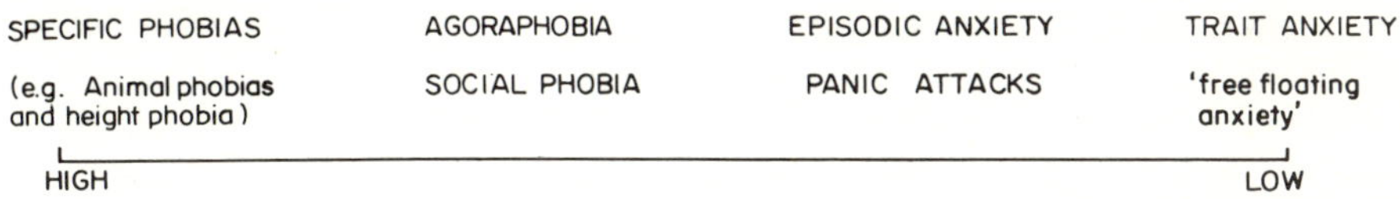


Figure 2 Specificity of external, contingent stimuli leading to anxiety

This approach is justified on clinical therapeutic grounds since there is now strong empirical evidence that psychological treatments based on the principle of exposure *in vivo* are increasingly effective as one moves towards the highly contingent end of this spectrum (Marks, 1981). Over 90% of patients with simple animal phobias can be cured using this method, and two-thirds of patients with agoraphobia or social phobia can likewise be helped to overcome their problem. On the other hand, it is not possible to use this method with the more common clinical anxiety states since, in most cases of anxiety neurosis, there are no external objects or situations which the patient can be encouraged to confront. Outcome research comparing behavioural treatments with other methods needs to take this diagnostic dimension into account before valid comparisons can be drawn. For example, Zitrin *et al.* (1978) compared behaviour therapy, supportive therapy, imipramine and placebo in 111 phobic patients. Imipramine was superior to placebo in those groups in which 'spontaneous' panic attacks could be identified, though in contrast to many other studies, behaviour therapy was no more effective than supportive psychotherapy, either in the treatment of agoraphobia, simple phobias, or 'mixed' phobias.

It is difficult to know what to make of these results. In the first place, diagnostic categorization is idiosyncratic, based on the subjective concept of spontaneous panics rather than on contingent anxiety. In the second place, the behavioural methods used during the 6-year course of the study were a heterogenous and unsystematic mixture of a group of powerful and weak behavioural techniques.

## PSYCHOLOGICAL METHODS OF REDUCING ANXIETY

These methods can be classified according to which of the three components of anxiety is the therapist's primary target.

**Methods aimed at behavioural change**

Exposure *in vivo* is the most thoroughly researched psychological method used in the management of anxiety. Its effectiveness in anxiety associated with simple phobias, agoraphobia, social phobia, and obsessive compulsive rituals, has been demonstrated in well designed controlled studies in many different centres, including London, Oxford, Holland, Greece and the United States (Marks, 1981). Treatment gains include not only a decrease in avoidance behaviour, but also a decrease in generalized anxiety and improvement in general functioning (Figure 3). Follow-up studies demonstrate that gains are maintained for up to 9 years (Munby and Johnston, 1980). Despite this being a symptom-orientated treatment *par excellence*, no evidence of symptom substitution has been reported. Treatment is as effective in the hands of specially trained nurse therapists, as when applied by psychiatrists or psychologists (Marks *et al.*, 1978).

The efficacy of exposure is well established, but the reasons why it is effective are unclear. Any attempt at providing a theoretical basis needs to take account of the following observations. First, equal improvement is found, whether the exposure is accompanied by high or low levels of arousal (Mathews *et al.*, 1974). Pairing the treatment with relaxation, as in the classical systematic desensitization method, or giving small doses of a minor tranquillizer as a premedication, neither improves nor impairs the results (Hafner and Marks, 1976). This makes the traditional learning theory explanations based on habituation and reciprocal inhibition untenable. Second, it has been demonstrated that a few long sessions, lasting 2 hours or more, produce a better outcome than the same account of treatment given in a greater number of short sessions (Stern and Marks, 1973). Apart from its theoretical interest, this finding leads to practical difficulties when therapists work in an inflexible system, which only allows appointments lasting less than an hour. Third, behavioural change precedes change in both physiological reactivity and in affect. Sometimes, as in the case of obsessional rituals, a period of several weeks may elapse between the successful interruption of neurotic patterns of behaviour and consequent decrease in associated ruminative thoughts and anxiety, a phenomenon termed 'cognitive lag'. Fourth, the treatment fails in up to a third of patients. Reasons for treatment failure can usually be identified. Associated psychiatric problems, in particular depression, may need attention before exposure can succeed. Sometimes the failure can be attributed to the patient's failure to comply fully with the programme. Alternatively, coexisting relationship problems undermine the effects of treatment (Hafner, 1977), or excessive use of alcohol or tranquillizers prevents change. However, there remains a small group of patients in whom failure cannot be explained.

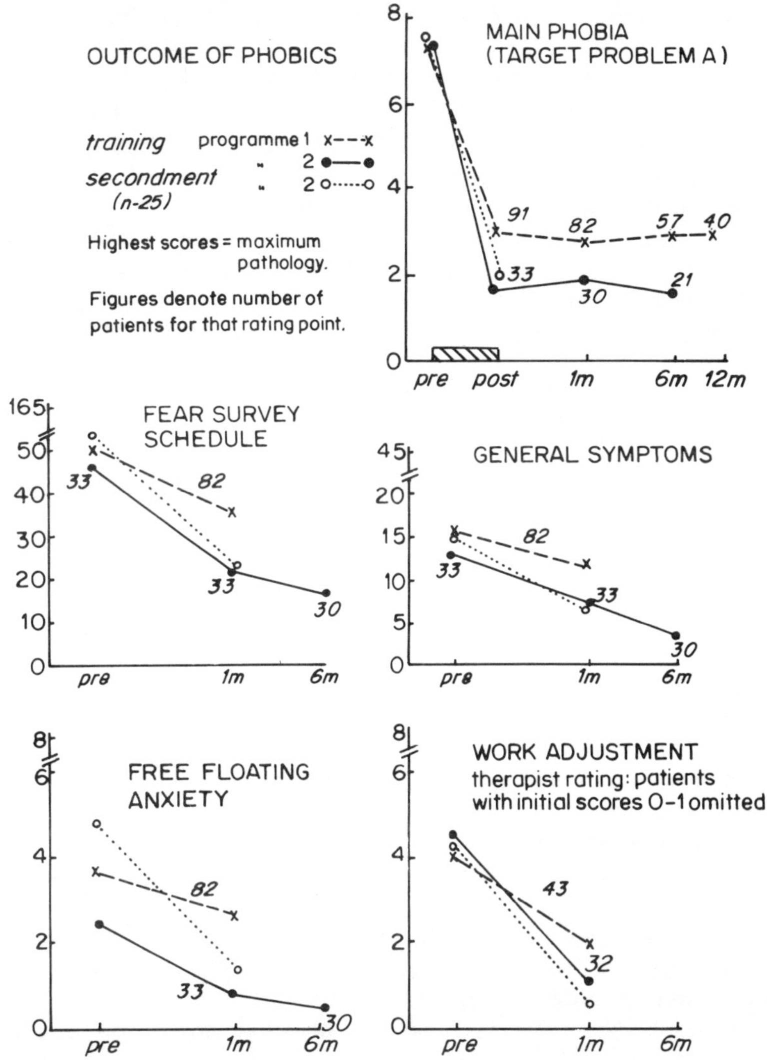


Figure 3 Outcome of phobics treated by nurse-therapists (Marks *et al.*, 1978)

## Methods aimed at inducing peripheral physiological change

The relaxation response, which involves a generalized reduction in multiple physiological systems (Benson, 1975) can be achieved by a wide variety of means. These include progressive muscular relaxation (Jacobsen, 1924), autogenic training (Schultz and Luthe, 1959), methods involving the induction of a variety of different fantasies (Singer, 1974), hypnosis (Barber and Hahn,

1963) and meditation techniques (Benson, 1975). In addition, changes in specific physiological systems can be achieved by biofeedback methods (Raskin *et al.*, 1973). During practice such methods produce a reduction both in physiological activity and in subjective anxiety. Patients usually find the procedures pleasant. When used as a control treatment drop-outs are rare! As far as lasting changes are concerned, a recent review pooled the results found in six controlled studies done in the past 10 years, all of which used the Spielberger measure of trait and state anxiety (Mathews, 1983). The change found in the relaxation groups was significantly greater than the change in control groups (Table 1). Unfortunately five out of the six studies were done on volunteer groups, for example, students with examination or speech anxiety.

Table 1 Spielberger trait anxiety scores

| | Pre | Post | Difference |
|---|---|---|---|
| Relaxation | 46.5 | 40.0 | 6.5 |
| Control | 45.4 | 43.0 | 2.4 |

From Mathews (1983). Data pooled from 6 controlled studies of relaxation.

The only study using a clinical population was done on inpatients with general anxiety symptoms (Townsend *et al.*, 1975). Biofeedback assisted relaxation was compared with group psychotherapy. Changes in scores were 5.3 and 2.5 respectively, a small but significant difference. This gives some substance to a clinical impression that relaxation produces a definite though small improvement in anxiety symptoms.

Several studies have failed to demonstrate consistent differences between the various methods of inducing relaxation. For example transcendental meditation produces similar results to muscular relaxation (Thomas and Abbas, 1978), as does biofeedback (Townsend *et al.*, 1975). Interestingly, prayer by itself was found to be significantly less effective than relaxation training. It had virtually the same effect on Spielberger's State-Trait Anxiety Inventory scores and on muscle tension scores as a control group (Elkins *et al.*, 1979). Though several different techniques have similar effects, the method of application appears to be important. Regular practice enhances beneficial effects (Lavallée *et al.*, 1976). Beiman *et al.* (1978) demonstrated that live relaxation was more effective than taped instructions, indicating that therapist factors may be more important than differences in technique.

Taken together, the evidence indicates that although various physiological variables may act as markers reflecting the depth of a state of relaxation, psychic factors must be taken into account if the phenomenon is to be fully understood. Important among these psychic factors is the patient's attitude towards treatment. Lavallée *et al.* (1976) allocated anxiety neurotics to diazepam or placebo drug regimens with or without feedback assisted relaxation training. Significant differences were confined to the follow-up period, during which the patients were encouraged to continue relaxation practice, but were also allowed diazepam as required. Those patients originally given placebo subsequently reported less anxiety, despite taking less medication (Figure 4). This group also reported more frequent relaxation practice. A plausible interpretation of these results is that benzodiazepines encourage continuing reliance on drugs, whereas placebo encouraged the patients to explore and practise alternative and possibly more effective self-management techniques.

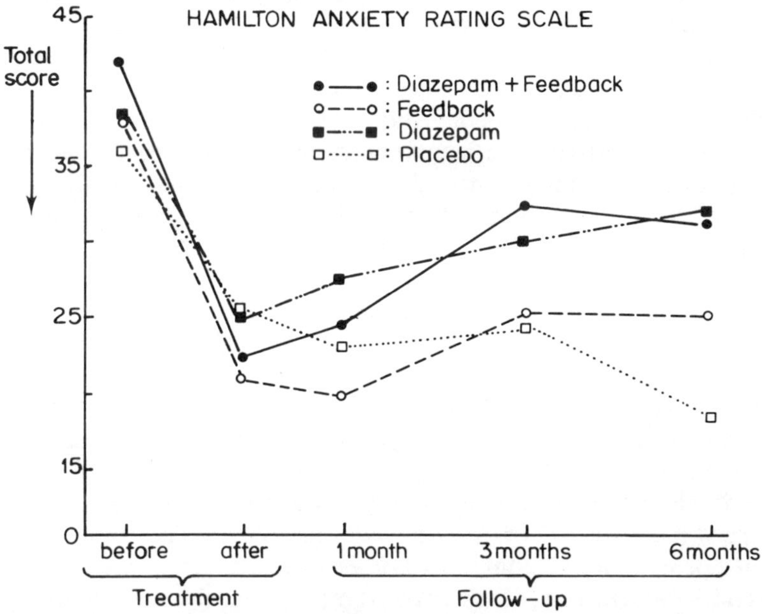


Figure 4 Mean total scores on Hamilton Anxiety Scale (Lavallée *et al.*, 1976)

## Methods aimed at inducing cognitive change

Many cognitive processes have been shown to be linked to emotional states. Examples include perception (Segal and Fusella, 1970), memory (Lloyd and Lishman, 1975), attitude (Schachter and Singer, 1962), apparent controllability (Seligman, 1975) and the amount of information available to the subject in stressful situations (Lazarus, 1971). A cognitively orientated therapist intentionally, directly, and overtly sets out to alter these and other cognitive processes. The aim is to correct misperception, misinterpretation, incompatible attitudes and counterproductive styles of thinking. Reduction of unpleasant affect or uncomfortable physiological sensations is not the primary target of therapy, and the emphasis is on coping with disabling symptoms, rather than eliminating them altogether.

In addition to the impetus given by empirical studies in cognitive psychology, a number of individuals have influenced the development of cognitive therapy. Beck emphasizes the mental constructs or 'schemata' which determine the way that patients perceive themselves, their past, and their future. In both anxiety and depression these are said to be either grossly biased or downright false. Studies of anxiety patients for example show that they report stereotyped intrusive thoughts concerning illness, death, attack, or social rejection, which have little or no basis in reality (Beck *et al.*, 1974). Beck advocates that the therapist helps the patient to challenge these schemata, partially through socratic argument and partially through carrying out homework tasks, designed to test their validity. Ellis (1962) focused on the irrational way that his patients thought about their lifestyles, their ambitions, and themselves. He forcefully pointed out the way in which anxiety, frustration, and unhappiness derived from inappropriate attitudes or beliefs. Meichenbaum (1977) stressed the importance of negative self-defeating thoughts. He encouraged his patients to modify their 'inner speech', and practise positive self-talk, even if at first this sounded artificial. At the same time negative thought patterns are disrupted using a range of thought-stopping techniques.

Certain factors are found in most cognitive therapeutic procedures. In the first place patients are asked to keep up a diary which records various aspects of their symptoms. The severity of symptoms is quantified, usually on a percentage scale. Nearly always some periodicity in symptoms is revealed. The patient learns to discriminate between different intensities of distress and is asked to mark a cut off point below which symptoms can be coped with (Figure 5). Note is made both of physical sensations and of the thoughts which accompany them, and if possible, the sequence of events is also noted. Events, thoughts, or sensations leading to a worsening of symptoms are entered on the diary and so are factors which make things easier. Diaries are discussed in detail with the therapist and are the basis for providing the patient with a framework for understanding the interaction between physical and psychological factors in the production of anxiety. Often panic attacks which appeared to the patient to come out of the blue can be shown to be related to covert physical or cognitive events. One patient with previously inexplicable episodes of shaking, sweating, and abdominal cramps was able to identify a slight tugging sensation in his groin which triggered the thought 'maybe I have got cancer'. This, in turn, was followed by an increasing state of physiological arousal and a cascade of anxiety-provoking thoughts. Similarly a nursing sister, who denied any psychological basis for 'cardiac symptoms' which had been extensively investigated by physicians, noted with surprise from her diary that her palpitations occurred whenever she was engaged in any activity related to her aged mother. Further discussion revealed that she had ample reasons

DIARY RECORD SHEET Please make an entry whenever you notice a definite increase in anxiety.

| Date / Time | Anxiety % | Activity: What you were doing at the time | Frightening feelings/thoughts Did you notice any bodily feelings, or thoughts ? | Coping method: Did you try any ? | Anxiety % after coping |
|---|---|---|---|---|---|
| | | | | | |

Figure 5 Diary record sheet

for feeling anxious about her mother, which she had previously denied.

Coupled with the task of collecting as much evidence as possible about symptoms, the patient is encouraged to try out a variety of methods of coping with symptoms when they arise. Some find it helpful to relabel the symptoms as 'anticipation' or 'excitement' rather than 'anxiety'. Positive self-statements and talking oneself through the state episode: 'I've done very well so far', and 'I know from experience that if I stick it out it won't last forever' are tried out in practice. Unrealistic beliefs are challenged: 'I can't expect everyone to approve of me all the time' and 'even if I do make a fool of myself it will not be the end of the world'. Patients are encouraged to face previously avoided situations and to test out whether the feared consequence will ensue. The post-coronary patient who fears any exertion will lead to a relapse is taken for a gentle run, just as the woman who is terrified of standing up to her overbearing husband is encouraged for once to be assertive. Patients may be asked to try deliberately to make their symptoms worse by an effort of will, a technique similar to paradoxical intention advocated by Frankl (1960). Exercises, including relaxation techniques, may be learnt as a means of cutting off the build-up of anxiety. Previous rehearsal of this procedure with artificially induced anxiety may be carried out in the clinic (Suinn and Richardson, 1971).

The methods described depend on the patient carrying out homework tasks between sessions. Within the treatment sessions, attention is paid to preparing the patient for these tasks and monitoring success and failure. Time is also spent helping the patient to re-evaluate the validity and implications of previous automatic styles of thinking. The main way of doing this is by using Socratic questioning and by examining the evidence collected by the patient. Descriptive pamphlets may be used in addition. However, practical 'experiments' include encouraging the patient to experience an attack of anxiety during the session. A clinical report (Bonn, 1973) suggests that an anxiety attack induced by a lactate infusion can be therapeutic. Unpublished reports indicate that anxiety simulated by overbreathing may be similarly helpful. Suinn and Richardson (1971) taught patients to induce anxiety using mental imagery and then to control this by using images which produce feelings of calm and mastery with or without relaxation.

Cognitive methods have been better evaluated in the treatment of depression than in anxiety. Rush and Beck (1977) compared cognitive therapy with imipramine in 41 outpatient depressives. The psychological treatment was found to be superior to pharmacological management and the results held up at 6-month follow-up. There are methodological objections to this study. For example, a marked imbalance between the amount of therapist time received by the two groups may have biased the outcome in favour of psychological treatment. However, the study has been influential and a major study in Edinburgh (Blackburn *et al.*, 1981) gives support for Beck's claims concerning the efficacy of cognitive methods as an acceptable and effective alternative or adjunct to drug treatment in outpatient depressive illness.

There are a number of *a priori* reasons for suggesting that anxiety should respond at least as well as depression to cognitive methods. Both ideation and patterns of behaviour are at least as important in the former as in the latter. Furthermore the anxiety itself acts as a powerful stimulus for the patient to look for and try out new forms of treatment. A pilot study on 12 patients with chronic anxiety (Mathews and Cobb, unpublished) showed that patients are usually easy to involve in a broad-based anxiety management package, and are prepared to carry out homework tasks. Worthwhile reductions in anxiety levels were produced following 8 × 1-hour treatment sessions, which were held at 6-month follow-up. Relaxation and cognitive methods were used in sequence in a crossover design, and the latter appeared to be the more powerful of the two.

Although a number of studies are planned or are in progress, there have been only two controlled studies looking at anxiety management methods in clinical populations. Woodward and Jones (1980) studied the treatment of 27 general anxiety outpatients selected from an NHS hospital waiting list. A no-treatment control group was compared to 'pure cognitive restructuring', 'modified systematic desensitization', and a combined treatment which they called 'cognitive behaviour modification'. This latter package contained relaxation, exposure, and cognitive elements. Four main stages in treatment were identified: preparing the patient; encouraging confrontation; teaching a

Table 2 Mean change scores for cognitive restructuring (CR), systematic desensitization (SD), and combined cognitive behaviour modification with no-treatment control group

| Dependent variable | CR ($n = 7$) (5 females, 2 males) | SD ($n = 7$) (4 females, 3 males) | CBM ($n = 6$) (3 females, 3 males) | Control ($n = 7$) (4 females, 3 males) |
|---|---|---|---|---|
| FSS | | | | |
| intensity | 2.7 | 8.57 | 12.3 | -3.3 |
| severity | 30.7 | 48.5 | 27.0 | 3.4 |
| Zung scale | 3.86 | 7.43 | 8.83 | 2.29 |
| Fear thermometer | 0.5 | 1.57 | 4.3 | 0.71 |
| Behaviour assessment | 2.86 | 2.71 | 4.17 | 0.43 |
| Diary | | | | |
| anxiety level | -0.84 | 1.67 | 1.43 | |
| thinking time | 5.85 | 13.82 | 5.86 | |

Woodward and Jones (1980).

variety of coping skills; and reinforcing effort and achievement. Therapist time was matched across the three groups (8 × 1¼ hours). All active treatments were superior to the control, and the combined treatment was significantly ($P < 0.01$) better than both other active treatments on the fear survey schedule (FSS) and superior to cognitive restructuring ($P < 0.01$) in terms of lowered subjective anxiety diary score (Table 2). Unfortunately, only the active groups were followed up and then for a mere 4 weeks, and the study lacks a placebo treatment. Nevertheless, the results are encouraging. Jannoun *et al.* (1982) used a time series design to study 27 anxiety state patients. The therapeutic procedure, in this case called 'anxiety management training', had as its main components self-monitoring, instruction booklets, muscle relaxation and cognitive control. All patients received five treatment sessions, each lasting 30–45 minutes, and patients were asked to practise for 30 minutes each day at home. Ratings by independent assessors after treatment and at 3 months follow-up showed significant and lasting treatment effects (Figure 6). However, as the authors point out, a time series design is not suitable, mainly because the effects of treatment are not immediate. The patients need time to absorb new ideas and to test them out in practice.

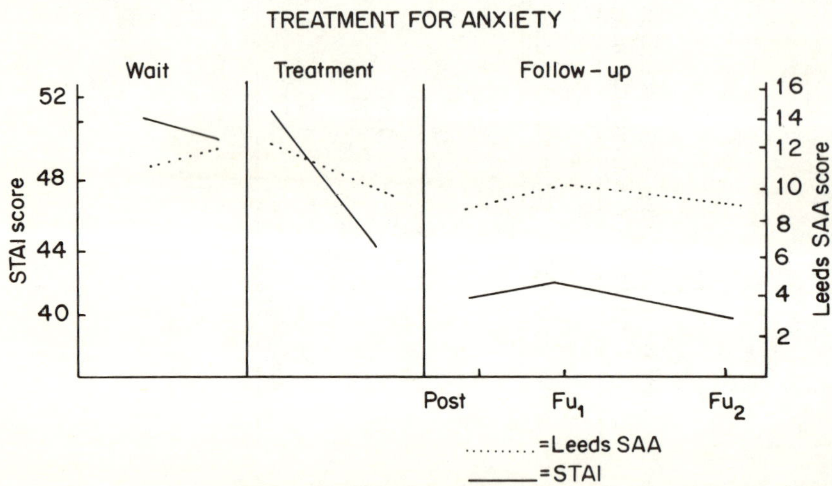


Figure 6 Average STAI (A-Trait) and Leeds SAA general ratings, during wait, treatment, and follow-up (Jannoun *et al.*, 1982)

In conclusion, psychological methods are well established in the treatment of conditions where anxiety is of a phobic type. As far as their role in more general forms of anxiety is concerned, psychological methods may be described as promising but unproven. Short-term treatment methods, involving 10 hours or less therapy time, and using skills that can be relatively quickly learnt by medical and paramedical staff, are at present in the process of development and evaluation.

## REFERENCES

Barber, T. X. and Hahn, K. W. (1963). Hypnotic induction and 'relaxation': an experimental study. *Arch. gen. Psychiat.*, **33**, 295–300.

Beck, A. T., Laude, R. and Bohnert, M. (1974). Ideational components of anxiety neurosis. *Arch. gen. Psychiat.*, **3**, 319–325.

Beiman, I., Israel, E. and Johnson, S. A. (1978). During-training and post-training effects on live and taped extended progressive relaxation, self relaxation and electromyogram feedback. *J. consult. clin. Psychol.*, **46**, 314–321.

Benson, H. (1975). *The Relaxation Response*, William Morris, New York.

Blackburn, I. M., Bishop, S., Glen, A. I. M., Whalley, L. J. and Christie, J. E. (1981). The efficacy of cognitive therapy in depression: a treatment trial using cognitive therapy and pharmacotherapy, each alone and in combination. *Brit. J. Psychiat.*, **19**, 181–189.

Bonn, J. A. (1973). Progress in anxiety states. *Proc. R. Soc. Med.*, **66**, 249–252.

Elkins, D., Anchor, K. N. and Sandler, H. M. (1979). Relaxation training and prayer behavior as tension reduction techniques. *Behavioral Engineering*, **5**, 81–87.

Ellis, A. (1962). *Reason and Emotion in Psychotherapy*, Lyle Short Press, New York.

Frankl, V. E. (1960). Paradoxical intention: a logotherapeutic technique. *Am. J. Psychotherapy*, **14**, 520–523.

Hafner, R. J. (1977). The husbands of agoraphobic women and their influence on treatment outcome. *Brit. J. Psychiat.*, **131**, 289–294.

Hafner, R. J. and Marks, I. M. (1976). Exposure in vivo of agoraphobia: The contribution of diazepam, group exposure and anxiety evocation. *Psychol. Med.*, **6**, 71–88.

Hamilton, M. (1959). The assessment of anxiety states by rating. *Brit. J. med. Psychol.*, **32**, 50–55.

Hodgson, R. and Rachman, S. (1974). Desynchrony in measures of fear. *Behav. Res. Ther.*, **12**, 319–326.

Jacobsen, E. (1924). The technic of progressive relaxation. *J. nerv. ment. Dis.*, **60**, 568–578.

Jannoun, L., Oppenheimer, C. and Gelder, M. (1982). Treatment for anxiety. *Behav. Ther.* **13**, 103–111.

Lang, P. (1971). The application of psychophysiological methods to the study of psychotherapy and behavior modification. Chapter 2 in: *Handbook of Psychotherapy and Behavior Change*, pp.75–125 (Eds. Bergin, A. E. and Garfield, S. L.), John Wiley, New York.

Lavallée, Y-J., Lamontagne, Y., Pinard, G., Annable, L. and Tetreault, L. (1976). Effects of EMG feedback, diazepam and their combination on chronic anxiety. *J. Psychosom. Res.*, **21**, 65–71.

Lazarus, A. A. (1971). *Behavior Therapy and Beyond.* McGraw-Hill, New York.

Leboeuf, A. and Lodge, J. (1980). A comparison of frontalis EMG feedback training and progressive relaxation in the treatment of chronic anxiety. *Brit. J. Psychiat.*, **137**, 279–284.

Lloyd, G. G. and Lishman, W. A. (1975). Effect of depression on the speed of recall of pleasant and unpleasant experiences. *Psychol. Med.*, **5**, 173–180.

Marks, I. M. (1981). *Cure and Care of Neuroses.* John Wiley, New York.

Marks, I. M., Bird, J. and Lindley, P. (1978). Psychiatric nurse therapy: developments and implications. *Behav. Psychother.*, **6**, 25–36.

Mathews, A. M. (1983). Anxiety and its management. In: *Current Themes in Psychiatry*, Vol. III. (Eds. Gaind, R. and Hudson, B.), Spectrum Publications, New York.

Mathews, A. M., Johnson, D. W., Shaw, P. M. and Gelder, M. G. (1974). Process variables and the prediction of outcome in behaviour therapy. *Brit. J. Psychiat.*, **125**, 256–264.

Meichenbaum, D. (1977). *Cognitive Behavior Modification. An Integrative Approach*, Plenum, New York.

Munby, M. and Johnston, D. W. (1980). Agoraphobia. The long-term follow-up of behavioural treatment. *Brit. J. Psychiat.*, **137**, 418–427.

Raskin, M., Johnston, G. and Rondestvedt, J. W. (1973). Chronic anxiety treated by feedback-induced muscle relaxation. *Arch. gen. psychiat.*, **28**, 263–267.

Rush, A. J. and Beck, A. J. (1977). Comparative efficacy of cognitive therapy and pharmacotherapy in the treatment of depressed outpatients. *Cognitive Therapy and Research*, **1**, 17–37.

Schachter, S. and Singer, J. E. (1962). Cognitive, social and physiological determinants of emotional state. *Psychol. Rev.*, **69**, 379–399.

Schultz, J. and Luthe, W. (1959). *Autogenic Training: a Psychophysiologic Approach in Psychotherapy*. Grune and Stratton, New York.

Segal, S. J. and Fusella, U. (1970). Influence of imaged pictures and sounds on detection of auditory and visual signals. *J. exp. Psychol.*, **83**, 458–464.

Seligman, M. (1975). *Helplessness*, Freeman and Co., San Francisco.

Singer, J. L. (1974). *Imagery and Daydream Methods in Psychotherapy and Behavior Modification*. Academic Press, New York.

Stern, R. S. and Marks, I. M. (1973). A comparison of brief and prolonged flooding in agoraphobics. *Arch. gen. Psychiat.*, **28**, 270–276.

Suinn, R. M. and Richardson, F. (1971). Anxiety management training: a non-specific behavior therapy program for anxiety control. *Behav. Ther.*, **2**, 498–510.

Thomas, D. and Abbas, K. A. (1978). Comparison of transcendental meditation and progressive relaxation in reducing anxiety. *Brit. med. J.*, **2**, 1749–1752.

Townsend, R. E., House, J. F. and Addario, D. (1975). A comparison of biofeedback-meditated relaxation and group therapy in the treatment of chronic anxiety. *Am. J. Psychiat.*, **132**, 598–601.

Woodwood, R. and Jones, R. B. (1980). Cognitive restructuring treatment. *Behav. Res. Ther.*, **18**, 401–407.

Zitrin, C. M., Klein, D. F. and Woerner, M. G. (1978). Behavior therapy, supportive psychotherapy, imipramine and phobias. *Arch. gen. Psychiat.*, **35**, 307–316.

## DISCUSSION

## CHAIRMAN: DR SUSAN IVERSEN

DR. A. J. ROSE: The average consultation time per annum of a patient on a GP's list is about 25 minutes. Obviously, this sort of treatment represents a fairly large increase in the amount of time that I am committing to at least that individual patient. Therefore, I was looking at the elements in which I might have the greatest success. Would you care to comment whether you think this is something you can dip into, and, if so, which bits are best to dip into?

DR. J. COBB: The average consultation time is 25 minutes, but how much of your time would the severe chronic anxiety patient take, and how many night calls might you have to do over the course of the 30 years that you are to have him in your practice? It might well be more than 3½ hours a year. It would certainly be more than 3½ hours over the course of 30 years.

The second point is that these methods are being used by nurse therapists and psychologists. It would not necessarily have to be the GP directly involved in treatment. The third point concerns how the GP deals with the beginning of an anxiety neurotic career—the first panic attack, for example. I would say that it is crucial how that first panic attack is dealt with. I would have thought that the patient's understanding of his own symptoms is a key thing—not understanding in the dynamic terms of Freud and so on, but in terms of simple body physiology, of thoughts, and of having some sort of model, thereby increasing their own controllability. Of course, if you give them a drug, you could argue that this would undermine that, because you are then reinforcing the attitude that there is something structurally wrong, that they have an illness and they need a drug for it. There is some work with agoraphobics that Marks and Ginsberg have done that looked at the time various staff, including general practitioners, spent with patients before and after a course of behavioural treatment. They also measured the time that relatives spent away from work with agoraphobics doing one thing or another for them before and after treatment, and there was a very clear and quite marked saving.

Benzodiazepines Divided
Edited by M. R. Trimble


# 5

# Controversies in Practice

ANDY J. ROSE

For the general practitioner the benzodiazepines are almost too good to be true. They are rapidly effective as tranquillizers and hypnotics and there is an approximately proportional dose–response ratio. They are very safe in overdosage. Occasionally their specific muscle relaxing properties are valuable and this effect is rarely a serious disadvantage. Long-term administration has never been encouraged, but it seems to produce few serious problems when it occurs.

Barbiturates were widely used before the benzodiazepines became available. The advantage of this change to the benzodiazepines is very clear with the benefit of hindsight, and if these nearly ideal drugs have come to be overused, because they are such an improvement, it can easily be understood. It is characteristic for anxious patients to demand treatment in a variety of ways, on repeated occasions, so putting pressure on the general practitioner. This pressure has often been met with a prescription for a benzodiazepine.

In the last 2 or 3 years the benzodiazepines have been subject to increased scrutiny by the medical profession (Committee on Review of Medicines, 1980) and by the lay public (Graham, 1981). Inevitably some people take up extreme positions, and it is common to find patients and doctors with firm views which conflict. It therefore seems appropriate to try to define the place for these drugs.

Anxiety is a frequently encountered condition in general practice. Much anxiety is normal, and much of it can be revealed as inappropriate. It is often possible to relieve symptoms by some very simple counselling. A difficult dilemma for the general practitioner occurs when a patient presents severe anxiety appropriate to the situation. This cannot be thought of as pathological, but it may be a poor response for the individual to make to his circumstances. Frequently it is not possible for the cause of the anxiety to be removed within the immediate or foreseeable future. The general practitioner is then faced with trying to help a patient complaining about a 'normal' situation. One of the remedies available is a minor tranquillizer and this may be the least problematic solution. It is certainly an easy short-term answer for the prescribing doctor. The long-term effects of this decision can be pharmacologically unsatisfactory, and degrade the doctor's role to that of a simple supplier with the patient controlling consumption with the doctors' unspoken blessing. Systems for giving repeat prescriptions can make this easier especially if they are not properly supervised. Fortunately or unfortunately, a casual approach to the use of these drugs frequently causes very little obvious harm as the drugs are so safe. However, the patient is only too aware of the ease with which they can be obtained, and often perceives this to be inversely proportional to the efficacy of the compounds. This behaviour therefore diminishes the stature of the drugs, as well as the nature of the doctor/patient relationship so the benefit to the patient is diminished too.

Although education and counselling are probably the best solution to anxiety when they are successful, failure is common and this does not encourage general practitioners to commit the large amounts of time required. The question therefore still remains as to the correctness of using these drugs for the treatment of 'normal' anxiety.

Pathological anxiety can occur as part of almost any psychiatric condition and the general practitioner must also be alert to the possibility of organic disease, in particular thyrotoxicosis presenting in this guise. Accurate diagnosis can be very difficult, and requires patience and sometimes specialist advice at an early stage. Treatment should be directed to any underlying pathology but additional treatment with benzodiazepines for anxiety may be helpful. Pathological anxiety can also exist alone and benzodiazepines are frequently used initially. When it comes to the point of prescribing a benzodiazepine the approach should be critical, as with any other drug. It is important to have a clear idea of the effect that is required for the individual patient. Insomnia and anxiety are inter-related, but some differential effect can be achieved by adjusting the dosage and time of administration. It is also important to choose a compound with a duration of action to suit the patient, and it may be possible to select the particular compound on the basis of other properties, for instance the degree of sedation.

The place of the short acting benzodiazepines for use as hypnotics seems logical. The idea of a rapidly metabolized compound which leaves no residual morning 'hangover' effect has been well accepted (Leading article, 1980). However, there have been reports of problems of depersonalization (Committee on Safety of Medicines, 1981) and there is some evidence of a persisting reduction in performance during the day following administration (Betts and Birtle, 1982). Short acting drugs have also been perceived to have advantages in the elderly, where metabolism and excretion may be delayed.

This approach is aimed at preventing unwanted accumulation of the active drug (Committee on Review of Medicines, 1980).

The long acting benzodiazepines permit less frequent administration, although there is no reason why smaller doses should not be given more frequently, if this meets the needs of the individual patient. It is also thought that more stable levels of the active drug may produce a more sustained relief of symptoms, which may suit many patients better than short pulses of relief which can be produced by the use of short acting agents. This phenomenon may be analogous to the situation of pain relief in the terminally ill, where it is found beneficial to use analgesics on a regular basis rather than as required (Dorr and Fritz, 1981). This approach permits long pain-free periods rather than allowing the pain to break through before further analgesia is given. A benzodiazepine with a prolonged duration of action may also mean that it is easier to stop treatment. The withdrawal of drug is more gradual, occurs over a longer period of time, and is therefore better tolerated (Tyrer *et al.*, 1981).

There is also information to suggest that some benzodiazepines cause less drowsiness than others when used in doses of similar potency (Rose and Kimber, 1980). This seems to be a particular area of controversy, but of great importance in practice.

It is difficult for the general practitioner to judge the value of all the data now accumulating on the benzodiazepines. Certainly the experience of the individual practitioner is not sufficient to confirm small differences between the compounds. In particular, much of the data relating to the different levels of drowsiness seems to come from normal individuals undergoing psychomotor testing (McEwan *et al.*, 1981) and it cannot be assumed that this can be applied to anxious patients in the clinical situation. However, if a real difference between the benzodiazeopines does exist, then it is important that it should be identified as many patients carry on skilled work requiring high levels of concentration and motor skill.

Clinical trials in general practice are difficult to conduct. It is hard to find interested doctors prepared to spend time on detailed work. It is difficult to achieve acceptable levels of standardization in diagnosis and in assessment, and even then it requires very large numbers of patients to show small differences between such drugs. However, it is important to seriously consider this approach as benzodiazepines are mainly prescribed in the United Kingdom by general practitioners and it would be of great value to study a situation as close to normal clinical practice as possible.

In this uncertain area, a common sense approach to prescribing is usually best, but it is important for general practitioners to recognize new coherent strands of opinion as they arise from amongst workers in the field. Expert opinion is often needed to contain non-expert uncertainty but the dialogue should also embody elements of teaching and learning. At the present time of increased interest in the benzodiazepines there seems to be a need to improve this dialogue. The vocabulary of discussion is important, and varies with the forum of debate. Many different words and expressions have overlapping meaning, and whilst we must be prepared to adjust our vocabulary to suit our audience, we must also spend time explaining what we mean so that there should be no misunderstanding. For example, one general practitioner may talk to another doctor about a 'short course of a benzodiazepine'. He may describe this to the patient as 'a short course of treatment with a mild tranquillizer' being careful to explain that 'mild' does not mean 'weak' and the patient may then read about 'chemical holidays on the National Health Service' in the press. It is important to explain and clarify our ideas so that any lack of precision is due to lack of knowledge and not failure to communicate accurately.

In the United Kingdom about 85% of benzodiazepines are prescribed by general practitioners. As suggested, these drugs have many attractions, but there is a great deal more to be learned about how to use them better. Statistics suggest that in recent years there has been a decline in the number of prescriptions issued in the United Kingdom for benzodiazepine tranquillizers, the overall fall being 16% from 1977 to 1981. This decline is due to general practitioners initiating treatment less frequently and the reduction has occurred mainly in the younger patients, below 30 years of age. It is of interest, however, that there are further data which may suggest that this fall is due to fewer patients presenting to their general practitioner, and that general practitioners are still prescribing benzodiazepine tranquillizers for the same proportion of patients presenting with anxiety needing treatment over this period of time. Whilst there are many possible explanations for this it suggests that prescribing habits may not be changing. Further work clarifying such issues is clearly needed.

## REFERENCES

Betts, T. A. and Birtle, J. (1982). Effect of two hypnotic drugs on actual driving performances next morning. *Brit. med. J.*, **285**, 852.

Committee on Review of Medicines (1980). Systematic review of the benzodiazepines. *Brit. med. J.*, **280**, 520–522.

Committee on Safety of Medicines (1981). Unexpected reactions to benzodiazepines. *Current Problems*, February, No. 5.

Dorr, R. T. and Fritz, W. L. (1981). Ancillary drug therapy—pain: In: *Cancer Chemotherapy Handbook*, Chapter 8, pp.169–170, Kimpton Medical, London.

Graham, J. (1981). The treachery of the tranquilliser. *Company*, May, 73.

Leading Article (1980). Hypnotics and hangover. *Brit. med. J.*, **280**, 743.

McEwen, J., Lawrence, J. R., Chamberlain, J. and Ings, R. M. J. (1981). The comparative clinical pharmacology of clobazam. *Clobazam: Royal Society of Medicine International Congress and Symposium Series*, **43**, 87–95.

Rose, A. J. and Kimber, G. (1980). A double-blind comparison of ketazolam given once each day with diazepam in divided doses and placebo in the treatment of anxiety. *Brit. J. clin. Pract.*, **34**, 107–113.

Tyrer, P., Rutherford, D. and Huggett, T. (1981). Benzodiazepines withdrawal symptoms and propranolol. *Lancet*, **i**, 520–522.

## DISCUSSION

## CHAIRMAN: DR SUSAN IVERSEN

PROFESSOR M. LADER: My first comment is with the 'prophylactic' use of benzodiazepines to prevent anxiety. One must distinguish between types of anxiety. It works well in patients with high, sustained levels of anxiety. With panic attacks, which come without much precipitation, the benzodiazepines are not very effective. With situational anxiety, where the patient can predict when the anxiety will be made worse, a short-acting drug is quite useful.

My question concerns your figures about prescribing. It is a mistake to take the figures for anxiety and tranquillizers in isolation. People present with what the general practitioner calls anxiety and gives an anxiolytic for, or with what he calls depression and gives an antidepressant for. A reciprocal relationship exists between them, especially in women where depressed women are as likely to be treated with a tranquillizer as they are with an antidepressant. The whole gamut of prescribing must be examined before any trends can be discerned about the totality of minor psychiatric disability.

PROFESSOR OSWALD: Dr. Rose referred to the relaxant properties of the benzodiazepines and said this is never a disadvantage. I wonder if we really know. Our muscles are strong if we exercise them, and our postural muscles are strong if we exercise them. If we relax them too much they may be less strong. There are an awful lot of middle-aged ladies around who complain of chronic back ache and also take diazepam all the time. This was the thought that came to me when we did a long-term study with 100 people, of whom 25 took placebo all the time and had no change in weight whatever; whereas the others who took either one or the other of two benzodiazepines in small doses each had a small loss of weight.

DR. D. A. W. JOHNSON: A number of years ago we looked at the prescribing habits of general practitioners in patients that they themselves had made the diagnosis of depression and we found that they used antidepressants and benzodiazepines almost interchangeably. We found that the longer the patient remained depressed, the more likely the patient was to receive either a non-therapeutic dose of the antidepressants—the dose of the antidepressant was actually reduced with time—or they were changed to a benzodiazepine. If we looked at the chronic depressives, people who had been depressed and under treatment for more than 3 months, in excess of half were on the benzodiazepines. We asked the general practitioners why this was taking place, and to a degree there was a failure of knowledge about the various drug groups, but more important was that, as the general practitioner saw it, the problem was of compliance, and side effects of medication causing a failure of compliance.

DR. A. CLARE: At the General Practice Research Unit we did a study, looking at people who are given a benzodiazepine for the first time. The great majority of these were clear of their symptoms and were off drugs within 3–4 weeks. We were interested in the small but cumulative percentage who stay on these drugs for 4–12 weeks, and then whose chances of being chronic long-term users by 12 months are very high indeed. We really do have to distinguish between the very small number who either abuse or chronically use, from the very, very large number who use in ways of which you and I might not necessarily morally approve, but who in terms of physical and mental health appear to be fairly unremarkable.

Benzodiazepines Divided
Edited by M. R. Trimble


# 6

# Implications of Benzodiazepine Prescribing

ROBERT N. STRAW

It is an axiom of pharmacotherapy that each patient be prescribed the proper drug in a suitable manner. This discussion will provide an overview of the benzodiazepines and how they differ in ways which are therapeutically meaningful. Also, it will address their apparent usage patterns and provide suggestions for factors to be considered which would minimize concerns regarding their misuse.

## CURRENTLY AVAILABLE BENZODIAZEPINES

As of this writing, 11 benzodiazepines are available for prescription within the United States (Table 1). While the labelling of most of these products restricts their usage to anxiety or insomnia, certain products have somewhat broader indications. For example, diazepam is also indicated as an adjunct for the relief of skeletal muscle spasm and in convulsive disorders, a rational extension of the pharmacological activity of all benzodiazepines.

Table 1 Benzodiazepines currently marketed in the United States

| Anxiolytics | Hypnotics |
|---|---|
| Alprazolam | Flurazepam |
| Chlordiazepoxide | Temazepam |
| Clorazepate | |
| Diazepam | |
| Halazepam | **Anticonvulsants** |
| Lorazepam | |
| Oxazepam | Clonazepam |
| Prazepam | |

Table 2 Examples of additional benzodiazepines marketed world-wide

| Anxiolytics | Hypnotics |
|---|---|
| Bromazepam | Cloxazolam |
| Camazepam | Estazolam |
| Clobazam | Flunitrazepam |
| Ketazolam | Nitrazepam |
| Medazepam | Triazolam |
| Nordiazepam | |
| Oxazolam | |
| Pinazepam | |

Outside the United States, at least an additional 13 compounds are commercially available (Table 2). Again, the majority of these products are primarily indicated as either anxiolytics or hypnotics. However, it should be noted that intercountry differences do occur with regard to indications or at least therapeutic usage. For example, oxazepam is used primarily as an anxiolytic in the United States whereas in some European countries it is more widely prescribed as a hypnotic.

## QUANTITATIVE DIFFERENCES AMONG BENZODIAZEPINES

Aside from relative potency, the primary differences among most of the benzodiazepines lies in their pharmacokinetic properties. Their onset and duration of action after single oral doses depend largely upon their absorption rate and rate and extent of distribution, respectively, whereas the rate and extent of accumulation during multiple dosage depend on elimination half-life and clearance (Greenblatt *et al.*, 1981). Representative drugs are presented in Table 3 in which they are classified as having either a long (elimination half-life usually greater than 24 hours), intermediate (half-life of 5–24 hours) or short (half-life of less than 5 hours) duration of action.

It is interesting to note that with the exception of flurazepam, all of the drugs classed as having long action are usually prescribed as anxiolytics and that all of the compounds within the short-acting class are prescribed as or have been studied as hypnotics. However, within the intermediate class some products are labelled as anxiolytics whereas others are used as hypnotics.

The therapeutic implications of half-life have been addressed by several authors. Compounds with shorter half-lives, and thus less likely to impair daytime function after a bedtime dose, are more rationally prescribed as hypnotics (see Solomon *et al.*, 1979; Hindmarch, 1980). On the other hand where anxiolytic activity is desired, drugs of a longer duration of action are more suitable (Lader, 1976). Indeed, the Committee on Review of Medicines

Table 3 Pharmacokinetic differences among benzodiazepines[a,b]

| Long | Intermediate | Short |
|---|---|---|
| Chlordiazepoxide | Alprazolam | Brotizolam |
| Clorazepate | Bromazepam | Midazolam |
| Clobazam | Camazepam | Triazolam |
| Diazepam | Estazolam | |
| Flurazepam | Flunitrazepam | |
| Ketazolam | Lorazepam | |
| Medazepam | Nitrazepam | |
| Prazepam | Oxazepam | |
| | Temazepam | |

[a] Classification refers to parent drug and biologically active metabolites.
[b] After Greenblatt *et al.* (1981).

has recently recommended (Anonymous, 1980a) that UK data sheets should contain such information as a guide to the prescribing physician.

From a therapeutic viewpoint, dosage regimens may also be used to appropriately mitigate certain side effects. For example, ketazolam, a long-acting benzodiazepine, given once daily at bedtime has been reported to be equal in efficacy to diazepam, given three times daily. However, in this dosage regimen, ketazolam produced a significantly lower incidence of drowsiness as compared to diazepam (Anonymous, 1980b).

## QUALITATIVE DIFFERENCES AMONG BENZODIAZEPINES

Aside from pharmacokinetic and potency differences, the view is frequently expressed that all benzodiazepines are the same. A review of the basic pharmacology of the older benzodiazepines (see Sternbach *et al.*, 1968) suggests that, with the exception of slight differences in ratios of activity in various animal models, such may well be the case. However, clinical data are insufficient to confirm or deny this hypothesis.

Recently, reports of at least semiqualitative differences among benzodiazepines have appeared. For example, it is usually considered that benzodiazepines are inappropriate as sole therapy in depression (Schatzberg and Cole, 1978; Johnson, chapter 18, this volume). Indeed, reports have been cited (Ananth and Ghadiran, 1980) that diazepam may induce depression. However, Feighner (1982) has recently reported that alprazolam, a triazolobenzodiazepine, 'offers clinical efficacy comparable to standard antidepressants, often with significant improvement in the first week of treatment' in outpatients with depression defined by the Feighner criteria (Feighner *et al.*, 1972). Further, Sethy and Hodges (1982) have reported that desipramine and alprazolam are active in a rat model thought to correlate with antidepressant activity, whereas diazepam was not. Alprazolam has also been reported to be an efficacious treatment for the relief of panic and phobic disorders (Chouinard *et al.*, 1982; Sheehan, 1982a) which have traditionally been treated with antidepressant drugs (Sheehan, 1982b).

Cohn *et al.* (1983) have reported that adinazolam, another triazolobenzodiazepine, possesses significant antidepressant activity in inpatients meeting DSM-III criteria for major depression. This compound is also active in animal models thought to correlate with antidepressant activity (Hester *et al.*, 1980).

A third triazolobenzodiazepine, estazolam, has been reported by Lingjaerde (1982) to be effective in the treatment of auditory hallucinations as well as bringing an overall improvement in the global state of schizophrenics. However, at least some patients in this study received concurrent neuroleptics. Preliminary data from Jimerson *et al.* (1982) have shown at least some antipsychotic effects for very high (250–300 mg/day) doses of diazepam.

Finally Ro 15-1788, an imidazobenzodiazepine, has been reported to be a 'potent antagonist' of the central effects of sedative benzodiazepines (Darragh *et al.*, 1981a). Ro 15-1788 does not itself possess demonstrable activity (Darragh *et al.*, 1981b).

Collectively, these reports demonstrate at least semiqualitative differences of newer benzodiazepine analogues from older drugs. Such differences may lead to broader clinical utility.

## CURRENT PATTERNS OF USAGE

Although intercountry differences exist, benzodiazepines are widely prescribed throughout most Western countries (for review see Bellantuono *et al.*, 1980). After peaking in 1973, a tendency for decreased use has appeared (Rickels, 1980).

Several surveys have addressed the issue of usage patterns. With regard to age, Greenblatt *et al.* (1975) have reported that 40% of the use is within the age range of from 40 to 59 years, Lasagna (1977) has reported 28% within the range of 20–39 years and Achong *et al.* (1978) have reported that 21% is in geriatric (i.e. over 65 years of age) patients. A recent review of usage in a Canadian family medicine centre reports greater usage in geriatrics than the previous surveys (Rosser, 1980). There is general agreement that benzodiazepines are more widely used in females than in males.

In 1974, the review of Balter *et al.* found that 10–17% of the population of nine European countries admitted to the use of benzodiazepines within the previous year. The aforementioned Canadian review (Rosser, 1980) reported approximately 10% of patients received a new prescription during the study year.

With regard to duration of usage, Balter's survey (1974) reported regular usage of at least one month's duration in from 3.4 to 8.6 of the total population and from 30–64% of benzodiazepine users. Rosser's (1980) more recent report supports the latter figures, especially in older patients.

Physician attitudes toward prescribing, especially in view of current controversies regarding misuse, have indicated that, overall, approximately 30% of physicians consistently prescribe benzodiazepines in patients with symptoms of anxiety while 20% are consistently against their use. The remaining 50% relate their usage to a case-by-case basis (Heiman and Wood, 1981).

## FACTORS TO CONSIDER PRIOR TO PRESCRIBING

### Diagnosis and the potential for presence of other psychopathology

Although 'insomnia' and 'anxiety' are widely used as diagnostic terms, each is far from being a single disease state. The Association of Sleep Disorders Centers (1979) has identified nine major distinctive categories of insomnia. The rational role of hypnotic drugs in their treatment is yet to be studied in at least some of these categories. For example, no studies have been published on the effects of hypnotics on respiration during sleep, opening to question their rational use in patients with sleep apnea (Dement *et al.*, 1982).

Further, insomnia is one of the most frequent symptoms of depression (Mezzich and Rabb, 1980). As depression is probably the most prevalent psychiatric illness, with a lifetime prevalence of 6–18% (Boyd and Weissman, 1981), it is likely that many patients who receive only hypnotics are, in fact, depressed and are being inappropriately treated.

With regard to anxiety, the problems of separating anxiety from depression are well recognized (for review see Klerman, 1980). With the exception of the evidence previously cited regarding the triazolobenzodiazepines, there is little to support the use of benzodiazepines in depressed patients. However, whether due to misdiagnosis or through inappropriate drug selection, they are being used. Keller *et al.* (1982) have reported that 19% of patients enrolled in the NIH Collaborative Study of the Psychobiology of Depression were receiving a minor tranquillizer as their most recent treatment prior to study entry. Just 3% of these patients were receiving intensive antidepressant treatment.

In addition to efficacy, patients with other psychiatric diagnoses are thought to be at risk for unusual adverse reactions. Hall and Kirkpatrick (1978) have reported that psychotic patients and those with borderline personalities are more likely to exhibit excitation syndromes with benzodiazepines.

Collectively, it appears that greater care must be used in diagnosis prior to prescribing a benzodiazepine. There is strong evidence to suggest that both hypnotic and anxiolytic benzodiazepines are being used in populations in which there is little evidence to support their use.

## Patient factors

### *Age*

It is well established that the elimination half-lives of most benzodiazepines are significantly longer in elderly patients (see Bellantuono *et al.*, 1980). Beyond that, there is a suggestion that 'receptor sensitivity' may be altered in these patients (Greenblatt and Shader, 1979). Further, geriatric patients also appear to be at greater risk for unusual side effects (Hall and Kirkpatrick, 1978). Thus, there is a clear need to use benzodiazepines with caution in this group.

### *Disease states*

Impairment of hepatic and/or renal function have been reported to prolong the half-life or to increase the incidence of side effects in patients receiving benzodiazepines (Bellantuono *et al.*, 1980). Both of these factors suggest increased caution in patients with such deficiencies.

### *Pregnancy/Lactation*

Although controversy exists, the prolonged use of benzodiazepines in the first trimester of pregnancy is generally not recommended because of a reported increased risk of congenital malfunctions (Bellantuono *et al.*, 1980).

As all benzodiazepines are likely to be excreted in breast milk, caution should again be exercised in their use during lactation. Especially with higher doses, symptoms of lethargy, failure to feed and weight loss have been reported in breast-fed infants (Patrick *et al.*, 1972).

## History of alcohol abuse

Although benzodiazepines have been widely used in the treatment of alcoholism, their use is somewhat controversial. In the treatment of acute withdrawal symptoms (e.g. seizures), the intravenous administration of a benzodiazepine is considered to be the treatment of choice (Greenblatt and Shader, 1975).

Many benzodiazepines have been studied for the treatment of withdrawal symptoms following the acute episode. The available evidence suggests that they are effective in relieving the acute anxiety that occurs during this period but that high doses are required (Greenblatt and Shader, 1974).

Benzodiazepines have failed to show any effect with regard to preventing relapses into drinking behaviour or in long-term behavioural adaptation (see Linnoila, this volume, chapter 21). As such, their chronic use can be questioned, especially in view of evidence that this population appears to be highly at risk with regard to abuse potential (Hollister, 1981).

**Duration of treatment**

Hollister (1980) has provided a succinct summary of the most rational approach to the length of treatment when he stated: 'In the interest of good medical care and to minimize risks of dependence, patients should be thoroughly selected for benzodiazepine administration, and drug therapy should be discontinued as soon as it is therapeutically practical to do so.' Rickels (1980) has expanded on this theme when he stated: 'Duration of treatment should be influenced by the duration of symptoms.' He went on to point out that many acutely anxious patients require treatment for only a few days or weeks whereas more chronically ill patients would be inadequately treated by such a course of therapy and may even require a 'form of maintenance treatment'.

There seems to be little doubt that the likelihood of dependence on benzodiazepines is influenced not only by dose but by the length of therapy. Long-term treatment even at 'therapeutic' doses have been reported to lead to well-documented evidence of withdrawal symptoms upon abrupt termination (see Lader, chapter 2, this volume). However, the time required to induce such dependence has not been established nor has objective criteria been developed which will enable the practitioner to clearly identify a potentially susceptible patient (Hollister, 1981).

With regard to long-term efficacy, several studies have demonstrated no tolerance development when benzodiazepines have been given for 6 months (see Fabre *et al.*, 1981; Oswald *et al.*, 1982). However, Solomon *et al.* (1979) have raised the question as to how representative clinical trial groups are to the real population, at least with regard to hypnotics.

Finally, it should be noted that although physiological and psychological dependence are usually associated in physicians' minds with benzodiazepine therapy, it is also recognized for other drugs such as tricyclic antidepressants. Physical dependence was recognized as a possible consequence of tricyclic therapy by approximately 35% of physicians surveyed by Heiman and Wood (1981) whereas psychological dependence was thought possible by 75% of the respondents. Thus, the possibility of 'abuse' of all psychotropics must be kept in mind.

## SUMMARY AND CONCLUSIONS

A number of benzodiazepines are currently available for prescribing. With regard to the older drugs, the chief therapeutic difference among them seems to be their duration of action. Those with short half-lives are more rationally used as hypnotics while those with a longer duration are more rationally used as anxiolytics. Recent evidence has suggested at least semiqualitative differences between some triazolo- and imidazo- benzodiazepines and the older drugs.

This may well lead to established clinical utility in other psychiatric conditions.

The rational use of these products can be assured by careful diagnosis, considering patient factors and minimizing the length of treatment. Such an approach will minimize concerns regarding their potential misuse.

## REFERENCES

Achong, M. R., Bayne, J. R., Gerson, L. W. and Golshani, S. (1978). Prescribing of psychoactive drugs for chronically ill elderly patients. *Can. Med. Ass. J.*, **118**, 1503–1508.

Ananth, J. and Ghadiran, A. M. (1980). Drug-induced mood disorders. *Int. Pharmacopsychiat.*, **15**, 59–73.

Anonymous (1980a). Systematic review of the benzodiazepines. *Brit. med. J.*, **1**, 910–913.

Anonymous (1980b). A double blind comparison of ketazolam given once each day with diazepam given in divided doses and placebo in the treatment of anxiety. *Brit. J. clin. pract.*, **34**, 107–113.

Association of Sleep Disorders Centers (1979). Diagnostic classification of sleep and arousal disorders. *Sleep*, **2**, 1–137.

Balter, M. B., Levine, J. and Manheimer, D. I. (1974). Cross-national study of the extent of anti-anxiety/sedative drug use. *New Engl. J. Med.*, **290**, 769–774.

Bellantuono, C., Reggi, V., Tognoni, G. and Garattini, S. (1980). Benzodiazepines: clinical pharmacology and therapeutic use. *Drugs*, **19**, 195–219.

Boyd, J. H. and Weissmann, M. M. (1981). Epidemiology of affective disorders. *Arch. gen. Psychiat.*, **38**, 1039–1046.

Chouinard, G., Annable, L., Fontaine, R. and Solyom, L. (1982). Alprazolam in the treatment of generalized anxiety and panic disorders: a double-blind placebo-controlled study. *Psychopharmacology*, **77**, 229–233.

Cohn, J. B., Feighner, J. P., Smith, W. T. and Pyke, R. E. (1983). Open-label studies of adinazolam in severe depression. *Psychopharmacol. Bull.*, in press.

Darragh, A., Lambe, R., and Brick, I. (1981a). Reversal of benzodiazepine-induced sedation by intravenous RO 15-1788. *Lancet*, **ii**, 1042.

Darragh, A., Scully, M., Lambe, R. and Brick, I. (1981b). Investigation in man of the efficacy of a benzodiazepine antagonist, RO 15-1788. *Lancet*, **ii**, 8–10.

Dement, W. C., Miles, L. E. and Carskadon, M. A. (1982). White paper on sleep and aging. *J. Am. Geriatric Soc.*, **30**, 25–50.

Fabre, L. F., McLendon, D. M. and Stephens, A. G. (1981). Comparison of the therapeutic effect, tolerance and safety of ketazolam and diazepam administered for six months to out-patients with chronic anxiety neurosis. *J. int. med. Res.*, **9**, 191–198.

Feighner, J. P. (1982). Benzodiazepines as antidepressants—a triazolobenzodiazepine used to treat depression. In: *Modern Problems of Pharmacopsychiatry*, Vol. 18, pp.196–212 (Ed. Ban, T. A.), Karger, Basel.

Feighner, J. P., Guze, S., Robins, E., Woodruff, R., Winokur, G. and Munoz, R. (1972). Diagnostic criteria for use in psychiatric research. *Arch. gen. Psychiat.*, **26**, 57–63.

Feurst, S. (1982). Personal communication.

Greenblatt, D. J. and Shader, R. I. (1974). *Benzodiazepines in Clinical Practice*, Raven Press, New York.

Greenblatt, D. J. and Shader, R. I. (1975). Treatment of the alcohol withdrawal syndrome. In: *Manual of Psychiatric Therapeutics*, pp.211–235 (Ed. Shader, R. I.), Little Brown, Boston.

Greenblatt, D. J. and Shader, R. I. (1979). Caution on use of benzodiazepines in the elderly. *New Engl. J. Med.*, **300**, 1054–1055.

Greenblatt, D. J., Shader, R. I., Divoll, M. S. and Harmatz, J. S. (1981). Benzodiazepines: a summary of pharmacokinetic properties. *Brit. J. clin. Pharmac.*, **11**, 11s–16s.

Greenblatt, D. J., Shader, R. I. and Koch-Weser, J. (1975). Psychotropic drug use in the Boston area. *Arch. gen. Psychiat.*, **32**, 518–521.

Hall, R. C. W. and Kirkpatrick, B. (1978). The benzodiazepines. *Am. Family Practitioner*, **17**, 131–134.

Heimann, E. M. and Wood, G. (1981). Patient characteristics and clinician attitudes influencing the prescribing of benzodiazepines. *J. clin. Psychiat.*, **42**, 71–73.

Hester, J. B., Rudzik, A. D. and Von Voigtlander, P. F. (1980). 1-(Aminoalkyl)-6-aryl-4H-s-triazolo[4,3a][1,4]benzodiazepines with antianxiety and antidepressant activity. *J. med. Chem.*, **23**, 392–402.

Hindmarch, I. (1980). Psychoactive function and psychoactive drugs. *Brit. J. clin. Pharmac.*, **10**, 189–209.

Hollister, L. E. (1980). Dependence on benzodiazepines. In: *Benzodiazepines: a Review of Research Results, 1980*, pp.70–82, (Eds. Saraza, S. I. and Ludford, J. P.), US Govt. Printing Office, Washington.

Hollister, L. E. (1981). Management of the anxious patient prone to drug abuse. *J. clin. Psychiat.*, **42**, 35–39.

Jimerson, D. C., Van Kammen, D. P., Post, R. M., Docherty, J. P. and Bunney, W. E. (1982). Diazepam in schizophrenia: a preliminary double-blind trial. *Am. J. Psychiat.*, **4**, 489–491.

Keller, M. B., Klerman, G. L., Lavori, P. W., Fawcett, J. A., Coryell, W. and Endicott, J. (1982). Treatment received by depressed patients. *J. Am. Med. Ass.*, **248**, 1848–1855.

Klerman, G. L. (1980). Anxiety and depression. In: *Handbook of Studies on Anxiety*, pp.145–164 (Eds. Burrows, G. D. and Davies, B.), Elsevier, Amsterdam.

Lader, M. (1976). Antianxiety drugs: clinical pharmacology and therapeutic use. *Drugs*, **12**, 362–373.

Lasagna, L. (1977). The role of benzodiazepines in nonpsychiatric medical practice. *Am. J. Psychiat.*, **134**, 656–658.

Lingjaerde, O. (1982). Effect of the benzodiazepine derivative estazolam in patients with auditory hallucinations. *Acta psychiat. scand.* **65**, 339–354.

Mezzich, J. E. and Rabb, E. S. (1980). Depressive symptomatology across the Americas. *Arch. gen. Psychiat.*, **37**, 818–823.

Oswald, I., French, C., Adam, K. and Gilham, J. (1982). Benzodiazepine hypnotics remain effective for 24 weeks.*Brit. med. J.*, **1**, 860–863.

Patrick, M. J., Tilstone, W. J. and Reavey, P. (1972). Diazepam and breast feeding. *Lancet*, **i**, 542–543.

Rickels, K. (1980). Benzodiazepines: clinical use patterns. In: *Benzodiazepines: a Review of Research Results, 1980*, pp.43–60 (Eds. Sarza, S. I. and Ludford, J. P.), US Govt. Printing Office, Washington.

Rosser, W. W. (1980). Patterns of benzodiazepine usage in a family medicine centre. *Can. Fam. Physician*, **26**, 718–720.

Schatzberg, A. F. and Cole, J. O. (1978). Benzodiazepines in depressive disorders. *Arch. gen. Psychiat.* **35**, 1359–1365.

Sethy, V. H. and Hodges, D. H. (1982). Role of $\beta$-adrenergic receptors in the antidepressant activity of alprazolam. *Res. Commun. Chem. Pathol. Pharmacol.* **36**, 329–332.

Sheehan, D. V. (1982a). Current perspectives in the treatment of panic and phobic disorders. *Drug Therapy*, pp.179–191.
Sheehan, D. V. (1982b). Panic attacks and phobias. *New Engl. J. Med.*, **307**, 156–158.
Solomon, F., White, C. C., Parron, D. L. and Mendelson, W. B. (1979). Sleeping pills, insomnia and medical practice. *New Engl. J. Med.*, **300**, 803–808.
Sternbach, L. H., Randall, L. O., Banziger, R. and Lehr, H. (1968). Structure-activity relationships in the 1,4 benzodiazepine series. In: *Drugs Affecting the Central Nervous System*, pp.237–264 (Ed. Burger, A.), Marcel Dekker, Inc., New York.

## DISCUSSION

## CHAIRMAN: DR SUSAN IVERSEN

DR. P. A. LASCELLES: I was surprised that you did not say very much about anticonvulsant use. I wondered whether that represents a difference in practice between the United States and this country, because I think many people would feel there are important uses for the benzodiazepines in status epilepticus, in myoclonic epilepsy in children, and particularly, so far as the 1,5-benzodiazepines are concerned, in seizures in adults.

DR. B. STRAW: The 1,5-benzodiazepines are not available in the United States. Clonazepam and diazepam are used in the United States.

DR. L. L. IVERSEN: You suggested that some of the new compounds such as alprazolam may act as antidepressants. This seems most likely to be due to some other activity that that compound possesses, however, rather than the fact that it belongs to the group of tranquillizers of benzodiazepine chemical class. In any group of psychopharmaceutical agents inevitably one comes across secondary pharmacological properties. Do you view it as being in that class, or do you really think it is a benzodiazepine that is somehow unique?

DR. B. STRAW: With regard to more traditional models of antidepressant activity such as reuptake blockade alprazolam looks like other benzodiazepines; it is essentially inactive. Some recent work has been done giving alprazolam along with reserpine, where it looks more like desipramine. With regard to adnizolam, this compound is in fact active in reuptake models.

PROFESSOR M. SANDLER: I wished to add to your list of indications for benzodiazepines the Lesch–Nyhan syndrome. This is a very interesting one, as a matter of fact, because hypoxanthenes and certain related compounds, which build up in this condition have a known affinity for benzodiazepine receptors. Thus, their occupants are likely to be displaced by benzodiazepines and this has, in fact, been used in treatment. The trouble is, that too high a dose is needed and side effects occur. I was wondering therefore whether Ro 15-1788 or some other effective benzodiazepine antagonist might just be indicated in this sort of patient.

PROFESSOR M. LADER: In the figures of the antidepressant actions of alprazolam and imipramine against placebo, in the course of the trial the Hamilton depression scores go down from about 26 at the start (which is not very high even to start with) to placebo scores of about 20 and active drug scores of about 15. There may be statistical significance—you had large *N*s—but I wonder if clinically the amount of improvement was worthwhile.

DR. D. A. W. JOHNSON: With regard to depression there are a number of reasons for criticizing those trials. First of all, the patients were clinically depressed at the end of the trial as well as at the beginning of the trial. The only difference between the antidepressant and the benzodiazepine was speed of response in, I think, the first 2 weeks when, of course, we would not expect the antidepressant to have any effect.

Secondly, the tricyclic dose in one of two trials which I was able to find was mean at 124.7, and in the other I was unable to discover the mean daily dose. Although the criteria used were the Feighner criteria, in the first trial they specifically excluded the more severely ill patients, and, as we all know, the severity of symptomatology at the beginning of a trial influences the chances of showing the difference between two drugs at the end of the trial.

There is no evidence to show that benzodiazepines have any effect in schizophrenia. There are many, many reasons for being extremely anxious that anybody reading the publication should pick up any idea that there were even suggestions or clues on the horizon that benzodiazepines should be used in schizophrenia for its antipsychotic effect.

Benzodiazepines Divided
Edited by M. R. Trimble


# 7

# Biochemical Characterization of Benzodiazepine Receptors

LESLIE L. IVERSEN*

## DISCOVERY OF BENZODIAZEPINE RECEPTORS IN THE BRAIN

Although the benzodiazepines have been in clinical use for over 20 years, it is only very recently that we have begun to understand the mechanisms by which they act in the brain. The discovery in 1977 by Squires and Braestrup in Copenhagen and Mohler and Okada in Basle, that mammalian brain possesses specific receptors for the benzodiazepines has produced a remarkable upsurge of research interest in these compounds. Both groups showed in these initial experiments, with the use of radiolabelled diazepam, that high affinity binding sites exist on cell membranes in mammalian CNS which recognize the benzodiazepines specifically. These binding sites appear to have pharmacological relevance, as the relative potencies of different benzodiazepines in competing for diazepam binding reflect accurately their potencies in various animal tests predictive of anxiolytic properties. All of the pharmacologically active benzodiazepines used clinically interact with the brain binding sites, and a number of different radioactively labelled benzodiazepines can be used as receptor ligands. The potent compound flunitrazepam has advantages over diazepam and is now widely used for this purpose.

The regional distribution of benzodiazepine receptors in brain has been mapped in detail by biochemical experiments, and also by radiographic mapping of binding sites in brain tissue sections (Young and Kuhar, 1980). Comprehensive reviews of benzodiazepine receptor properties can be found elsewhere (Braestrup and Nielsen, 1982b; Martin, 1983), and only a brief survey can be given here.

*In conjunction with A. Doble, C. L. Brown, and I. L. Martin

## INTERACTIONS OF BENZODIAZEPINES WITH GABA RECEPTORS IN BRAIN

Although there is no direct competition between benzodiazepines and GABA and related drugs for their receptors in brain, it is generally accepted that some interaction does exist. Benzodiazepines have been found to enhance the inhibitory synaptic actions of GABA in various regions of brain and spinal cord where GABA-ergic synapses occur. (For review see Costa *et al.*, 1978). It has been suggested that the benzodiazepine receptor binding site may be located in proximity to the chloride channel in cell membranes which is activated by occupation of GABA receptors (Figure 1). Receptor binding studies *in vitro* add some support to this hypothesis. Thus, a number of studies have shown that both GABA and chloride and related anions interact with the benzodiazepine binding sites in brain membranes, to enhance benzodiazepine binding. The action of both GABA and chloride is to increase the affinity of the binding sites for diazepam and related drugs. GABA and chloride exhibit a complex interaction, mutually enhancing each other's effects (Martin, 1983). The hypothesis that the benzodiazepine receptor represents part of a GABA receptor–chloride ionophore complex receives support from the observation that the ablity of a number of other anions to facilitate benzodiazepine binding is similar to the ease with which they can replace chloride in the production of inhibitory synaptic potentials in nerve cell membranes. In the presence of GABA the apparent MW of rat brain benzodiazepine receptors (estimated by a

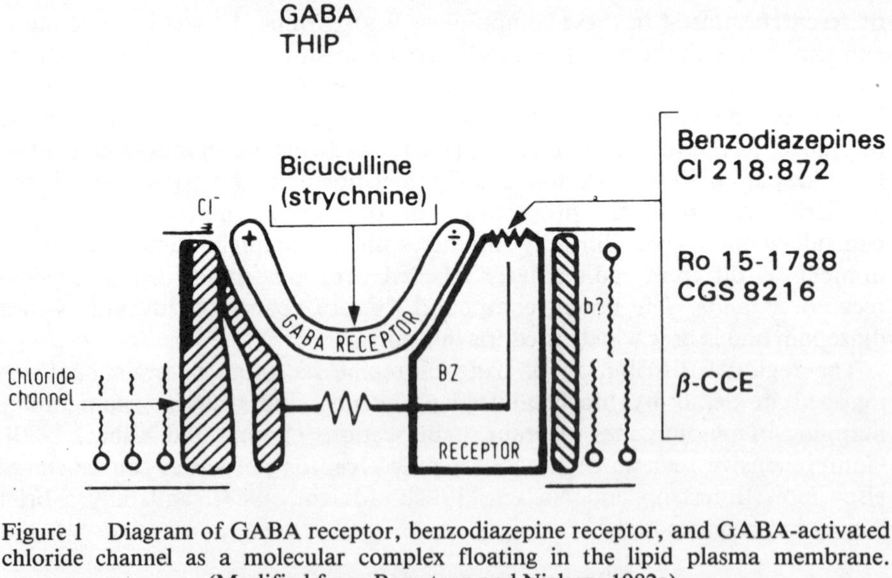


Figure 1 Diagram of GABA receptor, benzodiazepine receptor, and GABA-activated chloride channel as a molecular complex floating in the lipid plasma membrane. (Modified from Braestrup and Nielsen, 1982a)

radiation inactivation technique) decreased from 90,000–100,000 to 60,000–63,000 daltons, suggesting that GABA may act by promoting the disaggregation of a normally dimeric form (Doble *et al.*, 1982).

## RECENTLY DISCOVERED COMPOUNDS

There has been an intensive search for possible endogenous substances in brain which might normally act at benzodiazepine receptors, although if the benzodiazepine receptor does represent part of a chloride ion channel, it might be argued that such endogenous ligands need not exist. So far, such compounds have not been identified. Braestrup *et al.* (1980) described a novel compound, ethyl β-carboline-3-carboxylate (βCCE), which they isolated from human urine. This compound and related structures represent a novel class of substances which bind with high affinity to benzodiazepine receptors. It is now generally recognized that βCCE does not normally exist in human urine, but it represents a chemical artefact produced in the extraction procedure. βCCE has, nevertheless, proved to be a valuable experimental tool.

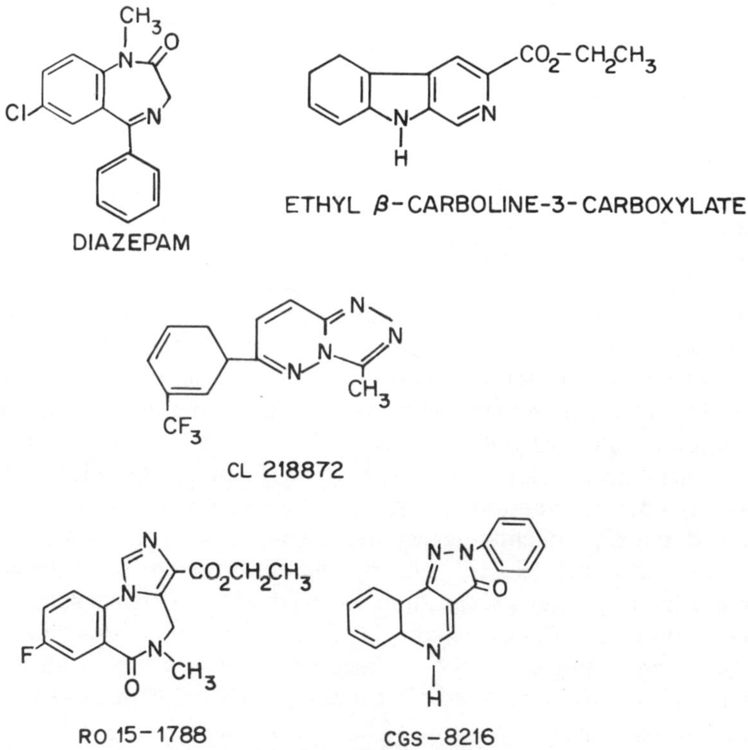


Figure 2 Structures of diazepam and some novel compounds which act on benzodiazepine receptors

Recent experiments in this laboratory and elsewhere have shown that radioactively labelled βCCE can be used as a ligand for benzodiazepine receptors in the brain. It exhibits a simple saturable binding curve, and the specific binding can be completely displaced with flunitrazepam or an excess of non-radioactive βCCE (Braestrup and Nielsen, 1981; Martin and Doble, 1983). The distribution of carboline binding sites in brain appears to mirror the distribution of benzodiazepine binding sites. Other recently discovered compounds (Figure 2) are the benzodiazepine antagonists CGS 8216 and Ro 15-1788, and the atypical triazolopyridasine CL 218872.

## MULTIPLE BENZODIAZEPINE RECEPTORS?

When βCCE is used to displace $^{3}$H-flunitrazepam binding, complex behaviour is observed in some regions of brain. In hippocampus, for example, as pointed out by Nielsen and Braestrup (1980) βCCE displaces $^{3}$H-flunitrazepam in an apparently multiphasic manner resulting in a shallow dose–response curve. If similar experiments were carried out in cerebellum, on the other hand, no such deviation from mass action occurred. Nielsen and Braestrup (1980) suggested that this might imply the existence of more than one type of benzodiazepine receptor binding site, distinguished by low and high affinity for βCCE. This appeared to support the similar suggestion made by Squires *et al.* (1979) who showed that the compound CL 218872 also exhibited shallow displacement curves when inhibiting $^{3}$H-flunitrazepam binding in rat brain membranes. It was suggested that the category of receptors present in cerebellum might represent a subtype (BZ1) and that the hippocampus contained a mixture of BZ1 and BZ2 subtypes. However, recent evidence from our own laboratory suggests that the two postulated receptor subtypes probably represent only different conformational and energy states of a single benzodiazepine receptor, possibly with differing linkages to a larger receptor/GABA/ionophore complex. This evidence is based on measurements of the on and off states of benzodiazepine and β-carboline binding (Doble *et al.*, 1982), Van't Hoff plots for benzodiazepine and carboline binding (Doble, 1983), and analysis of cooperativity phenomenon in binding experiments (Martin and Doble, 1983). Results of recent experiments suggest that the β-carboline and benzodiazepine binding sites, although closely related, can nevertheless be distinguished. When rat brain membrane preparations are exposed to flunitrazepam and then to ultraviolet light, flunitrazepam becomes covalently attached to the membranes and prevents the subsequent binding of radiolabelled benzodiazepines. However, β-carboline binding is virtually unaffected by such pretreatment (Brown and Martin, 1982). Benzodiazepines are still able to inhibit β-carboline binding in such photolabelled preparations, although higher concentrations are needed. In contrast, the potency of β-carboline derivatives and the benzodiazepine antagonist drugs Ro 15-1788 and

Table 1 Relative affinity of benzodiazepine receptor ligands in photoaffinity labelled and control rat hippocampal membranes

| Test drug | | Ratio of: $IC_{50}$ photoaffinity labelled / $IC_{50}$ control |
|---|---|---|
| Diazepam | | 30.1 ± 7.1* |
| Flunitrazepam | | 11.9 ± 2.5* |
| Ro 15-1788 | | 1.1 ± 0.1 |
| CGS 8216 | | 1.1 ± 0.1 |
| Methyl | | 1.1 ± 0.02 |
| Ethyl | β-carboline-3-carboxylate | 1.1 ± 0.1 |
| *N*-Propyl | | 1.0 ± 0.1 |
| CL 218872 | | 2.2 ± 0.03* |

*Significantly different from unity $P < 0.05$.
Potencies of drugs in inhibiting $^3$H-βCCE binding to rat brain membranes were measured in control preparations and after photolabelling benzodiazepine binding sites with flunitrazepam and exposure to UV light. Ratio of 1.0 indicates no change, and greater than 1.0 indicates a loss of potency after photolabelling (C. Brown and I. Martin—unpublished data).

CGS 8216 are not affected by the photolabelling procedure (Table 1). The possibility that this experimental procedure may be used as a means of distinguishing 'agonist' from 'antagonist' profiles in the benzodiazepine area is an intriguing one, and is being actively explored. The existence of separate binding sites for β-carbolines and benzodiazepine agonists in brain membranes may help to explain the complex interaction of these classes of compounds observed in competition experiments. The notion that more than one pharmacologically distinct category of benzodiazepine receptor may exist in brain, although an attractive one, remains unproven.

## CONCLUSIONS

The benzodiazepine receptor in brain appears to represent a component of the GABA receptor–chloride ionophore complex in neuronal membranes. It is not clear whether all GABA receptors are capable of modulation by benzodiazepines in the manner described; nor is it clear whether all benzodiazepine receptors in brain are coupled in this way to inhibitory synaptic mechanisms. Nevertheless, this represents a major step forward in our understanding of the mechanism of action of this important class of psychopharmacologically active agents. It is also believed that other compounds with similar psychopharmacological profiles, notably the barbiturates and ethanol may also act in some way to enhance the effectiveness of GABA at inhibitory receptors. However, neither barbiturates nor ethanol appear to act by the same mechanism which mediates benzodiazepine actions as there is no interaction of these classes of compounds in *in vitro* binding experiments.

## REFERENCES

Braestrup, C. and Nielsen, M. (1981). $^3$H-propyl β-carboline-3-carboxylate as a selective radioligand for the BZl benzodiazepine receptor subclass. *J. Neurochem.*, **37**, 333–341.

Braestrup, C. and Nielsen, M. (1982a). Anxiety. *Lancet*, **ii**, 1030–1034.

Braestrup, C. and Nielsen, M. (1982b). Benzodiazepine receptors. In: *Handbook of Psychopharmacology*, Vol. 17, pp.285–382 (Eds. Iversen, L. L., Iversen, S. D. and Snyder, S. H.), Plenum Press, New York.

Braestrup, C., Nielsen, M. and Olsen, C. E. (1980). Urinary and brain β-carboline-3-carboxylates as potent inhibitors of brain benzodiazepine receptors. *Proc. Natl Acad. Sci. USA*, **77**, 2288–2292.

Brown, C. L. and Martin, I. L. (1982). Photoaffinity labelling of the benzodiazepine receptor does not occlude the β-CCE binding site. *Brit. J. Pharmac.*, **77**, 312P.

Costa, E., Guidotti, A. and Toffano, G. (1978). Molecular mechanisms mediating the action of diazepam on GABA receptors. *Brit. J. Psychiat.*, **133**, 239–248.

Doble, A. (1983). Comparative thermodynamics of benzodiazepine receptor ligand interactions in rat neuronal membranes. *J. Neurochem.* (in press).

Doble, A., Martin, I. L. and Richards, D. A. (1982). GABA modulation predicts biological activity of ligands for the benzodiazepine receptor. *Brit. J. Pharmac.*, **76**, 238P.

Martin, I. L. (1983). The benzodiazepines and their receptor. In: *Cell Surface Receptors* (Ed. Strange, P. G.), Ellis Horwood, Colchester (in press).

Martin, I. L. and Doble, A. (1983). The benzodiazepine receptor in rat brain and its interaction with ethyl β-carboline-3-carboxylate. *J. Neurochem.* (in press).

Mohler, H. and Okada, T. (1977). Benzodiazepine receptor: demonstration in the central nervous system. *Science*, 198, 849–851.

Nielsen, M. and Braestrup, C. (1980). Ethyl β-carboline-3-carboxylate shows differential benzodiazepine receptor interaction. *Nature*, **286**, 606–607.

Squires, R. F., Benson, D. I., Braestrup, C., Coupet, J., Klepner, C. A., Myers, V. and Beer, B. (1979). Some properties of brain specific benzodiazepine receptors: New evidence for multiple receptors. *Pharmac. Biochem. Behav.* **10**, 825–830.

Squires, R. F. and Braestrup, C. (1977). Benzodiazepine receptors in rat brain. *Nature*, **266**, 732–734.

Young, W. S. and Kuhar, M. J. (1980). Radiohistochemical localisation of benzodiazepine receptors in rat brain. *J. Pharmac. exp. Ther.* **212**, 337–346.

## DISCUSSION

## CHAIRMAN: PROFESSOR MALCOLM LADER

PROFESSOR M. SANDLER: You mentioned rightly that GABA increases the affinity of benzodiazepine receptors for benzodiazepines. Is βCCE binding independent of GABA?

DR. L. L. IVERSEN: Yes. Dr. Ian Martin and others have argued that this might be another way of distinguishing the antagonist-type profile from the agonist profile.

PROFESSOR SANDLER: How do you fit it into the GABA scheme if GABA is independent?

DR. L. L. IVERSEN: We have already said that the carboline binding site appears to be a different one from the benzodiazepine site, but the two are still likely to be closely related because of the interaction that exists between carbolines and the benzodiazepines in binding studies. The reason for the fact that a GABA interaction exists for one and not the other site is unknown.

DR. FILE: I do not understand fully why, if you photoaffinity label receptors and you then reduce the binding to flunitrazepam and you do not to β-carboline, you say this shows different sites. It seems to me that because we know the structure of chlordiazepoxide is changed by UV light, exposure of the receptor to UV could change its physical properties in such a way that the benzodiazepines can no longer get at that site and bind but that the β-carbolines can get in.

DR. I. MARTIN: In the control procedure the membrane preparation is irradiated with UV light in the absence of flunitrazepam. You do not get a modification of the membrane itself, unless flunitrazepam is present during the photoactivation.

DR. FILE: So that excludes the structural change?

DR. MARTIN: That excludes the structural change in the membrane *per se*. It is important to point out that it is only certain benzodiazepines that can be used to 'phototag', if you like, the receptor.

DR. GRAY: Why could there not be interaction between the flunitrazepam and the membrane and the ultraviolet light?

DR. MARTIN: That is what we are saying.

DR. GRAY: But then the reason that you get the different binding would be, as Dr. File suggested, that you have a different physical structure. That would still leave open the possibility that before you have changed the physical structure because of this putative interaction between the light, the binding, the benzodiazepine, and the receptor, it might be the same recognition for all of the compounds.

DR. MARTIN: I think what we cannot say, at the moment, is how it has changed. All we can say is that we can modify the system such that part of it remains, as far as we can see, unaltered; and part of it is changed. We do not know whether it is a steric effect. When we photoaffinity label the system or the membrane with flunitrazepam we do not simply stick flunitrazepam on to its receptor. That is clear. I will not go into the details of why we know that, but we know we do not stick it on to the receptor in its on-confirmation. We insert, probably, a drug molecule fragment of flunitrazepam into the membrane matrix in such a way that we interfere with the access of certain compounds—in this case the benzodiazepines—but we do not interfere with the access of β-carbolines. That does not say that the β-carboline site is different from the flunitrazepam site. What it does say is that the recognition, or the access, properties are different. That is all we can say.

Benzodiazepines Divided
Edited by M. R. Trimble


# 8

# Animal Models of Anxiety

SUSAN IVERSEN

## INTRODUCTION

If one considers the behavioural basis of emotional behaviour, one recapitulates the history of animal psychology and learning theory. In the latter, behavioural responses are determined by the stimulus events of the environment. Psychologists use different words to describe the ways in which stimuli modify behaviour and to describe the different conditioning procedures which demonstrate that the presentation of meaningful stimuli or events cause long lasting changes in behaviour. Events may be pleasant or unpleasant or in other words reinforcing or punishing. If an animal makes a particular response that leads to reinforcement or punishment, the response is changed by that event. Reinforcers increase the probability of occurrence of the preceding response and punishers decrease it. Skeletal responses are readily modified in these ways and this provides the most reliable measures of *operant conditioning*, the term used to describe this particular procedure.

Reinforcers and punishers when presented also elicit responses. Food elicits salivation, electric shock to the hand leads to rapid withdrawal of the limb and a pain response, and the sight of an adversary provokes anger. These examples illustrate that the response profile elicited by meaningful stimuli include some easily identified skeletal (limb withdrawal) or autonomic responses (salivation) but usually, in addition, a range of ill-defined responses which in concert create a particular sensation. We have coined the term emotion for these broad constellations of responses elicited by events in the environment which concerns us. If one makes a list of generally accepted and distinguishable emotional states, it is long and variable. In fact, it is difficult to compile a list of 'the emotions', and even more difficult to state the spectrum of responses constituting a given state.

The problem of definition is matched only by the difficulty in measuring emotional states. The emotional responses elicited by events may also come to be modified by conditioning. The sight and smell of food elicits salivation; the so-called *unconditioned stimulus* elicits an *unconditioned response*. If neutral stimuli, which biologically are quite unable to elicit this autonomic response, say a bell, are regularly and precisely presented together with the food, after a number of conditioning trials, the bell, in the absence of food, will elicit salivation. A process of stimulus substitution has occurred, and we call this form of conditioning *classical* or *respondent conditioning*.

In theories which account for learned emotional responses in animals and man, classical conditioning plays a central role. If a rat learns at the sound of a buzzer to leap a hurdle and avoid an imminent electric shock, it is proposed that two sequential conditioning events occur. In the initial trials, the emotional response to the shock comes to be elicited by the preceding buzzer as a consequence of classical conditioning. Subsequently, conditioned emotional responses to the buzzer motivates the rat to make a specific response in order to reach a safe place. The shock-free environment acts as a reinforcer to strengthen the previous jumping response. There are of course a number of different theoretical formulations of the two-process models of learning, which are not of concern in this context (Mackintosh, 1974).

These introductory comments are presented to indicate that if one needs to manipulate and quantify emotional responses, there are a number of conditioning procedures and response measures which may be used. Weiskrantz (1968) provided a critical account of the various attempts to measure emotional behaviour, and pinpointed many of the theoretical and practical issues which have dogged this area of research over the years.

Since noxious stimuli are biologically so significant, ready to hand, and easy to automate in experimental situations, the study of the emotion of anxiety has figured prominently in this area of psychological research. The presentation of a noxious stimulus elicits a constellation of respondent effects, it also results in disruption of other ongoing behaviour.

Thus, if one wishes to quantify the anxiety induced by the presentation of a particular noxious stimuli either (a) the respondents associated with the emotional state or (b) the disruption of concurrent reinforced behaviour may be measured.

## CLASSICAL CONDITIONING AND ANXIETY

According to Liddell (1954) the foundations for the study of anxiety lie in the work of Freud and Pavlov. Pavlov himself had described a number of experimental situations in which classical conditioning led ultimately to profound emotional disturbance and disruption of normal behaviour. Dogs subjected to too difficult or prolonged conditioning developed chronic emotional disturbances, showing clear evidence of anxiety. For example, a dog was conditioned to respond to one visual pattern (circle) and not to another (ellipse). Later the circle became progressively similar to the ellipse until the discrimination became impossible. At this stage behavioural disorganizations occurred, termed by Pavlov 'experimental neurosis'. Liddell pursued these observations in sheep and goats introducing a wide range of technology for recording respondents (such as heart rate and respiration as well as bleating and skeletal responses) during the classical conditioning procedure and for long periods afterwards. Following the experience at regular intervals of unavoidable shock to the leg signalled with a buzzer, chronic changes in heart rate were observed. During the night, heart rate remained high and fluctuated in an abnormal fashion, rising to the slightest noise or disruption. The observation was made that sheep rendered neurotic in this way showed poor social behaviour in the flock, particularly when the latter was threatened by predators.

While extremely interesting, these techniques have not found widespread application as a model of anxiety. Respondents are difficult to measure, and extremely variable, both within and between individuals. It is notable that in the quote from Freud, with which Liddell introduces his paper, can be found the essence of the second principle which has proved germane to the development of animal models of anxiety—notably conflict between a desired goal and the aversive events which prevent the achievement of that goal. Freud wrote

> Goaded by the id, hemmed in by the superego, and rebuffed by reality, the ego struggles to cope with its economic task of reducing the forces and influences which work in it and upon it to some kind of harmony; and we may well understand how it is that we so often cannot repress the cry: 'Life is not easy'. When the ego is forced to acknowledge its weakness, it breaks out into anxiety: reality anxiety in the face of the external world, normal anxiety in the face of the superego, and neurotic anxiety in the face of the strength of the passions in the id.

Conflict disrupts behavioural organization, and measures of this disruption form the basis of the animal models of anxiety most commonly studied.

## DISRUPTION OF ONGOING BEHAVIOUR AS A MEASURE OF ANXIETY

### Behavioural suppression of operant behaviour induced by aversive stimuli

If an animal is trained to perform a given response for reinforcement and then periodically is simultaneously punished with an electric shock and at the same time rewarded for making that response, conflict exists. The learned response is disrupted. The shock may be programmed so that the response of the animal initiates the shock, or it may occur at set times irrespective of the behaviour of the animal. These procedures are termed immediate and adventitious punishment; immediate punishment disrupts behaviour to a greater degree than adventitious punishment. Skinner had, in the 1930s, pioneered the introduction of simple devices for recording skeletal responses, which for the first time permitted their precise quantification and visual representation on cumulative recorders.

In a classic paper in 1941, Estes and Skinner described a procedure involving signalled advantitious punishment. Rats were trained to press a lever for food on a fixed interval schedule of food presentation. When the behaviour generated by the reinforcement schedule had stabilized, an auditory signal was presented regularly every few minutes and the termination of the tone was associated with a shock to the feet, which was unavoidable and inescapable. Surprisingly, neither the onset of the tone nor the shock itself produced dramatic behavioural disturbances initially. However, with experience of the schedule controlling stimuli, responding on the lever during the tone progressively declined. Some typical response records from such an experiment are illustrated in Figure 1. The experimenters made a number of assumptions implicit in the title of their paper and wrote 'the principal result of the experiment was the conditioning of a state of anxiety to the tone, where the primary index was a reduction in the strength of a hunger-motivated lever-pressing behaviour'. They assumed that the conditioned anxiety responses caused the disruption of lever pressing. More likely, as Blackman (1972) has pointed out in an excellent critique of the so-called conditioned emotion response (CER), the behaviour conditioned to tone was freezing and was thus incompatible with active lever pressing. Despite the appeal of the CER pradigm, it has not been proved as useful as anticipated for screening anxiolytic drugs (Kelleher and Morse, 1964). The reasons for this are somewhat obscure (Blackman, 1972) probably relating to the contrast effects between the various elements of the schedule and the shock history of the subject. A number of laboratories are still persevering with CER techniques (see chapter 13) since a paradigm in which behaviour is disrupted by a signal associated previously with unpleasant events, rather than by the direct presentation of unpleasant events themselves, finds parallels in the aetiology of human anxiety. Emotion in man is frequently associated with the anticipation of events.

The CER technique was superseded as a model for evaluating anxiolytics by a procedure introduced by Geller and Seifter. This method is termed CONFLICT, and involves immediate punishment. Rats first learned to press a lever for a milk reward, presented on a variable interval (VI) (2 min) schedule for 1.25 h. When lever pressing rates had become stable, a tone was presented every 15 min for a 3 min duration. During these 'tone periods' the schedule

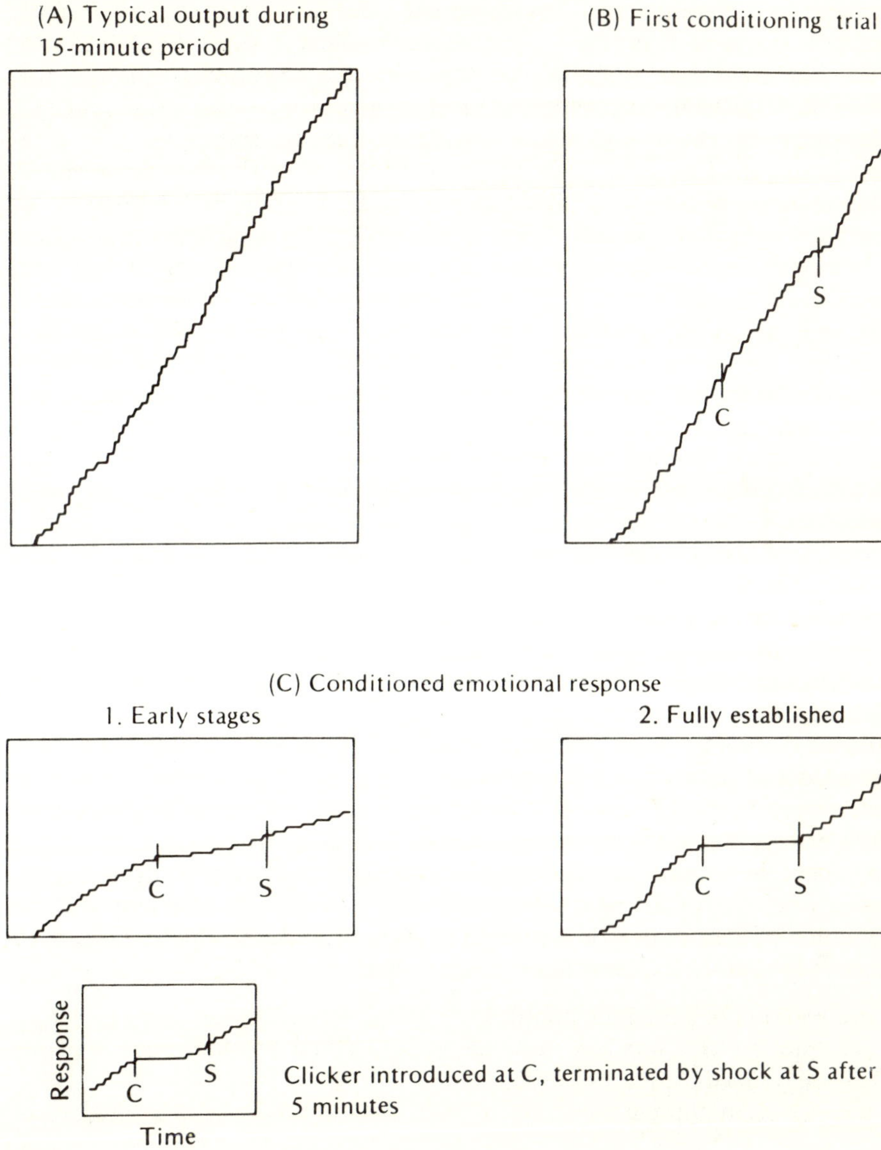


Figure 1 The conditioning of suppression during presentation of a preaversive auditory stimulus. Typical variable interval (VI) performance reinforced by food is presented in (A). (B) shows the effect of a brief shock (S) on this VI performance. ($C_1$) and ($C_2$) illustrate early and late conditioned suppression with progressively fewer responses emitted during the clicks. (Reproduced from Hunt and Brady, 1955)

changed to a continuous reinforcement schedule with every response rewarded. But in addition every response also resulted in shock (0.35–0.85 mA) to the feet. Behaviour stabilized quickly, with rats responding at a high rate during the VI schedule segments and barely at all during the alternate tone plus shock segment. Under high shock conditions, the rats responded only three times during the four tone + shock segments, and three shocks were received; but in presence of 10 mg/kg chlordiazepoxide, 56 shocks were tolerated by the same rat during those periods (Geller *et al.*, 1962). This dose dependent release of punished responding is typically seen with benzodiazepines. It has been observed in a number of species and on a variety of different multiple schedules involving conflict. The response suppression or behavioural inhibition associated with immediate punishment is reversed by anxiolytic drugs (barbiturates, meprobamate and benzodiazepines) in a dramatic and robust manner as illustrated in Figure 2, where the effect of 10 mg/kg pentobarbitone on punished responding in pigeons is studied. The *Geller Seifter* procedure is now the most commonly used screening test for novel anxiolytics.

Some conflict procedures which involve shorter training have become available, and currently punished drinking is finding widespread use. Here thirsty rats are trained to drink from a water spout which is subsequently connected to a shock generating circuit (Vogel *et al.*, 1971). Drinking now results in simultaneous punishment. This behavioural test is favoured since the drinking baseline does not require extensive training, and conflict can be introduced rapidly into the test situation. However, caution has been expressed about this test since benzodiazepines are reported to enhance to some extent the intake of water (Cooper and Francis, 1979) and food (Cooper, 1980), effects thought to be independent of their anxiolytic action. In conflict tests where the operant baseline involves unconditioned eating or drinking, the appetitive effects of the benzodiazepines are more likely to interfere with the evaluation of their anxiolytic action. In all these procedures which have proved sensitive to anxiolytics, three features are found:

1. presentation of a noxious stimulus;
2. presentation of a noxious stimulus brought about by the response of the animal (immediate punishment);
3. noxious event unpredictable.

## Disruption of unconditioned behaviour by aversive stimuli

It is striking that electric shock has figured prominently in the studies of anxiety in animals. The ease of presentation and the effectiveness of this stimulus encourage its use. However, it is clear that we should be attempting to find aversive events of more biological significance to the species being

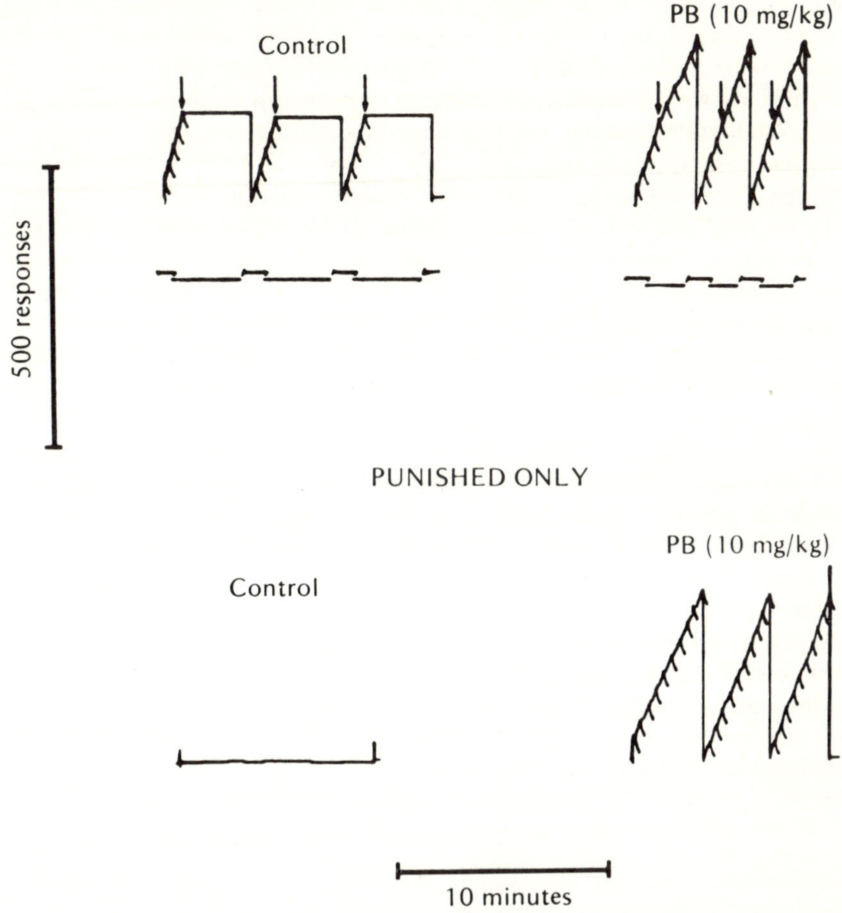


Figure 2 Effects of pentobarbitone (PB) on key pecking in the pigeon suppressed by punishment. Each frame shows a complete control session followed by a complete drug session. *Upper:* in non-punishment components (event record displaced upward), a 30-response, fixed-ratio schedule of food presentation was in effect in the presence of an orange light. The termination of each non-punishment component is indicated by a small arrow. In punishment components (event record displaced downward), a 30-response, fixed-ratio schedule was in effect in the presence of a white light; each of the first ten responses of each ratio produced a 35-ms electric shock of 6 mA, 60 cycles a.c. delivered through gold wire electrodes implanted around the pubis bones of the bird. The termination of each punishment component is indicated by the resetting of the pen to the bottom of the record. *Lower:* the punishment procedure was in effect throughout each session in the presence of a white light. Note that under both procedures, pentobarbitone attenuates the suppression of responding by punishment. (Reproduced from Kelleher and Morse, 1964)

investigated, and this is particularly important since animal models of anxiety are used for evaluating therapeutic methods of possible use in man. With this in view, File and Hyde (1978) have developed a test of social interaction in rats which has shown an interesting range of responsiveness to pharmacological agents. Male rates placed in a large arena indulge in social interaction responses. In highly unfamiliar and brightly lit arenas the level of interaction is low when compared to that in dimly lit familiar situations, presumably due to the anxiety induced by the former conditions. Chronic chlordiazepoxide and a number of other anxiolytic compounds significantly increase the low levels of social interaction in the unfamiliar bright arena. Novel highly illuminated environments also inhibit locomotion and exploration in rats and mice tested singly. Crawley and Goodwin (1981) have capitalized on this fact to develop a single trial test of anxiety in mice. A cage was divided by a partition into an area (2/3) brightly lit and a black unlit area (1/3). Movements between the two areas were recorded with photocells in the partition and general activity in the arenas with underlying movement detectors. Normal rats avoid the brightly lit arena, a spontaneous preference reversed by pretreatment with benzodiazepines. The increase in entries to the bright field under the drug was not secondary to a general increase in locomotor activity. Tye *et al.* (1975) described another simple test situation. Rats were trained to lever press for food, and when well trained entered the test box to find a bowl of free food on the back wall. Normal rats continue to press for food in the presence of this free food and do not approach the free food presumably because the novel food source generates anxiety. Rats pretreated with chlordiazepoxide (4–12 mg/kg) consume large quantities of the free food although their emission of lever presses for earned food does not increase.

### Behavioural disruption of respondent and operant responses by aversive stimuli

Anxiety as a state invokes changes not only in operant behaviour but also (and probably to a greater extent) in respondent behaviour. The animal tests of anxiety most favoured have, in a sense, taken the easy way out by using the suppression of a simple operant as an index of this complex state. When conflict paradigms were first under investigation some workers attempted to develop measures of anxiety which took account of the complexity of the response profile induced by aversive stimuli. Masserman and Pechtel (1956a,b) for example studied patterns of conflict in cats trained to drink milk and then puffed with air when they approached the bowl. Thirty-four rating scales were used in an attempt to define the behaviour in the conflict situation, but were so complex that they proved of little systematic use. Even with this degree of elaboration, Masserman and Pechtel (1956a) felt that their methods were inadequate for defining the effects of drugs and lesions on neurotic behaviour since they were measuring only the present behaviour of the cat and ignoring its past emotional heritage. They write: 'It is impossible to state the effects of any drug on any organism without considering the latter's genetic characteristics, past experiences, biological status, and perceptions, motivations toward, and evaluations of its current physical and social milieu.'

One cannot help but feel that it is time to take up again the challenge of devising methods for evaluating emotional responses which include measures of elicited autonomic responses to emotion-provoking stimuli. The considerable advances in psychophysiology and biofeedback technology may now make this worthwhile.

## Behavioural invigoration induced by aversive stimuli

Before concluding this resumé of animal tests of anxiety, it is important to stress that stimuli which are aversive do not necessarily or only result in suppression of ongoing behaviour. All the test situations described so far result in suppression or behavioural inhibition. However, aversive stimuli also lead to increases in arousal and attention. Non-reward is such an aversive stimulus, as originally described in the works of Amsel (1962) on frustrative effects of non-reward. It is Gray (1982 and page 101) who has developed the concept of frustration as an invigorating influence on behaviour, and has used these observations as a basis for a general theory of anxiety. If rats were exposed to partial reinforcement rather than continuous reinforcement in a straight runway task, their rate of extinction when reward is totally removed from the task is slower than that observed in rats who receive continuous reinforcement during the runway training. It is suggested that the experience of partial reward during learning creates frustration and subsequent invigoration of behaviour. Gray has many reasons to believe that the delayed extinction associated with partial reinforcement is an index of anxiety, since the extinction effect is abolished by treatment with anxiolytic drugs during the runway training. Whether or not the same brain circuitry mediates the arousing and inhibiting effects of anxiety as proposed by Gray remains to be seen. However, it is likely that the two response dimensions are related and that some anxiety-provoking stimuli activate the arousal dimension more than the response suppression dimension and vice versa. Although benzodiazepines influence both the arousal and the behavioural inhibition induced by anxiety, it has not been convincingly demonstrated that the identical brain circuitry is involved in these two effects. While the evidence for an involvement of the septo-hippocampal circuit in the partial reinforcement effect is compelling, it is, in my opinion, premature to associate immediate punishment with the identical CNS substrates.

## CONCLUDING STATEMENT

If one is seeking a behavioural test in animals with which to detect anxiolytics then success has been achieved. But if one is concerned to have tests which model more closely the human situation there is reason for disquiet. Human emotional behaviour is individual and environment specific, and as we see in the discussion of this paper, studies on the emotional behaviour of monkeys in social colonies emphasize this only too clearly. It may be misleading to depend solely on the emotional response of isolated animals in controlled conditions; the real world is not structured in this way. Perhaps we were wrong to isolate operant responses from the rich fabric of operant and respondent behaviour seen in complex behaviour, and we should again make serious attempts to relate autonomic changes with emotional experience.

Finally, it should be remembered that emotional responses in man are not predictable in terms of the input-out equation of the Skinnerian psychologist. Cognition plays an important role in the elaboration of emotional responses in man (Schachter and Singer, 1962), although it is difficult to evaluate complex factors of this kind. It would be premature to hope that any animal model can take full account of the human situation but it is important when describing models of precision and simplicity to at least be aware that at best we are teasing out markers of the rich fabric of emotional behaviour.

## REFERENCES


Amsel, A. (1962). Frustrative non-reward in partial reinforcement and discrimination learning: some recent history and a theoretical extension. *Psychol. Rev.*, **69**, 306–328.

Blackman, D. E. (1972). Conditioned anxiety and operant behaviour. In: *Schedule Effects: Drugs, Drinking and Aggression*, pp.26–49 (Eds. Gilbert, R. M. and Keehn, J. P.), University of Toronto Press, Toronto.

Cooper, S. J. (1980). Effects of chlordiazepoxide and diazepam on feeding performance in a food-preference test. *Psychopharmacology*, **69**, 73–78.

Cooper, S. J. and Francis, R. L. (1979). Water intake and time course of drinking after single or repeated chlordiazepoxide injections. *Psychopharmacology*, **65**, 191–195.

Crawley, J. and Goodwin, F. K. (1981). Preliminary report of a simple animal behaviour model for the anxiolytic effects of benzodiazepines. *Pharmac. Biochem. Behav.*, **13**, 167–170.

Estes, W. K. and Skinner, B. F. (1941). Some quantitative properties of anxiety. *J. exp. Psychol.*, **29**, 390–400.

File, S. E. and Hyde, J. R. G. (1978). Can social interaction be used to measure anxiety? *Brit. J. Pharmac.*, **62**, 19–24.

Geller, I., Kulak, J. T. and Seifter, J. (1962). The effects of chlordiazepoxide and chlorpzomazine on a punished discrimination. *Psychopharmacologia*, **3**, 374–385.

Gray, J. A. (1982). The neuropsychology of anxiety: An enquiry into the functions of the septo-hippocampal system. *The Behav. Brain Sci.*, **5**, 469–534.

Hunt, H. F. and Brady, J. V. (1955). Some effects of punishment and intermittent 'anxiety' on a simple operant. *J. comp. physiol. Psychol.*, **48**, 305–310.

Kelleher, R. T. and Morse, W. H. (1964). Escape behavior and punished behavior. *Fed. Proc.*, **23**, 808–817.

Liddell, H. S. (1954). Conditioning and emotions. *Scientific American*, 48–57.

Mackintosh, N. J. (1974). *The Psychology of Animal Learning*. Academic Press, London, New York, San Francisco.

Masserman, J. H. and Pechtel, C. (1956a). An experimental investigation of factors influencing drug action. *Psychiat. Res. Reports*. (April, 1956), 95–113.

Masserman, J. H. and Pechtel, C. (1956b). How brain lesions affect normal and neurotic behaviour. *Am. J. Psychiat.*, **112**, 865–872.

Schachter, S. and Singer, J. E. (1962). Cognitive, social and physiological determinants of emotional state. *Psychol. Rev.*, **69**, 379–399.

Tye, N. C., Nicholas, D.J. and Morgan, M.J. (1975). Chlordiazepoxide and preference for free food in rats. *Pharmac. Biochem. Behav.*, **3**, 1149–1151.

Vogel, J. R., Beer, B. and Gody, D. E. (1971). A simple and reliable conflict procedure for testing anti-anxiety agents. *Psychopharmacologia*, **21**, 1–7.

Weiskrantz, L. (1968). *Emotion. Analysis of Behavioural Change*, pp.50–90 (Ed. Weiskrantz, L.), Harper and Row, New York.

## DISCUSSION

## CHAIRMAN: PROFESSOR MALCOLM LADER

DR. J. HERBERT: I want to take up three points: they are, first the types of anxiety that we are talking about; second, the animal models that we can use; and, third, the question of the responses that we measure.

I thought one of the most important points Dr. Iversen made was to distinguish between two ways of measuring anxiety: the way in which the animal can identify a particular source of anxiety, for example a shock or whatever; and the other model (such as a novelty environment) in which the animal cannot. When we consider the mechanisms concerned with the processing of this information, we must take these two categories into account and suggest that they are somewhat different.

Animals normally live in groups and we can see that anxiety or a fear response has two kinds of function in animal societies. The first is to modify the animal's response to a source, which it knows from its experience is likely to prove aversive. In our studies on groups of monkeys, the most subordinate monkey in the group shows both the endocrinal and behavioural correlates which allow one to label it as 'anxious'. It does so because it knows that its group contacts are more dominant animals which, under certain circumstances, are going to attack it and, therefore, represent a source of possible injury or threat.

Its assessment and thus its behavioural response to a situation is, therefore, going to be such as to minimize punishment, bearing in mind that it has to do so and yet allow itself the opportunities to get the kind of things which it needs in order to maintain itself, particularly food and perhaps even mates. In other words, the animal is making an assessment on an immediate basis of what ethologists call 'cost' and 'benefit'. This interaction is one of the causes of 'anxiety' or 'fear'.

The second — which is also seen in animal studies under more natural conditions as well as in the laboratory — is a situation in which an animal is faced with an unfamiliar environment or situation. That means that the animal has insufficient information upon which to make a decision about what to do. This, as we all know, is highly anxiety-inducing, but it is different from the first situation. I think therefore, we should expect not only the behavioural strategies but also the neural mechanisms it uses to be different in the two situations. Behaviour in the second will be directed forward by information from its environment in order to allow it to assess the likelihood of any possible threat so that it may behave in a way which again minimizes the 'cost' and maximizes the 'benefit'.

We see these two mechanisms operating side by side in groups of animals. Work carried out for the last few years in our laboratory (principally by Dr. Keverne and his associates) has been directed towards this. I will briefly summarize it. Groups of monkeys, like groups of men or any other groups of animals, form dominance hierarchies. Dominance hierarchies occur within sexes as well as between sexes; the first is more obvious than the second.

The dominance hierarchies are stable and can be reproduced in the laboratory very easily. They represent a natural phenomenon. The result of being at the bottom of the dominance hierarchy is extremely important. First of all, there are marked behavioural changes. Such an animal shows reduced behaviour of certain categories: for example, less movement in the cage; less aggression, greatly reduced sexual activity. Other activies are heightened, for example, visual monitoring, which we find a very sensitive and a very interesting way of looking at behaviour.

In animal studies, most people have been interested in behavioural responses. This, of course, historically was not the case: Cannon for example was concerned with autonomic changes. More recently, this has been extended to a whole variety of neuroendocrine responses. Interest is focusing largely on three endocrinal systems, which are to some degree separate. The interesting thing is that they may show different kinds of responses to different sorts of anxiety; and, second, they may have different consequences for the behavioural response of the animal, because we are dealing now not only with a parameter which reflects the animal's central state, but which may also play a part in determining it.

The three systems I am referring to are the adrenal medullary system which has classically been of interest in this area and which is still difficult to study; the ACTH/cortisol system, which has recently become of great interest, because it is now recognized to be part of the pro-opiocortin system; and changes in prolactin. The last peptide—a large one—looks as if it is going to turn out to be a neuropeptide, but a neuropeptide with a difference. Thus it is produced peripherally and gets into the brain extraordinarily easily, very surprising for a molecule of such a size; furthermore it has a marked effect on behaviour.

THE CHAIRMAN: You discussed Schachter's work. We all quote this and like to believe in it. In the original publications the significant results are sparse and not always convincing.

DR. S. IVERSEN: You are absolutely right. If you look at the small print and particularly if you look at the responses to placebo treatment in those experiments, the simple story begins to come undone. I suspect that is because we are focusing on one aspect of a broad response range to that particular drug and there is going to be an cnormous variation in the biological base in any individual coming into a drug state. So there is an enormous range of emotional tone in subjects in such an experimental situation which can surely account for these variations in the placebo response, let alone the response under the drugged condition.

THE CHAIRMAN: He also used the wrong drug. Caffeine might have been more appropriate.

DR. J. GRAY: There has been one attempt to replicate the original Schachter study, and another which tried to match its essential features by using hypnosis to induce, by post-hypnotic suggestion, a state of unexplained arousal. Neither of these experiments came up with the original Schachter finding, so I think one has to be cautious.

PROFESSOR OSWALD: You have talked about anxiety. I wondered if there were any modern developments in studying aggression with benzodiazepines in animal research.

Dr. S. FILE: There have not been very many studies recently. High doses, given acutely, which are simply sedative and reduce anything you like to measure, lower aggression. We have looked recently at chronic administration of low doses of chlordiazepoxide (the original benzodiazepine that was claimed to reduce aggression). We put drugged animals into a long-established colony of 12 male rats which had been living together for several months, and had a clearly established hierarchy, that attacked all intruders. We looked at the behaviour of this colony towards undrugged animals, animals given acute low doses of benzodiazepines and chronic treatment. The chronically treated animals were free to run around the colony and were attacked less. They did not show more aggression towards the resident rats, but there was something in their behaviour which inhibited overt biting attacks by the residents. They were able to walk over several residents without being attacked, to go to the prime sites and were not chased off. So, I think that some of the changed aggression in drugged animals, or people, may be in response to different behaviours emitted towards them.

DR. M. SCHMUTZ: We have had, for a long time, an animal model with freely moving cats that have implanted electrodes in the perifornical area of the hypothalamus. By intensifying the electrical stimulus gradually we can induce a 'rage reaction': the cat behaves as if it was confronted with a dog, showing wide pupils, piloerection and attacking behaviour. In this animal model, benzodiazepines such as diazepam increase the threshold level for the rage reaction.

Benzodiazepines Divided
Edited by M. R. Trimble


# 9

# Gamma-aminobutyrate, the Benzodiazepines and the Septohippocampal System

JEFFREY A. GRAY*

The last decade has seen an explosion of research regarding the mode of action of the benzodiazepines. This paper is directed to a question that is at once more limited and broader: where and how in the brain do antianxiety drugs (including the benzodiazepines) act so as to induce anxiety?

This question is more limited, because it seeks to delineate only those sites and modes of action that mediate reduction in anxiety, as distinct from the various other effects of these drugs (e.g. anticonvulsant, muscle-relaxant or sedative effects). But the limitation on the question does not make it easier to answer—on the contrary, it acquires an added dimension of difficulty precisely because of the need to segregate those neurophysiological, neurochemical, and behavioural changes produced by the benzodiazepines which are related to anxiety reduction from those which are not.

Our question is also broader than the usual one, because it is addressed to the site and mode of action of other drugs, besides the benzodiazepines, which similarly reduce anxiety. These include the barbiturates, meprobamate and alcohol, as well as newly synthesized drugs such as the triazolopyridazines. A comparative review of the effects of the barbiturates, alcohol, and the benzodiazepines shows that, across a wide variety of tests used to assess anxiety in animals and across a wide range of species from fish to monkeys, these different classes of drug produce a remarkably similar pattern of behavioural change (Gray, 1977). This similarity of effect legitimizes a search for a common mode of neural action. At the same time, it aids in the segregation of the antianxiety effects of the benzodiazepines from other kinds

*In association with Stella Quintero and Jane Mellanby.

of effect. As a simple example: the benzodiazepine receptor discovered by Braestrup and Squires (1977) and Möhler and Okada (1977) does not bind barbiturates, meprobamate or alcohol, so occupancy of this receptor cannot be a prerequisite of antianxiety action (Gray, 1979).

A better case can be made for enhancement of the effects of the inhibitory transmitter, $\gamma$-aminobutyrate (GABA), as the common path for antianxiety action. Both the benzodiazepines and the barbiturates produce this type of effect in electrophysiological and biochemical experiments (Barker and Ransom, 1978; Olsen, 1981), as does ethanol (Nestoros, 1980; Ticku, 1980).

However, the behavioural effects of the antianxiety drugs are too specific easily to be explained by a *general* facilitation of GABA-ergic transmission in the brain. These drugs have been studied in a great variety of behavioural paradigms. It is possible to fit most of the reported findings into a reasonably simple summary (but one which is derived from a relatively complex branch of the theory of learning). This summary states that the antianxiety drugs block behavioural responses to conditioned stimuli associated with punishment, to conditioned stimuli associated with the omission of anticipated reward ('frustrative non-reward'), and to novel stimuli (Gray, 1977). Conversely, the antianxiety drugs do not affect behavioural responses to other kinds of stimuli, including unconditioned punishment or unconditioned non-reward. The specificity of this pattern of behavioural change suggests that it is controlled by an equally specific functional system within the brain. Yet GABA-ergic neurons are found throughout the central nervous system, including the spinal cord, as are benzodiazepine receptors. Thus the most likely result of a general facilitation of GABA-ergic transmission would be to inhibit neuronal firing (on average) throughout the whole neuraxis, giving rise perhaps to sedation or a lowered probability of convulsions. If we are to find, rather, a substrate for the specifically antianxiety action of the benzodiazepines we must seek for a specialized system in the brain which (a) is activated by the anxiogenic stimuli listed above, and (b) is subject to GABA-ergic inhibitory control.

## THE SEPTOHIPPOCAMPAL SYSTEM

Direct electrophysiological or biochemical approaches cannot easily be applied in this search, since they omit the important behavioural dimension by which such a specialized system must be defined. Instead, one must resort to more indirect approaches. One such approach is to seek similarities between the profile of behavioural change seen after administration of antianxiety drugs, on the one hand, and after various interventions in the brain, on the other. If a brain intervention produces a profile closely similar to the antianxiety profile, then this suggests that the intervention is interrupting the function of a system which is normally active during stages of anxiety. Conversely, a profile which is the polar opposite of that seen after antianxiety drug administration would suggest that the intervention is causing such a system to be active. Application of these arguments to the available data converges upon the septohippocampal system as a site of particular interest for the neuropsychology of anxiety (Gray, 1970, 1982a). Lesions to either the septal area or the hippocampal formation produce a behavioural syndrome which is remarkably similar to that seen after administration of antianxiety drugs (Gray, 1977, 1982a; Gray and McNaughton, 1983). Conversely, although there is much less evidence, stimulation of the septal area (in a manner which mimics the normal, physiological control exerted by this region over the hippocampal theta rhythm) produces a pattern of behavioural change opposite to that produced by antianxiety drugs (Gray, 1982a; Holt and Gray, 1982). On this basis, then, one may propose the hypothesis that the septohippocampal system plays a central role in mediating anxiety, and that the antianxiety drugs reduce anxiety by dampening activity in this system.

This hypothesis is in no way incompatible with the evidence that benzodiazepines and barbiturates enhance GABA-ergic transmission. There are at least three ways in which such an enhancement could reduce septo-hippocampal function. First, the hippocampus itself has an extensive, intrinsic GABA-ergic interneuronal system (Storm-Mathisen, 1978). Second, the septohippocampal system receives an important serotonergic input from the raphe nuclei. A considerable body of evidence implicates these ascending serotonergic neurons in anxiety and antianxiety drug action (Graeff and Schoenfeld, 1970; Stein *et al.*, 1973). There are GABA receptors located both on the cell bodies of these neurons (Belin *et al.*, 1979; Gallager, 1978) and presynaptically on their terminals in the forebrain (Bowery *et al.*, 1980). Third, the septohippocampal system also receives an important noradrenergic input from the locus coeruleus. Again, there is much evidence implicating this pathway in anxiety and antianxiety drug action (Lidbrink *et al.*, 1973; Gray *et al.*, 1975; Redmond, 1979; Gray, 1982a). And again there are GABA receptors both on the cell bodies of these neurons (Iversen and Schon, 1973; Guyenet and Aghajanian, 1977) and the forebrain terminals (Bowery *et al.*, 1980; Fung and Fillenz, pers. comm.).

More specific hypotheses as to the functions of the septohippocampal system and its serotonergic and noradrenergic afferents in anxiety have been presented elsewhere (Gray, 1982a,b). These hypotheses also allot functions to the Papez circuit (from hippocampus to subiculum, thence to anterior thalamus and mammillary bodies, thence to cingulate cortex, and thence to entorhinal cortex and back to hippocampus); and to the prefrontal cortex (which in primates projects to the entorhinal cortex and also directly to the hippocampal formation).

In very general terms the resulting theory holds that the septohippocampal system and the associated Papez circuit functions as a comparator; that is, it generates (in the light of past stimulus–stimulus and response–stimulus regularities) predictions as to the next expected event and compares such predictions to actual events. If there is a mismatch between prediction and actual event, or if the predicted event is aversive, the septohippocampal system takes over control of behaviour, interrupts ongoing behaviour patterns ('behavioural inhibition'), and generates a search for alternative behaviour patterns. An increase in anxiety, on this theory, reflects increased activity in the septohippocampal system with one or both of two consequences: an increased scan of environmental events for mismatch (as defined above); and an increased likelihood of behavioural inhibition and associated behavioural changes. Clinically, the first of these consequences map roughly onto obsessional symptoms, and the second onto phobic symptoms.

The ascending noradrenergic and serotonergic fibres are held to facilitate the passage of information from the entorhinal cortex through the septohippocampal system, in accord with electrophysiological evidence (Segal, 1977a,b), leading under appropriate circumstances to an increase in anxiety. The primary antianxiety action of benzodiazepines, barbiturates, and other drugs with similar clinical and behavioural effects is then seen to consist in a reduction of activity in these monoaminergic pathways (Lidbrink *et al.*, 1973; Stein *et al.*, 1973; Gray *et al.*, 1975; Redmond, 1979).

The prefrontal cortex is allotted two functions in the theory. It provides the comparator with information about ongoing motor programmes (necessary for prediction); and in man it provides a route for verbally coded neocortical control over the predictive and search functions of the septohippocampal system. This type of descending control is of particular importance for some of the cognitive symptoms of anxiety, as in for example the obsessional syndrome. Section of the fibres which mediate such descending control is held responsible for the success of prefrontal and cingulate lesions in the therapy of drug-resistant anxiety states (Powell, 1979).

This is an excessively condensed summary of a complex theory, but it must suffice. The details of the theory are in any case unimportant for understanding the particular experiments we shall recount here, which have been concerned with a more empirical level of analysis.

## THE EXPERIMENTS

We have used psychopharmacological methods to ask whether antianxiety drugs act via enhancement of GABA transmission. As noted above, the specifically antianxiety action of these drugs appears to consist in a blockade of behavioural responses to stimuli associated with punishment, stimuli associated with non-reward, and novel stimuli (Gray, 1977). Accordingly, we studied responses of all three kinds in rats injected with a benzodiazepine (chlordiazepoxide HCl) or a barbiturate (amylobarbitone Na); we compared the effects of these anxiolytics to those produced by GABA agonists; and we tested whether GABA antagonists would block any effects obtained with either the anxiolytics or the GABA agonists.

A similar strategy was followed in electrophysiological experiments. In these we used free-moving male rats chronically implanted with a stimulating electrode in the septal area (which contains the pacemaker cells controlling the hippocampal theta rhythm) and a recording electrode in the hippocampal formation.

In such a preparation, stimulation of the septal area at a frequency within the naturally occurring range of theta frequencies (about 6–12 Hz) drives hippocampal theta at the stimulation frequency. If one now measures the threshold current able to produce this effect, there is a minimum threshold at a frequency of 7.7 Hz (James *et al.*, 1977). This minimum disappears after treatment with barbiturates, benzodiazepines, or alcohol (McNaughton *et al.*, 1977), in each case because the threshold for driving theta is selectively increased at 7.7 Hz. It is not possible to mimic this effect with a range of pharmacological and hormonal interventions affecting cholinergic, serotonergic, dopaminergic, or adrenocortical function (McNaughton *et al.*, 1977; Valero *et al.*, 1977). The effect is mimicked, however, by pharmacological blockade of noradrenergic transmission (McNaughton *et al.*, 1977) or destruction (using 6-hydroxydopamine) of the dorsal ascending noradrenergic bundle, which carries afferents from the locus coeruleus to the septohippocampal system (Gray *et al.*, 1975; McNaughton *et al.*, 1977). Thus it is likely that the antianxiety drugs abolish the 7.7-Hz minimum threshold in the 'theta-driving curve' by reducing noradrenergic input to the septohippocampal system.

Evidence that the lack of a 7.7-Hz minimum is connected to the emotional effects of the antianxiety drugs comes from a study of the Maudsley Reactive and Non-reactive strains of rat, selectively bred by Broadhurst (1975) for high and low emotionality, respectively. Like several other rat strains we have studied, the Reactive animals display the 7.7-Hz minimum; this is absent, however, in the Non-reactive strain (Drewett *et al.*, 1977). The Non-reactive strain also has more benzodiazepine binding sites, especially in the hippocampus and hypothalamus, than the Reactive strain (Robertson *et al.*, 1978). It is not known, however, whether this observation is connected to the strain difference in septal driving of hippocampal theta.

As well as testing the general proposition that antianxiety drugs act by enhancement of GABA transmission, our experiments, both behavioural and electrophysiological, were directed to a more specific issue. Recent research demonstrates the existence of two types of GABA receptor. The classical $GABA_A$ receptor responds to muscimol as agonist and bicuculline as antagonist. Bowery *et al.* (1980), however, have described a novel $GABA_B$ receptor which does not respond to these compounds, but is instead sensitive to baclofen (as agonist). The novel receptor is apparently located presynaptically on forebrain terminals of both noradrenergic and serotonergic neurons. If these receptors are important in antianxiety action, we might therefore expect to mimic the behavioural and electrophysiological effects of anxiolytics with baclofen, and not to be able to block them with bicuculline. If, however, $GABA_A$ receptors are important, we should be able to mimic anxiolytic effects using muscimol and block them with bicuculline.

Besides these drugs, we also studied a fourth GABA-related compound, picrotoxin. This is a less specific GABA antagonist than is bicuculline. It perhaps acts by shutting the chloride channel thought to be opened by GABA in the post-synaptic membrane (Braestrup and Nielsen, 1980). Thus picrotoxin might be expected to reverse anxiolytic effects whether these are produced at the $GABA_A$ or the $GABA_B$ receptor. Furthermore, recent evidence (Olsen, 1981) suggests that barbiturates and picrotoxin bind to a common 'picrotoxinin' receptor. If this hypothesis is correct, the behavioural and electrophysiological effects of amylobarbitone should be particularly susceptible to blockade by picrotoxin.

It would be nice to begin expounding the results of our experiments with a resounding statement of general principles. Unfortunately, they are too complex to permit any such statement. Different patterns of drug action emerged in each of the paradigms we studied. But it should be emphasized that these differences appeared only in the experiments on GABA agonists and antagonists. As is usual in studies of the anxiolytic drugs themselves (e.g. Gray, 1977), the pattern of change produced by these substances was consistent both across paradigms and between drugs.

## ELECTROPHYSIOLOGICAL RESULTS

The predictability of the effects of the anxiolytics themselves was confirmed in a study of the influence of meprobamate on the theta-driving curve, i.e., on the function relating threshold septal stimulating current (able to drive the hippocampal theta rhythm) to stimulation frequency (Figure 1). We have previously reported that amylobarbitone, chlordiazepoxide, diazepam, and ethyl alcohol (all in low doses at which antianxiety behavioural effects predominate over other kinds of drug effect) eliminate the 7.7-Hz minimum in this function by raising the threshold selectively at this frequency (McNaughton *et al.*, 1977). Figure 1 shows the identical effect for meprobamate. Thus the correlation between this electrophysiological change and anxiolytic action remains good (the effect is not produced by a range of drugs without anxiolytic behavioural action: McNaughton *et al.*, 1977).

Given this close correlation between abolition of the 7.7-Hz minimum in the theta-driving curve and anxiolytic action, one can now ask whether the same change is produced by GABA agonists. Muscimol indeed has this effect, over a wide range of doses (0.000125–0.20 mg/kg), with a maximum at the very low

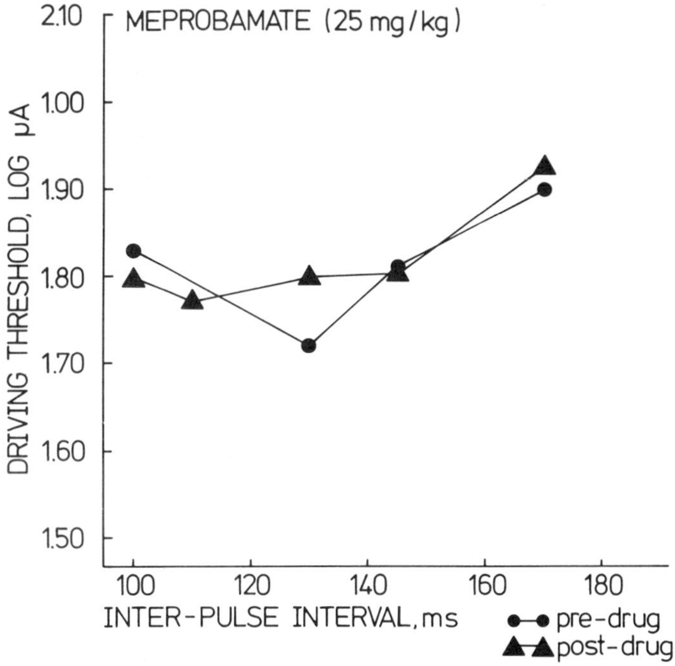


Figure 1 Thresholds for septal driving of hippocampal theta rhythm as a function of stimulation frequency in free-moving male rats: effect of meprobamate (25 mg/kg i.p.). Note the characteristic minimum threshold at the inter-pulse interval of 130 ms (7.7-Hz) in the pre-drug curve; and the elimination of this 7.7-Hz minimum by meprobamate

dose of 0.00125 mg/kg (Mellanby *et al.*, 1981; see Figure 2). (The doses given, throughout the paper, are for intraperitoneal injection.) This result is important, not only in its own right, but also in demonstrating that systemic injection of muscimol even in very low doses affects the brain. Earlier work had suggested that very little muscimol reaches the brain after systemic injection (Baraldi *et al.*, 1979; Maggi and Enna, 1979), thereby offering a ready explanation for negative results with this route of administration. In the light of our findings (Figure 2), this argument is untenable. Unlike muscimol, however, baclofen (in doses from 0.125 to 2 mg/kg) had no significant effect on the shape of the theta-driving curve. These results, then, suggest that, if anxiolytics block the 7.7-Hz minimum by enhancing GABA transmission, they do so at the $GABA_A$ receptor. This inference, in its turn, weakens the possibility that the anxiolytic effect on the theta-driving curve is due to an action on the presynaptic receptors located by Bowery *et al.* (1980) on the forebrain terminals of monoaminergic neurons, since these are of the $GABA_B$ variety.

If muscimol affects the theta-driving curve by an action at the $GABA_A$ receptor, its action should be blocked by bicuculline. As shown in Figure 3,

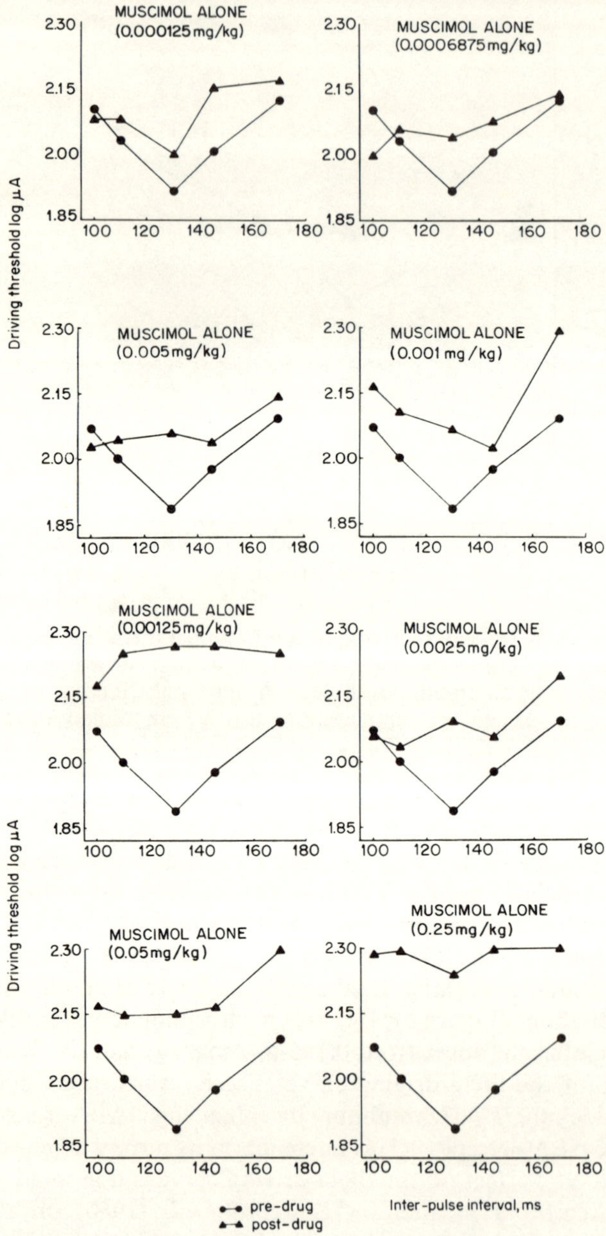


Figure 2 Thresholds for septal driving of hippocampal theta rhythm as a function of stimulation frequency: effects of muscimol (0.000125–0.25 mg/kg)

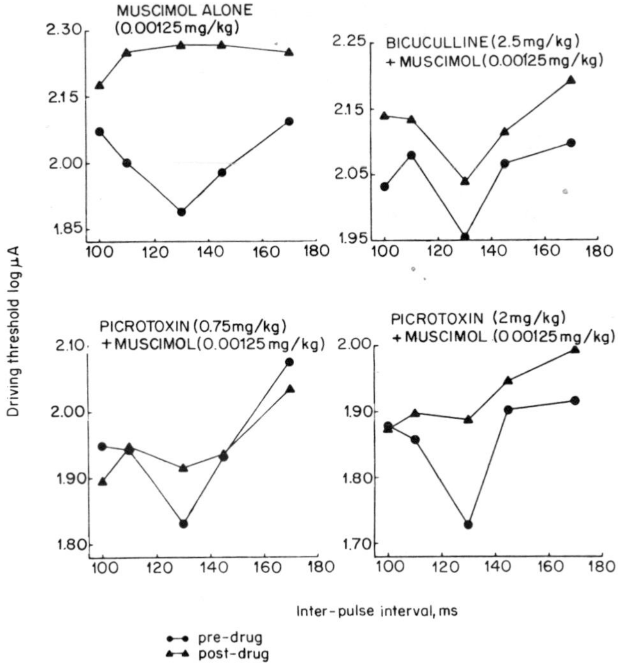


Figure 3 Thresholds for septal driving of hippocampal theta rhythm as a function of stimulation frequency: effect of muscimol (0.00125 mg/kg) blocked by bicuculline (2.5 mg/kg) but not by picrotoxin (0.75 and 2 mg/kg)

this prediction is confirmed. Somewhat surprisingly, however, the less specific GABA antagonist, picrotoxin (in doses up to 2 mg/kg i.p.) failed to alter the effect of muscimol. Neither antagonist affected the theta-driving curve when given on its own.

If the antianxiety drugs alter the theta-driving curve by the same mechanism as does muscimol, their effects too might be expected to be antagonized by bicuculline but not by picrotoxin. We tested this prediction by combining each of three antianxiety drugs, chlordiazepoxide (5 mg/kg), amylobarbitone (15 mg/kg) and meprobamate (25 mg/kg), with each of the two GABA antagonists, bicuculline (up to 2.5 mg/kg) and picrotoxin (up to 2 mg/kg). Adding muscimol to the three anxiolytics, we have a four × two table into which we can insert 'yes' if the GABA antagonist blocks the elimination of the 7.7-Hz minimum in the theta-driving curve and 'no' if it does not. There are four possible patterns which can emerge from this exercise. Table 1 shows that our experiments demonstrated all four, a different pattern for each anxiolytic and none of these like muscimol. Figure 4 illustrates some of the data on which this table is based.

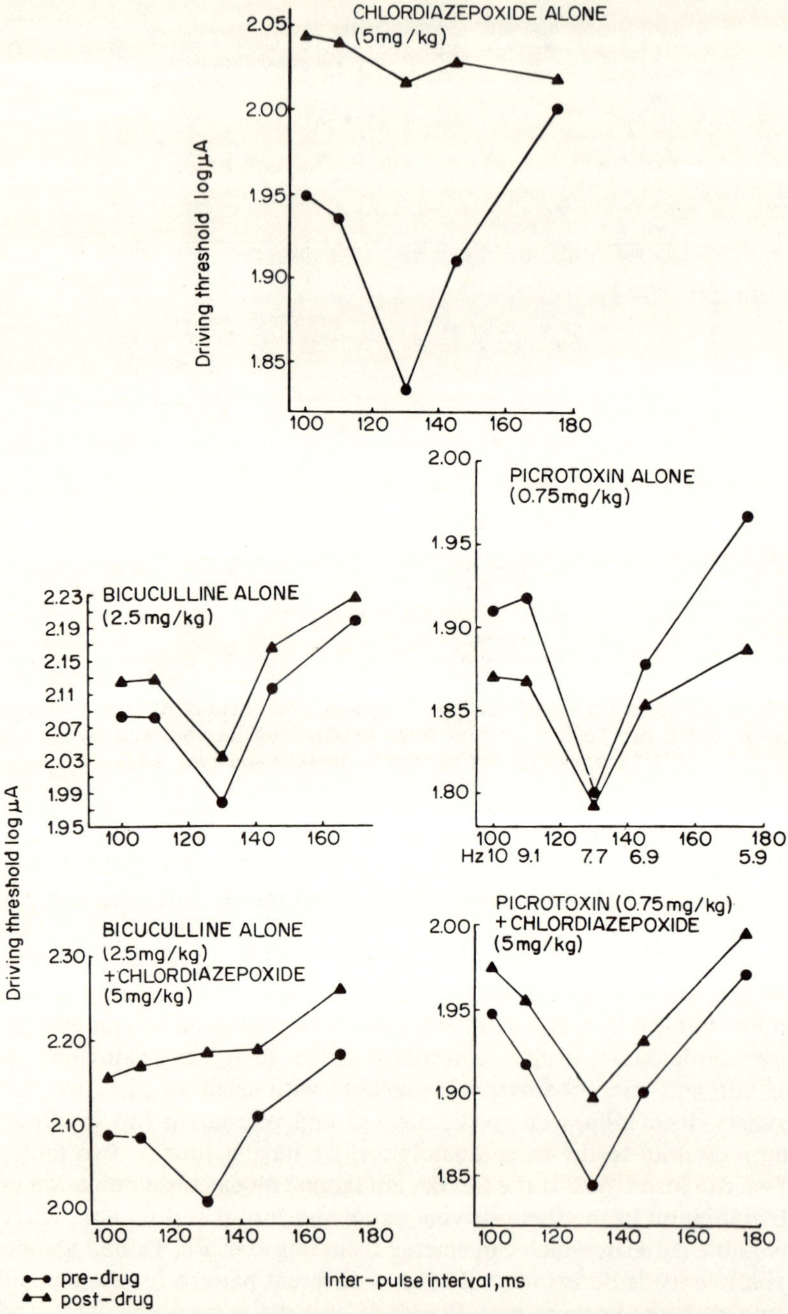


Figure 4(a) Thresholds for septal driving of hippocampal theta rhythm as a function of stimulation frequency: effect of chlordiazepoxide HCl (5 mg/kg) blocked by picrotoxin (0.75 mg/kg) but not by bicuculline (2.5 mg/kg)

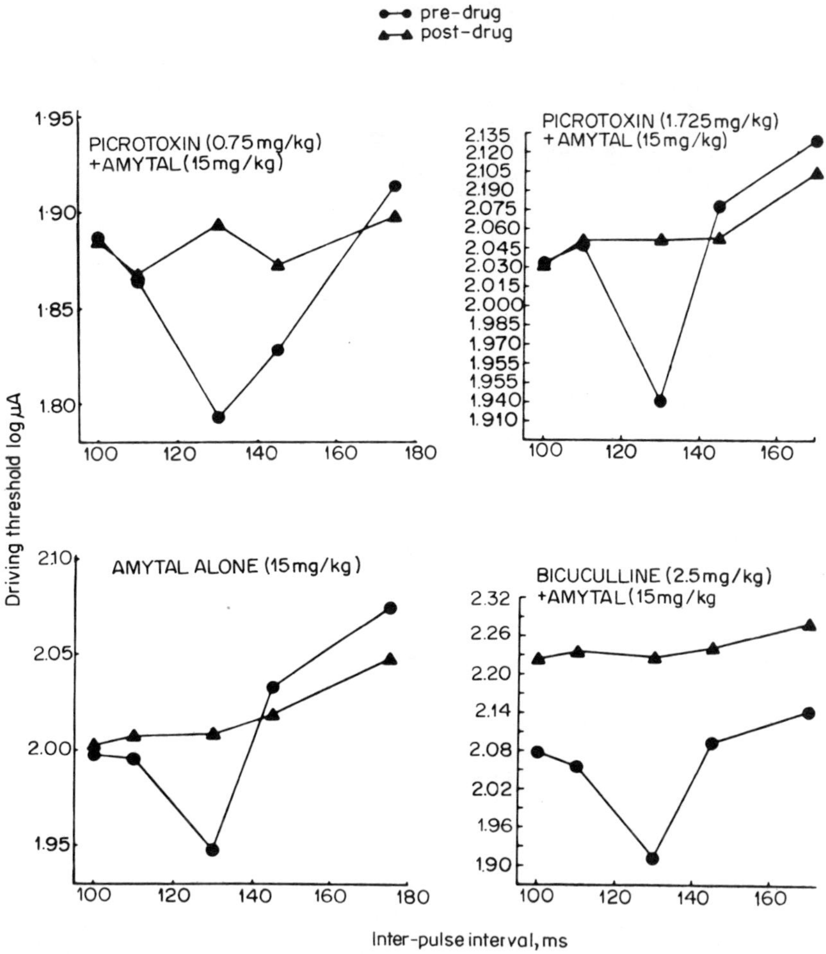


Figure 4(b) Thresholds for septal driving of hippocampal theta rhythm as a function of stimulation frequency: effect of amylobarbitone Na (Amytal, 15 mg/kg) not affected by picrotoxin (0.75 and 1.725 mg/kg) or bicuculline (2.5 mg/kg)

Table 1 The capacity of the GABA antagonists, bicuculline and picrotoxin, to antagonize ('Yes') the elimination of the 7.7-Hz minimum in the theta-driving curve produced by anxiolytics or muscimol. All injections intraperitoneal; doses in parentheses (mg/kg)

| | Chlordiazepoxide (5) | Amylobarbitone (15) | Meprobamate (25) | Muscimol (0.00125) |
|---|---|---|---|---|
| Bicuculline (2–2.5) | No | No | Yes | Yes |
| Picrotoxin (0.75) | Yes | No | Yes | No |

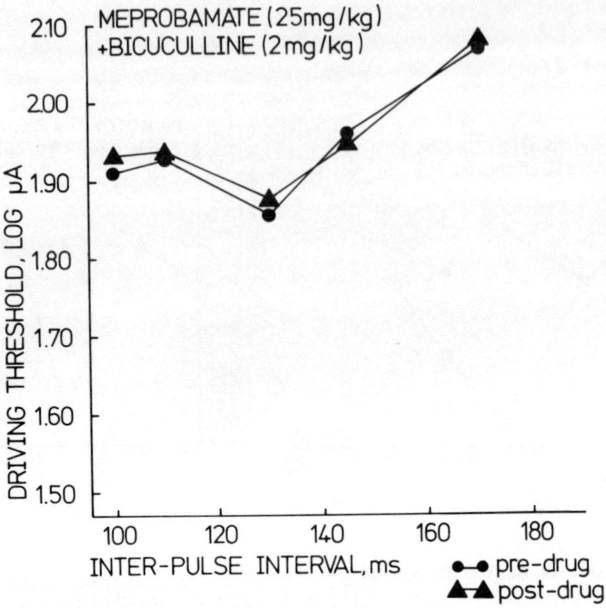


Figure 4(c) Thresholds for septal driving of hippocampal theta rhythm as a function of stimulation frequency: effect of meprobamate (25 mg/kg) blocked by bicuculline (2 mg/kg)

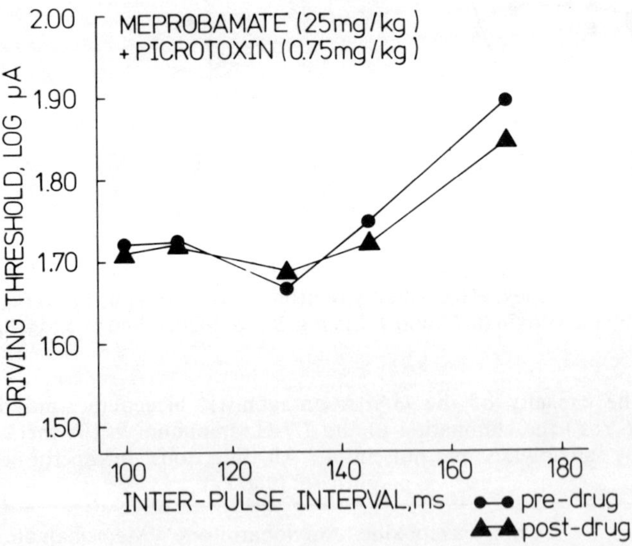


Figure 4(d) Thresholds for septal driving of hippocampal theta rhythm as a function of stimulation frequency: effect of meprobamate (25 mg/kg) blocked by picrotoxin (0.75 mg/kg)

## BEHAVIOURAL RESULTS

### Response to novelty

The effects of drugs on the theta-driving curve have in the past been a good guide to their effects on behaviour (McNaughton *et al.*, 1977). Thus, given the findings summarized above, we might expect that:

1. the behavioural effects of chlordiazepoxide would be blocked by picrotoxin but not by bicuculline;
2. the effects of amylobarbitone would not be blocked by either GABA antagonist;
3. muscimol but not baclofen would have anxiolytic-like behavioural effects; and
4. the effects of muscimol would be blocked by bicuculline but not by picrotoxin. (Similar predictions can be made for meprobamate, but we have not yet tested this drug further.)

In a first look at some of these predictions we made use of a simple test of response to novelty, i.e. to stimulus change. The rat is placed in the stem of a T-maze separated by glass partitions from the two arms, of which one is black and one white. After 3 minutes the rat is removed, one of the arms is changed so that they are now both white or black, the partitions are taken out, and the rat is returned to the stem of the T-maze. Normal rats tend (with about 75% probability) to enter the changed arm. Amylobarbitone abolishes this tendency, the drugged rat choosing at random between the two arms (Ison *et al.*, 1966). We have demonstrated the same effect after 5 mg/kg chlordiazepoxide (Table 2). A similar change is also seen after destruction of the fornix-fimbria,

Table 2 Percentage of animals choosing the changed arm in a test of response to stimulus change in the T-maze under various drug treatments. All injections intraperitoneal; doses in parentheses (mg/kg)

| Drug treatment | Percentage choice |
|---|---|
| Saline | 75 |
| Acidic saline[1] | 69 |
| Chlordiazepoxide (15) | 47* |
| Chlordiazepoxide (15) + bicuculline (2) | 53* |
| Chlordiazepoxide (15) + picrotoxin (0.75) | 64 |
| Muscimol (0.01) | 58 |
| Muscimol (0.25) | 49† |
| Muscimol (0.25) + bicuculline (2) | 44† |
| Muscimol (0.25) + picrotoxin (0.75) | 71 |

[1]Control for bicuculline.
*Different from controls at $P<0.05$.
†Different from controls at $P<0.005$.

which connects the septal area and the hippocampal formation (Gaffan, 1972); and also after destruction of the dorsal ascending noradrenergic bundle (Owen, 1979), removing the source of noradrenergic innervation of the septohippocampal system. Furthermore, in animals in which the dorsal bundle has been destroyed, there is no effect of amylobarbitone on this behaviour (Owen, 1979), though this may simply reflect the fact that the animal's responses are already at chance level. Thus there is some reason to think that abolition by anxiolytic drugs of the response to stimulus change, like the effect of these drugs on the theta-driving curve, is due to an impairment in the noradrenergic input to the septohippocampal system.

The first of the predictions listed above is that picrotoxin but not bicuculline will block the behavioural effects of chlordiazepoxide. This prediction was confirmed: the response to stimulus change (see Table 2) under chlordiazepoxide (47%) was significantly lower than the saline control level (75%) and unaltered by combining bicuculline with chlordiazepoxide (53%); but picrotoxin, which had no effect on its own (78%), increased the rate of response to stimulus change under chlordiazepoxide to a level (64%) which no longer differed significantly from control. A further prediction was that muscimol would act like chlordiazepoxide. This prediction was also confirmed. But to get a clear-cut result it was necessary to use a dose (0.25 mg/kg) 200 times larger than the most effective dose in the theta-driving experiments (0.00125 mg/kg). This large dose significantly reduced the response to stimulus change to 49%; a dose of 0.01 mg/kg reduced the response to 58%, a result which just failed to reach conventional levels of statistical significance when tested against controls. In the theta-driving experiments, the effect of muscimol was blocked by bicuculline, but not by picrotoxin. The final result we tested, therefore, was that the same pattern would emerge in the T-maze experiments. The results, however, were exactly the opposite: the combination of muscimol (0.25 mg/kg) and bicuculline left the choice of arm at random levels (44%), but combining muscimol with picrotoxin restored the response to 71%, not significantly different from control levels. These results are summarized in Table 3.

With the exception of the last result, these findings in the T-maze were encouraging for the hypotheses we were testing. And even the last result

Table 3 The capacity of the GABA antagonists, bicuculline and picrotoxin, to antagonize ('Yes') the reduction of the response to stimulus change produced by chlordiazepoxide or muscimol. All injections intraperitoneal; doses in parentheses (mg/kg)

| | Chlordiazepoxide (5) | Muscimol (0.25) |
|---|---|---|
| Bicuculline (2) | No | No |
| Picrotoxin (0.75) | Yes | Yes |

(blockade of the effect of muscimol by picrotoxin but not by bicuculline), while discrepant with our electrophysiological findings, at least agreed with the pattern of antagonism seen with chlordiazepoxide (Tables 1 and 3).

**Response to stimuli associated with punishment**

The response to stimulus change has the virtue that it is easy to measure. But it is not widely accepted as a good behavioural test of anxiolytic action. A test with better credentials and good face validity is the suppression of food-rewarded bar pressing which occurs during a stimulus signalling that bar pressing may also be followed by foot shock (Geller and Seifter, 1960). The problem with these experiments is that they are extremely time-consuming. However, we have been able to gather data relevant to several of the predictions listed above.

In our particular version of the Geller–Seifter schedule (Rawlins *et al.*, 1980), rats are trained in Skinner boxes to bar press for sucrose delivered on a random-interval (RI) schedule with a mean interreinforcement time of 64 seconds (RI-64). After stable responding is achieved, each 40-minute session is interrupted by three intrusion periods, each 3 minutes long and signalled by a tone. During the intrusion period, bar pressing continues to be reinforced with sucrose as before, but in addition an independent RI-64 schedule programmes 0.5-second foot shocks which are also contingent upon bar pressing. Shock intensity is individually adjusted for each animal to produce similar levels of suppression of barpressing during intrusion periods (at about 45–50% of baseline response). Only after stable levels of responding both during baseline (no tone, no shock) and intrusion periods (tone, shock) have been attained do drug trials begin. Each animal acts as it own control, receiving drug or vehicle on different days according to various balanced schedules (e.g., drug–saline–saline–drug). Drug-produced changes in baseline rates are controlled for statistically; to do this, we use analysis of covariance in which response rates during intrusion periods are the variate and rates during the 3 minutes before intrusion periods are the covariate.

Both chlordiazepoxide (5 mg/kg) and amylobarbitone (15 mg/kg) disinhibited responding suppressed by the threat of foot shock, a well-known effect of both benzodiazepines and barbiturates (Gray, 1977). The specificity of the chlordiazepoxide effect was verified by administration of the recently developed benaodiazepine receptor antagonist, Ro 15-1788 (Haefely *et al.*, 1981). This drug (1.0 mg/kg) significantly, though not totally, reversed the disinhibitory effect of chlordiazepoxide (Figure 5). However, the putative endogenous ligand for the benzodiazepine receptor, ethyl-$\beta$-carboline-3-carboxylate (Braestrup and Nielsen, 1980), in a dose of 0.5 mg/kg, had no effect on response suppression either alone or in combination with chlordiazepoxide.

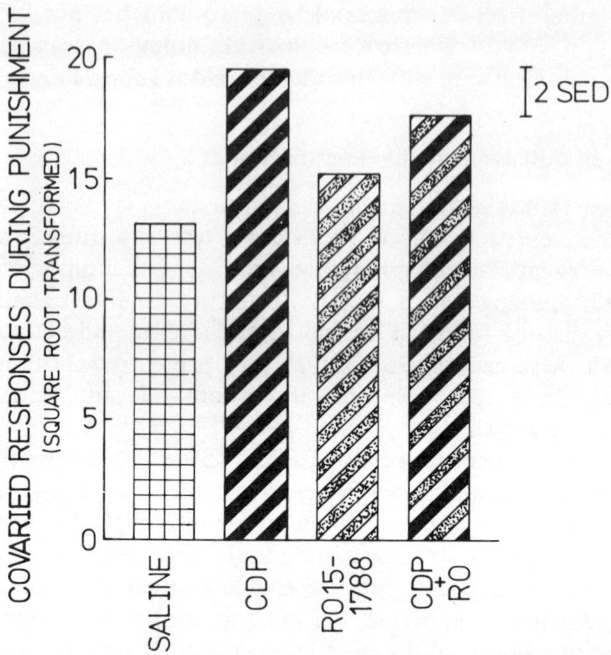


Figure 5 Bar pressing rates during punishment periods (covaried on unpunished response rates) after treatment with saline, chlordiazepoxide (CDP, 5 mg/kg), Ro 15-1788 (1.0 mg/kg), or the two drugs combined. The same animals were tested under all conditions. Bar marker: 2 standard errors appropriate for comparisons between any two means

We first tried to mimic the disinhibitory effects of chlordiazepoxide and amylobarbitone using muscimol in a range of doses (0.0025, 0.01, and 0.25 mg/kg) which were clearly effective in the theta-driving and/or T-maze experiments. At no dose was there any significant change in any aspect of the animals' responding. We next tried baclofen, at 0.125, 1, and 2 mg/kg. There was a small indication of an effect (insignificant) at 1 mg/kg. We therefore repeated the experiment at this dose, and obtained a small but significant disinhibition (Figure 6). In a third experiment rats were given saline, muscimol (0.00125 mg/kg), baclofen (1 mg/kg), muscimol + baclofen, or saline, each animal receiving every drug condition in a quasi-random order over each block of 4 days. The results are shown in Figure 6. There was a clear disinhibition of punished responding only in the muscimol + baclofen conditions. Muscimol by itself was without effect, replicating our earlier findings; but baclofen by itself was also without effect, contradicting our previous finding that this drug caused significant disinhibition. Given the size of the group (18), the combined effect of muscimol + baclofen is almost certainly reliable. Any effect that

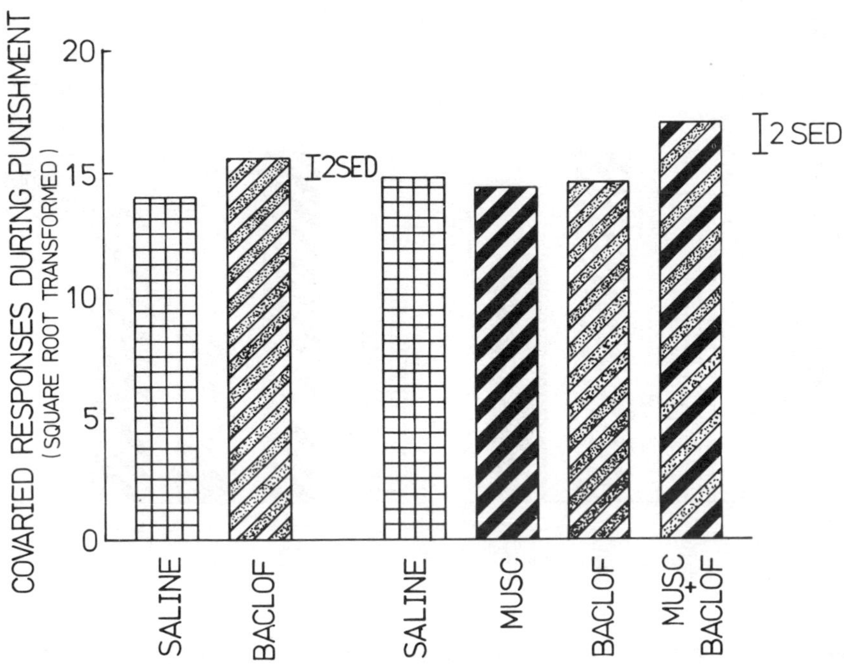


Figure 6 Bar pressing rates during punishment periods (covaried on unpunished response rates). Left-hand pair of histograms: effect of baclofen (1 mg/kg). Remaining four histograms: effects of muscimol (0.00125 mg/kg), baclofen (1 mg/kg) or the two drugs combined. Bar markers as for Figure 5, referring to histograms to their left

baclofen has on its own, however, is fragile; and muscimol on its own seems completely to lack disinhibitory properties in our version of the Geller–Seifter paradigm.

The results with the combination of muscimol and baclofen suggest that disinhibition of punished responding requires an action at both $GABA_A$ and $GABA_B$ receptors. If so, one might expect to be able to block the effects of chlordiazepoxide in this paradigm by antagonizing GABA transmission at either receptor. This expectation was confirmed using the $GABA_A$ antagonist, bicuculline (1.75 mg/kg; see Figure 7). The less specific antagonist, picrotoxin (0.75 mg/kg), however, failed to block the disinhibitory effect of chlordiazepoxide, although on its own this drug significantly increased the degree of response suppression during intrusion periods (Figure 8). The latter observation confirms reports from Soubrié's laboratory (Soubrié *et al.*, 1978, 1979) that this drug has effects opposite in sign to those of the anxiolytics in several behavioural paradigms, including the suppression of bar pressing by foot shock.

In the punishment experiments, then, the disinhibitory effect of chlordiazepoxide was blocked by bicuculline, not by picrotoxin. But this pattern is

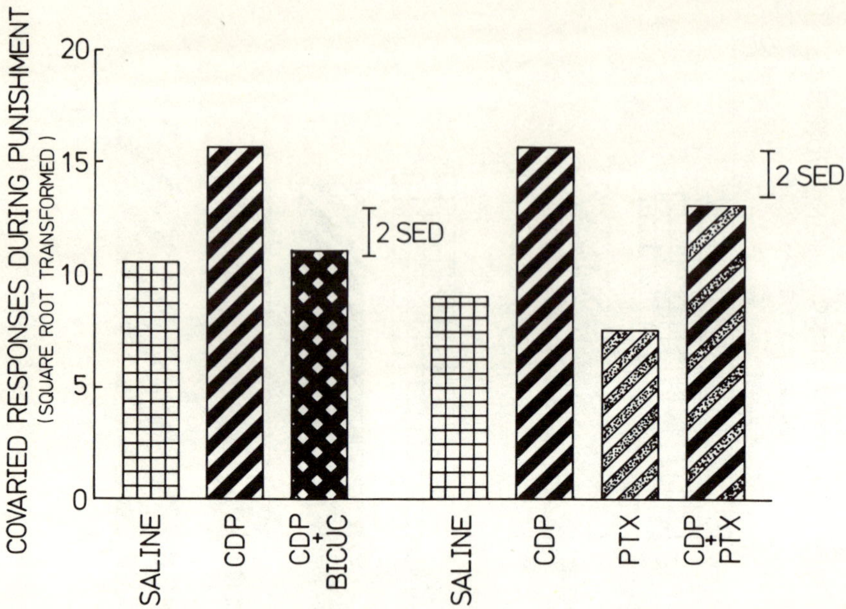


Figure 7 Bar pressing rates during punishment periods (covaried on unpunished response rates). Left-hand three histograms: effect of chlordiazepoxide (CDP, 5 mg/kg) blocked by bicuculline (1.75 mg/kg). Right-hand four histograms: effects of chlordiazepoxide, picrotoxin (PTX, 0.75 mg/kg) or the two drugs combined. Bar markers as for Figure 5, referring to histograms to their left

exactly the reverse of the one observed in the theta-driving and T-maze experiments, in which picrotoxin but not bicuculline blocked the effects of chlordiazepoxide. It is particularly surprising to find this reversal in a paradigm in which muscimol, supposedly the agonist at the receptor at which bicuculline is an antagonist, lacks effect; especially since in the theta-driving and T-maze experiments muscimol *did* have an anxiolytic-like effect. This confusing set of results is not clarified when we attempt to block the effects of the combination of muscimol and baclofen in the punishment paradigm. For our preliminary results suggest that bicuculline *fails* to alter the effects of the GABA agonist cocktail, while picrotoxin *blocks* them. These early findings are at least consistent, however, with the evidence (see above) that, if either GABA agonist has a disinhibitory effect on its own in the punishment paradigm, it is baclofen, not muscimol.

The blockade by bicuculline of the effect of chlordiazepoxide in the punishment experiment is in agreement with the general hypothesis that an enhancement of GABA transmission underlies anxiolytic behavioural action. If this hypothesis is applicable to all anxiolytic action, not just to the

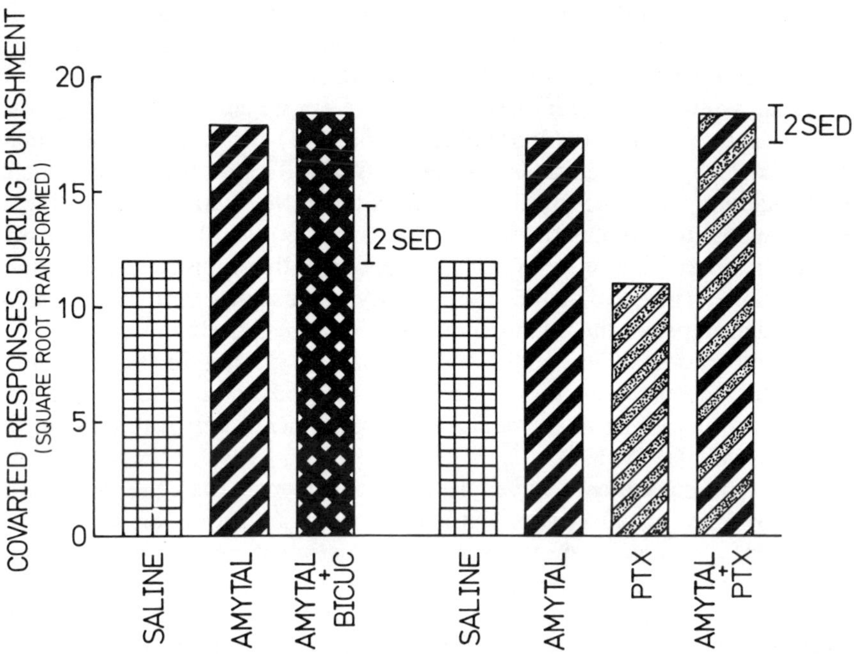


Figure 8 Bar pressing rates during punishment periods (covaried on unpunished response rates). As Figure 7, but for amylobarbitone (Amytal; 15 mg/kg) in place of chlordiazepoxide

benzodiazepines, we would expect that the disinhibitory effects of amylobarbitone in the punishment paradigm would also be susceptible to blockade at least by bicuculline. However, neither this drug nor picrotoxin altered the capacity of amylobarbitone to increase response rates suppressed by punishment (Figures 7 and 8). These findings are consistent with the results of the theta-driving experiments (Table 1); here too neither GABA antagonist altered the effects of amylobarbitone.

## CONCLUSIONS

The patterns of results obtained in our three experimental paradigms are clearly too various to permit a single, unified answer to the questions to which this paper has been addressed. They do, however, permit a number of conclusions relevant to particular hypotheses. We summarize these conclusions here.

First, our electrophysiological experiments with meprobamate extend to an anxiolytic of a class not previously studied in this way: the correlation between abolition of the 7.7-Hz minimum in the theta-driving curve and antianxiety behavioural action (McNaughton *et al.*, 1977). This observation is therefore consistent with the central role allotted to the septohippocampal system in anxiety and antianxiety action by Gray (1982a,b).

Second, a number of our observations are consistent with the hypothesis (Costa and Greengard, 1975; Haefely *et al.*, 1981) that the benzodiazepines affect anxiety by enhancing GABA transmission. These observations include the blockade of the effect of chlordiazepoxide on the theta-driving curve and on the response to stimulus change by picrotoxin; and the blockade of the effect of this benzodiazepine on response suppression in the punishment experiment by bicuculline. They also include the capacity of muscimol to mimic the effects of benzodiazepines in the theta-driving and T-maze experiments; the capacity of the combination of muscimol and baclofen to do this in the punishment experiment; and the capacity of picrotoxin to produce an effect opposite to that of benzodiazepines in the punishment experiment, confirming the reports of Soubrié *et al.* (1978, 1979).

Third, our experiments have yielded no evidence that the barbiturate, amylobarbitone, produces anxiolytic effects via an action on GABA-ergic mechanisms. Neither in the theta-driving experiment nor in the punishment experiment (a well-established test of anxiolytic action) was the effect of this drug blocked by either bicuculline or picrotoxin in doses which were effective against chlordiazepoxide, muscimol or the muscimol-plus-baclofen combination in the same experiments. This is unlikely to be due to our particular doses of amylobarbitone (15 mg/kg) and chlordiazepoxide (5 mg/kg). Although the complexity of our experimental designs precluded the study of a range of doses of these drugs, as would obviously have been desirable, the doses we chose are about equally effective in a wide variety of behavioural tasks (Gray, 1977), give rise to similar changes in our electrophysiological tests (McNaughton *et al.*, 1977), and produced comparable degrees of release of punished responding in the experiments described here. Thus, though barbiturates, like benzodiazepines, enhance GABA-ergic transmission (Olsen, 1981), it seems unlikely that this effect underlies their anxiolytic properties. If this conclusion is correct, it implies that, though enhanced GABA-ergic transmission may underlie the anxiolytic effects of the benzodiazepines, it is not a prerequisite for anxiolytic action in general. Klepner *et al.* (1979) came to a similar conclusion from studies which demonstrate the existence of two types of benzodiazepine receptor, only one of which is apparently associated with GABA receptors. Indeed, these authors propose that anxiolytic action is unrelated to enhanced GABA transmission even in the case of the benzodiazepines.

Fourth, our results are in clear contradiction of the hypothesis (Olsen, 1981) that barbiturates produce their effects by binding to the same receptor as picrotoxin. Neither in the electrophysiological nor in the behavioural experiments did we find any effect of picrotoxin on the response to amylobarbitone, even though in some of the same experiments the same dose of picrotoxin clearly blocked responses to chlordiazepoxide, meprobamate or muscimol.

Fifth, our limited observations on meprobamate are consistent with a role for enhanced GABA transmission in the effects of this compound, since its effects on the theta-driving curve were reversed by either picrotoxin or bicuculline.

Finally, our observations offer no support for the notion that anxiolytic action is related specifically to one or other of the two types of GABA receptor described in previous research (e.g. Bowery *et al.*, 1980). The experiments we directed to this issue have produced a bewildering variety of results. In the theta-driving experiments we could produce an anxiolytic-like effect using muscimol but not baclofen; and we could block the effect of muscimol with bicuculline but not picrotoxin. This is consistent with an action at the classical $GABA_A$ receptor. But we could block the effect of chlordiazepoxide on the theta-driving curve only with picrotoxin, not bicuculline, suggesting that this benzodiazepine acts on a different type of receptor. In the T-maze experiments, we could again mimic the action of anxiolytics using muscimol (we have not yet studied baclofen in this paradigm); but this effect was blocked by picrotoxin, not by bicuculline, in the case of both muscimol and chlordiazepoxide. This pattern of results is not consistent with an action of either drug at the $GABA_A$ receptor. Finally, in the punishment experiments, we could mimic anxiolytic action reliably only by combining muscimol and baclofen. This result suggests that action at both $GABA_A$ and $GABA_B$ receptors is necessary for an anxiolytic behavioural effect; although the unreliable effect obtained with baclofen on its own, the complete lack of effect of muscimol on its own, and our preliminary findings that the effects of the agonist cocktail can be blocked by picrotoxin but not by bicuculline are consistent with a greater role for $GABA_B$ than $GABA_A$ receptors. This last inference is, however, contradicted by the results obtained in the punishment paradigm with chlordiazepoxide: for the first time the effects of this drug were reversed by bicuculline, not by picrotoxin, suggesting a predominant role for $GABA_A$ receptors.

At the beginning of this paper we identified a problem with the GABA hypothesis of antianxiety action: enhancement of GABA transmission throughout the brain is too general a mechanism to produce the highly specific behavioural changes which constitute reduced anxiety (Gray, 1977, 1979). One way to add the missing ingredient of specificity would be to find a subset of receptors through which anxiolytics act. This strategy has been advocated previously by Klepner *et al.* (1979), in the context of benzodiazepine receptors. These workers distinguished between two types of benzodiazepine receptor and presented evidence that anxiolytic action is linked to only their type I receptor (which is unrelated to GABA receptors). A weakness of this hypothesis, however, is that type I receptors are found particularly in the cerebellum, a region which on other grounds is most unlikely to play a role in anxiety (Gray, 1982a). We have examined here a second possibility: that anxiolytic action might be tied to enhanced transmission only at the $GABA_A$ or the $GABA_B$ receptor. In the light of our results, this hypothesis could now be sustained only if we chose to link anxiolytic action exclusively to one or other of the paradigms we have studied. There are at present no grounds for adopting this strategy. Thus, to the extent that anxiolytic action depends on enhanced GABA transmission at all (and this hypothesis is in any case contradicted by our findings with amylobarbitone), it seems that such enhancement must occur at both (at least) types of GABA receptor to produce the full spectrum of anxiolytic effects.

Perhaps we are wrong to seek for the specificity of antianxiety action in the pharmacological characteristics of the anxiolytic drugs themselves. An interesting alternative possibility has been suggested by Haefely (1980), who pointed out that GABA-ergic cells frequently appear to play a critical role in negative feedback loops. These cells are often activated by firing in long-axoned neuronal pathways and provide recurrent inhibition to keep that firing within bounds. This type of system operates, for example, in the hippocampus, where recurrent inhibition is probably provided by GABA-ergic basket cells. In such a feedback loop, the GABA-ergic neurons would fire only if the principal cells for which they provide feedback are themselves excited. If we now assume that the anxiolytic effects of the benzodiazepines are due to an enhancement of the post-synaptic action of GABA, as proposed for example by Guidotti *et al.* (1978), this enhancement can only take place at synapses where GABA transmission is occurring; and this transmission can in turn take place (on the arguments advanced above) only in systems where the related principal cells are themselves firing. In this way, benzodiazepines would selectively dampen activity in anxiety-related brain systems, not because these drugs have a special affinity for such systems, but because it is in these systems that (given appropriate anxiogenic stimulation) neuronal firing of a kind with which they interact is currently taking place. (Parallel arguments can be produced to account for the other effects produced by the benzodiazepines, e.g. anticonvulsant action.)

If it is correct that the hippocampus plays an important role in anxiety, as proposed by Gray (1982a,b), the foregoing arguments lead one to expect the benzodiazepines to enhance recurrent inhibition in this structure. Haefely *et al.* (1981) review several studies in which such effects have been demonstrated. A further possibility is that benzodiazepines might enhance GABA-ergic transmission in the larger feedback loop comprising the hippocampal formation and the septal area. Operation of this loop has been implicated in some of the behavioural (Gray *et al.*, 1978) and electrophysiological (Rawlins *et al.*, 1979) effects of the anxiolytic drugs; and there is evidence for a

GABA-ergic synapse in the hippocamposeptal limb of the loop (McLennan and Miller, 1974).

These suggestions are obviously at present only tentative. For the moment, we must conclude that the basis for the specificity of the antianxiety action of the benzodiazepines and other anxiolytic drugs remains an open question.


## ACKNOWLEDGEMENTS

The research reported in this paper was supported by the UK Medical Research Council. S.Q. held a scholarship from the Fundacion Gran Mariscal de Ayacucho, Venezuela. We were greatly helped in the behavioural testing by R. Lawson and S. Henney, and in the electrophysiological testing by H. Nordeen. We are grateful to Dr. Ian Martin, of the Neurochemical Pharmacology Unit, Cambridge, for donating the ethyl-β-carboline-3-carboxylate, and to Dr. W. Haefely, Hoffman-La Roche, Basel, for donating the Ro 15-1788. Other drugs were donated by Eli Lilly & Co., Basingstoke (amylobarbitone sodium); Roche Products Ltd, Welwyn Garden City (chlordiazepoxide HCl); Sigma, Poole, Dorset (muscimol); and Ciba Laboratories (baclofen).


## REFERENCES


Baraldi, M., Grandison, L. and Guidotti, A. (1979). Distribution and metabolism of muscimol in the brain and other tissues of the rat. *Neuropharmacology*, **18**, 57–62.

Barker, J. L. and Ransom, B. R. (1978). Pentobarbitone pharmacology of mammalian central neurones grown in tissue culture. *J. Physiol. Lond.*, **280**, 355–372.

Belin, M. F., Aguera, M., Tappaz, M., McRae-Deguerce, A., Bobillier, P. and Pujol, J. F. (1979). GABA-accumulating neurons in the nucleus raphe dorsalis and periaqueductal gray in the rat: a biochemical and autoradiographic study. *Brain Res.*, **170**, 279–297.

Bowery, N. G., Hill, D. R., Hudson, A. L., Doble, A., Middlemiss, D. N., Shaw, J. and Turnbull, M. (1980). Baclofen decreases neurotransmitter release in the mammalian CNS by an action at a novel GABA receptor. *Nature, Lond.*, **283**, 92–94.

Braestrup, C. and Nielsen, M. (1980). Benzodiazepine receptors. *Arzneimittelforsch*, **30**, 852–857.

Braestrup, C. and Squires, R. F. (1977). Specific benzodiazepine receptors in rat brain characterized by high-affinity $^{3}$H-diazepam binding. *Proc. Natl Acad. Sci. USA*, **74**, 3805–3809.

Broadhurst, P. L. (1975). The Maudsley reactive and nonreactive strains of rats: a survey. *Behav. Genet.*, **5**, 299–319.

Costa, E. and Greengard, P. (eds.) (1975). *Mechanism of Action of Benzodiazepines*, Raven Press, New York.

Drewett, R. F., Gray, J. A., James, D. T. D., McNaughton, N., Valero, I. and Dudderidge, H. J. (1977). Sex and strain differences in septal driving of the hippocampal theta rhythm as a function of frequency: effects of gonadectomy and gonadal hormones. *Neuroscience*, **2**, 1033–1041.

Gaffan, D. (1972). Loss of recognition memory in rats with lesions of the fornix. *Neuropsychologia*, **10**, 327–341.

Gallager, D. W. (1978). Benzodiazepines: potentiation of a GABA inhibitory response on the dorsal raphe nucleus. *Eur. J. Pharmac.*, **49**, 133.

Geller, I. and Seifter, J. (1960). The effects of meprobamate, barbiturates, D-amphetamine and promazine on experimentally induced conflict in the rat. *Psychopharmacologia*, **1**, 482–492.

Graeff, F. G. and Schoenfeld, R. I. (1970). Tryptaminergic mechanisms in punished and nonpunished behavior. *J. Pharmac. exp. Ther.*, **173**, 277–283.

Gray, J. A. (1970). Sodium amylobarbital, the hippocampal theta rhythm and the partial reinforcement extinction effect. *Psychol. Rev.*, **77**, 465–480.

Gray, J. A. (1977). Drug effects on fear and frustration: possible limbic site of action of minor tranquilizers. In: *Handbook of Psychopharmacology*, pp.433–529 (Eds. Iversen, L. L., Iversen, S. D. and Snyder, S. H.), Plenum Press, New York.

Gray, J. A. (1979). Anxiety and the brain: not by neurochemistry alone. *Psychol. Med.*, **9**, 605–609.

Gray, J. A. (1982a). *The Neuropsychology of Anxiety: an Enquiry into the Functions of the Septo-Hippocampal System*, Oxford University Press, Oxford.

Gray, J. A. (1982b). Précis of Gray's 'The Neuropsychology of Anxiety: An Enquiry into the Functions of the Septo-Hippocampal System'. *Behav. Brain Sci.*, **5**, 469–534.

Gray, J. A., Feldon, J., Rawlins, J. N. P., Owen, S., and McNaughton, N. (1978). The role of the septo-hippocampal system and its noradrenergic afferents in behavioural responses to nonreward. In: *Functions of the Septo-Hippocampal System*, pp.275–300 (Eds Elliott, K. and Whelan, J.), Elsevier, Amsterdam.

Gray, J. A. and McNaughton, N. (1983). Comparison between the behavioural effects of septal and hippocampal lesions: a review. *Neurosci. Biobehav. Rev.*, in press.

Gray, J. A., McNaughton, N., James, D. T. D. and Kelly, P. H. (1975). Effect of minor tranquillisers on hippocampal theta rhythm mimicked by depletion of forebrain noradrenaline. *Nature*, **258**, 424–425.

Guidotti, A., Toffano, G. and Costa, E. (1978). An endogenous protein modulates the affinity of GABA and benzodiazepine receptors in rat brain. *Nature, Lond.*, **275**, 553–555.

Guyenet, P. G. and Aghajanian, G. K. (1977). ACh, substance P and metenkephalin in the locus coeruleus: pharmacological evidence for independent sites of action. *Eur. J. Pharmac.*, **53**, 319–328.

Haefely, W. (1980). Paper delivered at the *World Congress of Biological Psychiatry*, Göteborg, Sweden.

Haefely, W., Pieri, L., Polc, P. and Schaffner, R. (1981). General pharmacology and neuropharmacology of benzodiazepine derivatives. In: *Handbook of Experimental Pharmacology*, pp.10–262 (Eds. Hoffmeister, F. and Stille, G.), Springer-Verlag, Berlin.

Holt, L. and Gray, J. A. (1982). Septal driving of the hippocampal theta rhythm produces a long-term, proactive and non-associative increase in resistance in extinction. *Quant. J. exp. Psychol.*, in press.

Ison, J. R., Glass, D. H. and Bohmer, H. M. (1966). Effects of sodium amytal on the approach to stimulus change. *Proc. Am. Psychol. Ass.*, **2**, 5–6.

Iversen, L. L. and Schon, F. (1973). The use of radioautographic techniques for the identification and mapping of transmitter-specific neurons in CNS. In: *New Concepts of Transmitter Regulation*, pp.153–193 (Eds. Mandell, A. and Segal, D.), Plenum Press, New York.

James, D. T. D., McNaughton, N., Rawlins, J. N. P., Feldon, J., and Gray, J. A. (1977). Septal driving of hippocampal theta rhythm as a function of frequency in the free-moving male rat. *Neuroscience*, **2**, 1007–1017.

Klepner, C. A., Lippa, S. A., Benson, D. I., Sano, M. C., and Beer, B. (1979). Resolution of two biochemically and pharmacologically distinct benzodiazepine receptors. *Pharmac. Biochem. Behav.*, **11**, 457–462.

Lidbrink, P., Corrodi, H., Fuxe, K., and Olson, L. (1973). The effects of benzodiazepines, meprobamate, and barbiturates on central monoamine neurons. In: *The Benzodiazepines*, pp.203–223 (Eds. Garattini, S., Mussini, E. and Randall, L. O.), Raven Press, New York.

Maggi, A. and Enna, S. J. (1979). Characteristics of muscimol accumulation in mouse brain after systemic administration. *Neuropharmacology*, **18**, 361–366.

McLennan, H. and Miller, J. J. (1974). Gamma-aminobutyric acid and the inhibition of the septal nuclei of the rat. *J. Physiol., Lond.*, **237**, 625–633.

McNaughton, N., James, D. T. D., Stewart, J., Gray, J. A., Valero, I. and Drewnowski, A. (1977). Septal driving of hippocampal theta rhythm as a function of frequency in the male rat: effects of drugs. *Neuroscience*, **2**, 1019–1027.

Mellanby, J., Gray, J. A., Quintero, S., Holt, L. and McNaughton, N. (1981). Septal driving of hippocampal theta rhythm: a role for gamma-aminobutyrate in the effects of minor tranquilizers. *Neuroscience*, **6**, 1413–1421.

Möhler, H. and Okada, T. (1977). Benzodiazepine receptor: demonstration in the central nervous system. *Science, NY*, **198**, 849–851.

Nestoros, J. N. (1980). Ethanol selectively potentiates GABA-mediated inhibition of single feline cortical neurons. *Life Sci.*, **26**, 519–523.

Olsen, R. W. (1981). GABA-benzodiazepine-barbiturate receptor interactions. *J. Neurochem.*, **37**, 1–13.

Owen, S. (1979). Investigations of the role of the dorsal ascending noradrenergic bundle in behavioural responses to nonreward and novelty in the rat. Unpublished D.Phil. thesis, University of Oxford.

Powell, G. (1979). *Brain and Personality*, Saxon House, London.

Rawlins, J. N. P., Feldon, J. and Gray, J. A. (1979). Septo-hippocampal connections and the hippocampal theta rhythm. *Expl. Brain Res.*, **37**, 49–63.

Rawlins, J. N. P., Feldon, J., Salmon, P., Gray, J. A. and Garrud, P. (1980). The effects of chlordiazepoxide HCl administration upon punishment and conditioned suppression in the rat. *Psychopharmacology*, **70**, 317–322.

Redmond, D. E., Jr. (1979). New and old evidence for the involvement of a brain norepinephrine system in anxiety. In: *Phenomenology and Treatment of Anxiety*, pp.153–203 (Eds. Fann, W. G., Karacan, I., Pokorny, A. D. and Williams, R. L.), Spectrum, New York.

Robertson, H. A., Martin, I. L. and Candy, J. M. (1978). Differences in benzodiazepine receptor binding in Maudsley reactive and Maudsley nonreactive rats. *Eur. J. Pharmac.*, **50**, 455–457.

Segal, M. (1977a). The effects of brainstem priming stimulation on interhemispheric hippocampal responses in the awake rat. *Expl. Brain Res.*, **28**, 529–541.

Segal, M. (1977b). Changes of interhemispheric hippocampal responses during conditioning in the awake rat. *Expl. Brain Res.*, **29**, 553–565.

Soubrié, P., Thiébot, M. H. and Jobert, A. (1978). Picrotoxin-diazepam interaction in a behavioural schedule of differential reinforcement of low rates. *Experientia*, **34**, 1621–1622.

Soubrié, P., Thiébot, M. H. and Simon, P. (1979). Enhanced suppressive effects of aversive events induced in rats by picrotoxin: possibility of a GABA control on behavioral inhibition. *Pharmac. Biochem. Behav.*, **10**, 463–469.

Stein, L., Wise, C. D. and Berger, B. D. (1973). Anti-anxiety action of benzodiazepines: decrease in activity of serotonin neurons in the punishment system. In: *The Benzodiazepines*, pp.299–326 (Eds. Garattini, S., Mussini, E. and Randall, L. O.), Raven Press, New York.

Storm-Mathisen, J. (1978). Localization of putative transmitters in the hippocampal formation, with a note on the connections to septum and hypothalamus. In: *Functions of the Septo-hippocampal System*, pp.49–79 (Eds. Elliott, K. and Whelan, J.), Ciba Foundation Symposium 58.

Ticku, M. K. (1980). The effects of acute and chronic ethanol administration and its withdrawal on GABA receptor binding in rat brains. *Brit. J. Pharmac.*, **70**, 403–410.

Valero, I., Stewart, J., McNaughton, N. and Gray, J. A. (1977). Septal driving of the hippocampal theta rhythm as a function of frequency in the male rat: effects of adreno-pituitary hormones. *Neuroscience*, **2**, 1029–1032.

## DISCUSSION

## CHAIRMAN: PROFESSOR MALCOLM LADER

DR. M. SCHMUTZ: I have two comments regarding the differences between barbiturates and benzodiazepines in respect to GABA-related compounds: I think we can say that we have, on the one hand, the benzodiazepine–GABA receptor complex and, on the other hand, a so-called picrotoxin receptor at which barbiturates have been claimed to bind. This picrotoxin receptor is considered to be associated with the chloride channel. Between the picrotoxin receptor site and the benzodiazepine receptor site there is coexistence but no direct interaction. So drugs that antagonize the activity of benzodiazepines do not necessarily have to antagonize the activity of barbiturates.

DR. GRAY: This is correct. We have sometimes been able to block the effect of chlordiazepoxide with bicuculline and not with picrotoxin. We have at other times been able to block the effects of chlordiazepoxide with picrotoxin and not with bicuculline. We have not been able to block the effects of sodium amylobarbitone with either picrotoxin or bicuculline, in doses which are clearly effective in the relevant experiment against chlordiazepoxide. We have sometimes been able to reverse the effect of muscimol with bicuculline, as you would expect, and not with picrotoxin but we have sometimes been able to reverse the effect of muscimol with picrotoxin and not with bicuculline. So I would love it if our results fitted that nice scheme, picrotoxin going with barbiturates on the one hand and bicuculline going with chlordiazepoxide on the other. It does not work out that way. We get every possible combination, except that we can never block the barbiturate effect.

DR. SCHMUTZ: A second comment: it is known that at low doses the barbiturates have a GABA-enhancing effect, as have the benzodiazepines, but at higher doses and unlike the benzodiazepines they also have a stabilization effect on membranes.

DR. GRAY: In all of these experiments the dose of sodium amytal has been 15 mg/kg, which is towards the low end of the behaviourally effective range. You could go lower, but you would begin to get quite fragile effects. It is true that the barbiturates do not have the range of doses that you can work on with the benzodiazepines.

DR. L. L. IVERSEN: I wondered also whether dose might be important in determining some of your results with bicuculline and picrotoxin, because they seem to be all one-dose level experiments. Unless you are comparing picrotoxin and bicuculline doses which at least have similar ratios to the convulsive dose, then I do not think it is really a fair comparison.

DR. GRAY: The problem with working with these compounds in behavioural experiments is that you need to know what they do on their own. If you use them on their own, you cannot push the dose up very much because the animals have convulsions and die.

Perhaps Stella Quintero would like to say what ranges of doses of the two antagonists were used?

MS STELLA QUINTERO: When I was doing the theta driving test, which was the first thing we tried—because it was a quick way of checking whether there was something promising there or not—I tried different doses of picrotoxin and different doses of bicuculline. Those doses were published (Mellanby *et al.*, 1981). Convulsive effects with picrotoxin started at 2 mg/kg. With bicuculline similar effects occurred, so the level of the dosage was reduced so as to produce no convulsions.

DR. GRAY: They are about the highest doses we can use.

DR. IVERSEN: The choice of muscimol as a GABA agonist in your studies is perhaps a little strange, because it does not penetrate well into the CNS even though you observe some effects on hippocampus, and on behaviour at remarkably low doses. One still has to ask whether these are the central effects. I wondered if you had tried the newer compound, THIP, for which there is much better evidence that it really does penetrate the CNS and is a direct GABA-mimetic.

DR. GRAY: We have not used any other agonists.

Benzodiazepines Divided
Edited by M. R. Trimble


# 10

# Behavioural Actions of Benzodiazepine Antagonists

SANDRA E. FILE

## INTRODUCTION

Benzodiazepine antagonists have been so named because although they displace $^{3}$H-benzodiazepines from their binding sites, they lack benzodiazepine-like actions and, rather, are able to reverse the behavioural and electrophysiological effects of the benzodiazepines (Braestrup *et al.*, 1980; Tenen and Hirsch, 1980; Bernard *et al.*, 1981; Hunkeler *et al.*, 1981; Czernik *et al.*, 1982). This chapter will be concerned with three such compounds, whose structures are given in Figure 1: ethyl β-carboline-3-carboxylate (βCCE); Ro 15-1788 (an imidazodiazepine); and CGS 8216 (a pyrazoloquinoline). The binding of these antagonists differs from that of benzodiazepine 'agonists' in that it is not enhanced by GABA, but is either little changed, or is decreased (Marengos and Patel, 1981; Mohler and Richards, 1981; Czernik *et al.*, 1982).

It has been suggested, at least for Ro 15-1788 (Hunkeler *et al.*, 1981), that this compound is a pure antagonist, lacking any intrinsic behavioural effects, and acting simply to reverse the actions of the benzodiazepines. As will be seen from the following sections this is not the case: all three antagonists have intrinsic actions and, at least in some respects, they differ from each other. Thus, it can no longer be assumed that they will be inert when given alone, and they cannot be used interchangeably on the assumption that the results will be the same regardless of the antagonist selected. This chapter will also demonstrate that the antagonists do not reverse all the behavioural effects of chlordiazepoxide, but that some are left unchanged and some are enhanced. Finally, some examples will be given of the interactions that can occur when two antagonists are combined. The data to be discussed will be drawn from three behavioural tests measuring convulsions, anxiety, and exploration and motor activity.

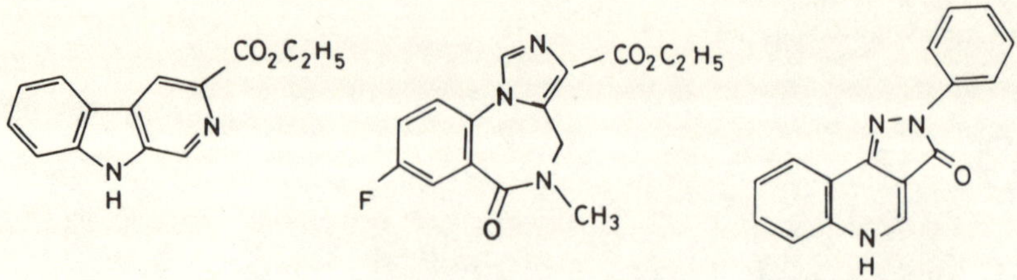

βCCE RO 15-1788 CGS 8216

Figure 1 Chemical structure of three benzodiazepine 'antagonists'

The route of administration of the benzodiazepine antagonists is important. The β-carbolines are rapidly metabolized (Simonsen *et al.*, 1982) and hence massive doses need to be given by any route other than intravenous. Even with i.v. injection their short half-life necessitates immediate testing and the use of tests of short duration. Ro 15-1788 also has a relatively short half-life, but can be, and usually is, administered intraperitoneally. As will be seen in the following section, at high doses the actions of this drug become benzodiazepine-like and so attention must be paid to the particular dose used when interpreting results. In contrast to the others, CGS 8216 is particularly long-acting; it can be given intraperitoneally.

## CONVULSIONS

The first reports of intrinsic actions of benzodiazepine antagonists came from studies on convulsions. Ethyl β-carboline-3-carboxylate (βCCE) was found to be proconvulsant in mice, rats, and baboons (Oakley and Jones, 1980; Cepeda *et al.*, 1981; Cowen *et al.*, 1981). Other carbolines, e.g. methyl β-carboline-3-carboxylate (βCCM) and methyl 6,7-dimethoxy-4-ethyl β-carboline-3-carboxylate (DMCM) have been found to be frank convulsants (Jones and Oakley, 1981; Braestrup *et al.*, 1982). Intriguingly it was reported that low doses of Ro 15-1788 were able to antagonize the proconvulsant action of βCCE, as well as antagonizing the anticonvulsant action of diazepam (Nutt *et al.*, 1982). This provided the first clue to the fact that the actions of benzodiazepine antagonists were more complex, and more interesting, than had at first been suspected. It has been suggested (Nutt *et al.*, 1982; Petersen *et al.*, 1982) that the benzodiazepine receptor has two states, each leading to a behavioural consequence. In one state the agonist leads to an anticonvulsant action, in the other the agonist produces a convulsant effect. Ro 15-1788 is an antagonist for both these states (see Figure 2). One exception to the proposed model comes from the reported potentiation of isoniazid-induced seizures by Ro 15-1788 (Corda *et al.*, 1982).

In high doses the effect of Ro 15-1788 changes and it becomes benzodiazepine-like (Dantzer and Perio, 1982; Nutt *et al.*, 1982) and therefore this compound

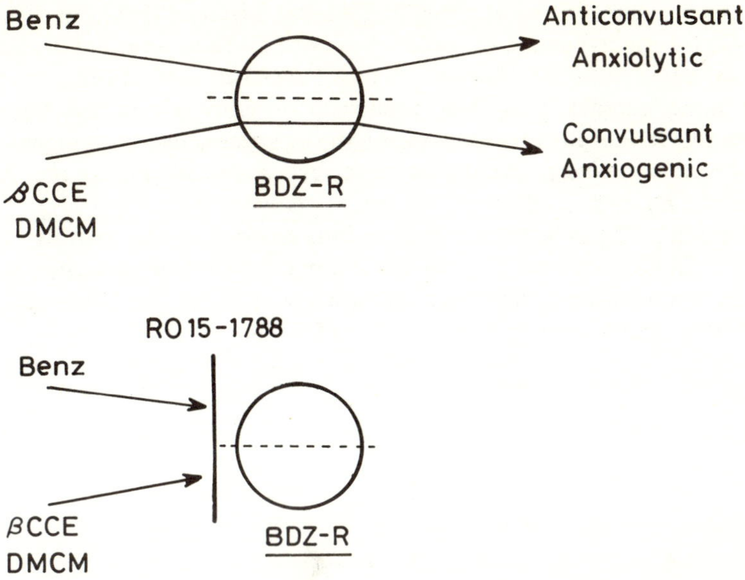


Figure 2 Schematic illustration of the benzodiazepine receptor complex (BDZ-R) which has two conformational states or binding sites, each with a behavioural outcome. The benzodiazepines induce a state with the behavioural consequences of anticonvulsant and anxiolytic activity, whereas the β-carbolines βCCE and DMCM induce a state leading to anxiogenic and proconvulsant (βCCE) or convulsant (DMCM) actions. Ro 15-1788 is able to block the behavioural effects of both classes of drug

is probably a partial agonist. It is therefore essential to take careful note of the dose of Ro 15-1788 used in any studies, and to be aware that effects at high doses may be due to a benzodiazepine-like action. A similar caution applies to βCCM. In low doses (<25 mg/kg) it is convulsant, but as the dose is increased from 25 to 50 mg/kg there is a reducing convulsant effect. Thus with an increase in dose βCCM is able to antagonize its own convulsant effect, which can also be antagonized by βCCE, Ro 15-1788, and CGS 8216 (Skolnick, 1982), as well as by propyl β-carboline-3-carboxylate and diazepam (Jones and Oakley, 1981).

## ANXIETY

The anxiolytic actions of the benzodiazepines are well documented and do not need rehearsing here. βCCE, Ro 15-1788, and CGS 8216 have all been reported to antagonize the anxiolytic actions of the benzodiazepines (Bernard *et al.*, 1981; Hunkeler *et al.*, 1981; Brown and Johnson, 1982; Petersen *et al.*, 1982). However, this is not surprising, since each of these antagonists in low doses has been found, in the social interaction test, to be anxiogenic in rats when given alone (File *et al.*, 1982a; File and Lister, 1983a). A $\beta$-carboline, FG 7142, the methyl amide of $\beta$CCE, has been given to human volunteers and produced anxiety attacks (Dorow, cited by Braestrup *et al.*, 1982).

The same interaction as was reported for convulsions has been found between $\beta$CCE and Ro 15-1788. Although the latter is itself anxiogenic, in low doses it is able to reverse the anxiogenic effects of $\beta$CCE (File *et al.*, 1982a), as well as the anxiolytic effect of diazepam (Hunkeler *et al.*, 1981). Thus the model in Figure 2 can be extended to include anxiogenic and anxiolytic effects.

Both CGS 8216 and Ro 15-1788 are anxiogenic when given alone, and when given in combination their effects are additive (Figure 3). This suggests that CGS 8216 is acting in a similar way to Ro 15-1788.

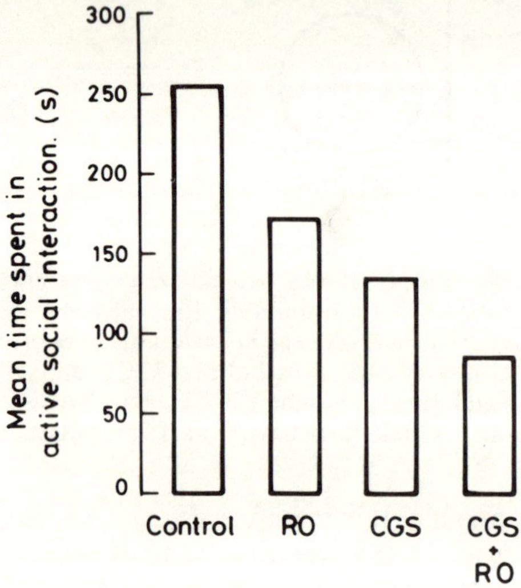


Figure 3 In the social interaction test (see File, 1980), anxiogenic actions are revealed by a decrease in the time spent by pairs of male rats in active interaction. The mean time spent in social interaction was significantly reduced by 10 mg/kg Ro 15-1788 (RO) and by 10 mg/kg CGS 8216 (CGS). The combination of these two drugs (CGS + RO) led to an even greater anxiogenic effect. Both drugs were given i.p., Ro 15-1788 was injected 30 min and CGS 8216 60 min before test

## EXPLORATION AND MOTOR ACTIVITY

The experiments to be described in this section all come from the holeboard test. A holeboard is a wooden box with four holes in the floor, under which objects can be placed. The number of head-dips made, and the time spent head-dipping into the holes, provide a measure of directed exploration (File and Wardill, 1975). This can be measured independently from locomotor activity and rears, which are measured by the interruption of infrared photobeams in the walls of the box.

Typically, with acute administration, even low doses of benzodiazepines reduce exploratory head-dipping, locomotor activity, and rearing in the rat (File, 1982). Ro 15-1788 (4–20 mg/kg) and CGS 8216 (3–20 mg/kg) reverse the sedative effects of chlordiazepoxide, reflected in decreases in locomotor activity and rearing, without significant effects on their own, i.e. they behave as classical antagonists (File *et al.*, 1982b; File and Lister, 1983b). In contrast to the other two antagonists, βCCE (2 mg/kg) when given alone produces a small reduction in locomotor activity and a marked reduction in rears. When combined with chlordiazepoxide the effects of the two drugs were not additive, nor was there mutual antagonism of their effects (File and Lister, 1982).

The pattern of results for exploratory behaviour is different and reveals a particularly challenging set of interactions. It also illustrates clearly that the actions of the three antagonists are not the same as each other.

First, βCCE (1 and 2 mg/kg) significantly reduces head-dipping, as does an acute dose of chlordiazepoxide (5 mg/kg). In combination, the drugs do not antagonize each other's effects, and nor are their effects additive (File and Lister, 1982).

In marked contrast, Ro 15-1788 (4–20 mg/kg) significantly increases exploratory head-dipping. In combination with chlordiazepoxide, rather than a mutual antagonism of effects, there was a further elevation of head-dipping (File *et al.*, 1982b).

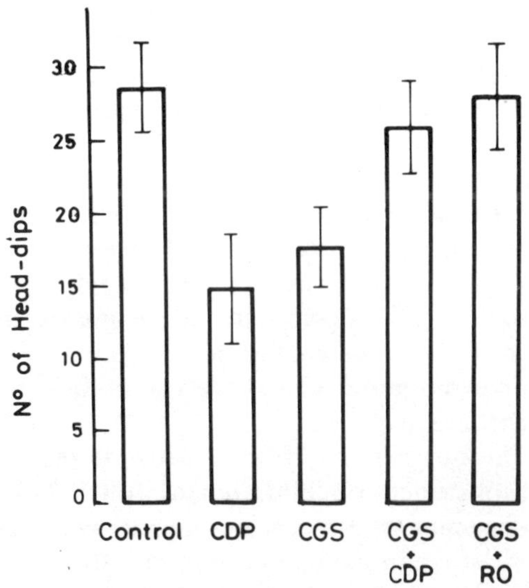


Figure 4 Mean (±s.e.m.) number of head-dips made by rats tested for 7.5 min in a holeboard, 30 min after i.p. injection of 5 mg/kg chlordiazepoxide (CDP) or 60 min after i.p. injection of CGS 8216 (CGS). For the groups given both CGS 8216 and CDP (CGS + CDP) or CGS 8216 and Ro 15-1788 (CGS + RO) the CGS 8216 was given 60 min before test and the other drugs 30 min before

Third, CGS 8216 reduces head-dipping when given alone, and in combination with chlordiazepoxide these effects are reversed, as they are equally well by Ro 15-1788 (see Figure 4). A summary of the effects of the three antagonists alone, and in combination with chlordiazepoxide on head-dipping and motor activity is given in Table 1.

Table 1 Summary of the effects of three benzodiazepine antagonists (βCCE, Ro 15-1788 and CGS 8216) alone and in combination with chlordiazepoxide (CDP 5 mg/kg) on motor activity and head-dipping in the holeboard test

| | βCCE | | CGS 8216 | | Ro 15-1788 | |
|---|---|---|---|---|---|---|
| | Alone | + CDP | Alone | + CDP | Alone | + CDP |
| Motor activity | (↓) | No change | = | Antag. CDP | = | Antag. CDP |
| Head-dipping | (↓) | No change | ↓ | Mutual antag. | ↑ | Enhancement of RO |

## SUMMARY AND CONCLUSIONS

Several points emerge from the behavioural experiments described above. One is that all three of the benzodiazepine antagonists possess intrinsic actions and that although there are some similarities (e.g. all are anxiogenic), there are also marked differences in their respective actions. Some of these actions of the antagonists may reflect antagonism of an endogenous ligand or ligands that either provide a background tone in the system or are released in response to the test situation.

Alternatively, some of the behavioural actions may reflect an agonist action at a benzodiazepine receptor. Certainly the interactions that have emerged so far among the antagonists themselves and between the antagonists and chlordiazepoxide call into question the simple concept of a clear division of agonists and antagonists at a single benzodiazepine receptor. The model illustrated in Figure 2, that can explain the various actions on anxiety, does not hold for the results on exploration. This suggests that these two behaviours are controlled by different receptors.

The question of the number of different benzodiazepine receptors is far from settled. The displacement of $^{3}$H-diazepam by CL 218,872 revealed two subclasses of benzodiazepine CNS receptors (Klepner *et al.*, 1979), of different affinities, but each sensitive to nanomolar concentrations of drug. However, there is controversy over whether the binding of βCCE reveals one or two classes (Nielsen and Braestrup, 1980; Marengos and Patel, 1981). In addition to this question of subclasses of receptor sensitive to nanomolar concentrations of benzodiazepines, there has been a recent report (Bowling and DeLorenzo, 1982) of a binding site sensitive to micromolar concentrations. This latter receptor can be distinguished by pharmacological and binding characteristics from the nanomolar CNS receptors and from the peripheral-type of binding site. The behavioural relevance of the micromolar and peripheral-type (now also found in rat cortex, Schoemaker *et al.*, 1981) receptors is not yet established; but the effects of Ro 5-4864, a ligand for these receptors, but not for the nanomolar CNS receptors, suggest they should not be ignored (File and Mabbutt, 1983).

## REFERENCES


Bernard, P., Bergen, K., Sobiski, R. and Robson, R. D. (1981). CGS 8216 (2-phenylpyrazolo[4,3-c]quinolin-3(5H)-one), an orally effective benzodiazepine antagonist. *The Pharmacologist*, **23**, 150.

Bowling, A. C. and DeLorenzo, R. J. (1982). Micromolar affinity benzodiazepine receptors: identification and characterisation in central nervous system. *Science*, **216**, 1247–1250.

Braestrup, C. and Nielsen, M. (1981). [3H]propyl β-carboline-3-carboxylate as a selective radioligand for the BZl benzodiazepine receptor subclass. *J. Neurochem.*, **37**, 333–341.

Braestrup, C., Nielsen, M. and Olsen, C. E. (1980). Urinary and brain β-carboline-3-carboxylates as potent inhibitors of brain benzodiazepine receptors. *Proc. Natl Acad. Sci. USA*, **77**, 2288–2292.

Braestrup, C., Nielsen, M. and Petersen, E. N. (1982). Interaction of convulsive ligands with benzodiazepine receptors. *Science*, **216**, 1241–1243.

Brown, C. L. and Johnson, A. M. (1982). Ethyl β-carboline-3-carboxylate reverses the effects of benzodiazepines in a test for detecting anxiolytic activity. *Brit. J. Pharmac.*, **75**, 43.

Cepeda, C., Tanaka, T., Besselievr, R., Potier, P., Naquet, R. and Rossier, J. (1981). Proconvulsive effects in baboons of β-carboline, a putative endogenous ligand for benzodiazepine receptors. *Neurosci. Letters*, **24**, 53–57.

Corda, M. G., Costa, E. and Guidotti, A. (1982). Specific proconvulsant action of an imidazodiazepine (Ro 15-1788) on isoniazid convulsions. *Neuropharmacology*, **21**, 91–94.

Cowen, P. J., Green, A. R., Nutt, D. J. and Martin, I. L. (1981). Ethyl β-carboline carboxylate lowers seizure threshold and antagonizes flurazepam-induced sedation in rats. *Nature*, **290**, 54–55.

Czernik, A. J., Petrack, B., Kalinsky, H. J., Psychoyos, S., Cash, W., Tsai, C., Rinehart, R. K., Granat, F. R., Lovell, R. A., Brundish, D. E. and Wade, R. (1982). CGS 8216: receptor binding characteristics of a potent benzodiazepine antagonist. *Life Sci.* **30**, 363–372.

Dantzer, R. and Perio, A. (1982). Behavioural evidence for partial agonist properties of Ro 15-1788, a benzodiazepine receptor antagonist. *Eur. J. Pharmacol.*, **81**, 655–658.

File, S. E. (1980). The use of social interaction as a method for detecting anxiolytic activity for chlordiazepoxide-like drugs. *J. Neurosci. Methods*, **2**, 219–238.

File, S. E. (1982). Development and retention of tolerance to the sedative effects of chlordiazepoxide: role of apparatus cues. *Eur. J. Pharmac.*, **81**, 637–643.

File, S. E. and Lister, R. G. (1982). βCCE and chlordiazepoxide reduce exploratory head-dipping and rearing: no mutual antagonism. *Neuropharmacology*, **21**, 1215–1218.

File, S. E. and Lister, R. G. (1983a). Quinolines and anxiety: anxiogenic effects of CGS 8216 and partial anxiolytic profile of PK 9084. *Pharmac. Biochem. Behav.* (In press.)

File, S. E. and Lister, R. G. (1983b). Ro 15-1788 and chlordiazepoxide each reverse the reduction in exploration caused by CGS 8216. *Brit. J. Pharmac.* (in press.)

File, S. E., Lister, R. G. and Nutt, D. J. (1982a). The anxiogenic action of benzodiazepine antagonists. *Neuropharmacology*, **21**, 1033–1037.

File, S. E., Lister, R. G. and Nutt, D. J. (1982b). Intrinsic actions of benzodiazepine antagonists. *Neurosci. Letters*, **32**, 165–168.

File, S. E. and Mabbutt, P. S. (1983). Behavioural effects of Ro 5-4864, a ligand for the micromolar benzodiazepine receptor. *Brit. J. Pharmac.* (In press.)

File, S. E. and Wardill, A. G. (1975). Validity of head-dipping as a measure of exploration in a modified holeboard. *Psychopharmacologia*, **44**, 53–59.

Hunkeler, W., Mohler, H., Pieri, L., Polc, P., Bonetti, E. P., Cumin, R., Schaffner, R. and Haefely, W. (1981). Selective antagonists of benzodiazepines. *Nature*, **290**, 514–516.

Jones, B. J. and Oakley, N. R. (1981). The convulsant properties of methyl β-carboline-3-carboxylate in the mouse. *Brit. J. Pharmac.*, **74**, 884–885.

Klepner, C. A., Lippa, A. S., Benson, D. I., Sano, M. C. and Beer, B. (1979). Resolution of two biochemically and pharmacologically distinct benzodiazepine receptors. *Pharmac. Biochem. Behav.*, **11**, 457–462.

Marengos, P. J. and Patel, J. (1981). Properties of [3H] β-carboline-3-carboxylate ethyl ester binding to the benzodiazepine receptor. *Life Sci.*, **29**, 1705–1714.

Mohler, H. and Richards, J. G. (1981). Agonist and antagonist benzodiazepine receptor interaction in vitro. *Nature*, **294**, 763–765.

Nielsen, M. and Braestrup, C. (1980). Ethyl β-carboline-3-carboxylate shows differential benzodiazepine receptor interaction. *Nature*, **286**, 606–607.

Nutt, D. J., Cowen, P. J. and Little, H. J. (1982). Unusual interactions of benzodiazepine receptor antagonists. *Nature*, **295**, 436–437.

Oakley, N. R. and Jones, B. J. (1980). The proconvulsant and diazepam-reversing effects of ethyl β-carboline-3-carboxylate. *Eur. J. Pharmac.*, **68**, 381–382.

Petersen, E. N., Paschelke, G., Kehr, W., Nielsen, M. and Braestrup, C. (1982). Does the reversal of the anti-conflict effect of phenobarbital by βCCE and FG 7142 indicate benzodiazepine receptor mediated anxiogenic properties? *Eur. J. Pharmac.* (in press).

Schoemaker, H., Bliss, M. and Yamamura, H. I. (1981). Specific high-affinity saturable binding of [$^3$H] Ro 5-4864 to benzodiazepine binding sites in the rat cerebral cortex. *Eur. J. Pharmac.*, **71**, 173–175.

Simonsen, H., Nielsen, M. and Braestrup, C. (1982). Peripheral metabolism of β-carboline-carboxylic acid esters. *Acta pharmacol. toxicol.*, **50**, 89–92.

Skolnick, P. (1982). Antagonists—β-carbolines, inosine. Paper read at *Pharmacology of Benzodiazepines* conference NIH, April 1982.

Tenen, S. S. and Hirsch, J. D. (1980). β-carboline-3-carboxylic acid ethyl ester antagonises diazepam activity. *Nature* **288**, 609–610.

## DISCUSSION

## CHAIRMAN: PROFESSOR MALCOLM LADER

DR. M. SCHMUTZ: First, I think it is fascinating that you could show that the benzodiazepine receptor complex is probably not as simple as people generally think.

Second, probably one could simplify a little bit. We have now heard about benzodiazepine receptor agonists, antagonists, and I have heard also about contra-agonists. Is it not the case that we have a receptor complex and that we have a broad variety of drugs binding to that receptor complex? These drugs can be anxiolytic, anxiogenic, convulsants, or anticonvulsants; they can do anything, when they bind. If they are agonists I think they are all agonists to some extent, because they simply bind. They are only antagonists when they displace another drug that has first been bound, or has bound, to the receptor. It is probably artificial to construct agonists, antagonists, and contra-agonists in this case.

DR. FILE: I should like to say several things. First of all, I did say that antagonists were discovered because they displaced tritiated benzodiazepines from their binding sites; I did not say they bound to those binding sites. Until you have radiolabelled the compounds you really cannot say that it is binding to that receptor and, therefore, we do not know whether they are agonists or antagonists. The classification of these compounds into 'agonists' and 'antagonists' was based on a really rather arbitrary distinction as to whether or not GABA enhanced their binding or their ability to displace benzodiazepines. The agonists as we know them have their binding to their receptor enhanced by GABA, whereas antagonists do not. That was a neat and a very helpful working hypothesis. Our results in anxiety would at least agree with putting them into two different categories like that. We would not put them into the same clusters on the basis of their effects on exploration. So you have to say that they are working at a different population of benzodiazepine receptors or a different subtype, but we have no evidence for different subtypes yet.

DR. L. IVERSEN: I agree with what Dr. Schmutz said. If the benzodiazepine binding site is a part of a chloride ion channel, there is no reason at all why there has to be an endogenous ligand. There are precedents for this: tetrodotoxin and tetrachotoxin are drugs which block sodium channels in excitable membranes, but we do not think of endogenous ligands for such drug receptors, unless it is sodium. When dealing with that sort of drug receptor, the whole concept of agonists and antagonists, and whether they do anything at all to the normal animal becomes problematic. It may be that antagonists will not do much unless the agonist drug is also present. Perhaps some of our confusion here arises because we are thinking about benzodiazepine receptors as if they were ordinary receptors for some transmitter, which they may not be.

DR. FILE: I think you are absolutely right that if there is not an endogenous transmitter or ligand you would not expect a proper competitive antagonist to have any behavioural effect. Our reason for being interested in them to start with was that, if we do get behavioural effects—as we clearly do—that is indirect evidence that there is either an endogenous ligand or there is background tone in the system. Background tone in the system could be provided by levels of something like GABA, which is not necessarily an endogenous ligand for the benzodiazepine receptor but alters the coupling of that receptor to another receptor like GABA.

THE CHAIRMAN: There is another explanation, of course: we always think of these drugs as having been pure in their actions, but I do not know of any drug that is pure in its action and it could thus be having an independent action elsewhere.

DR. FILE: For Ro 15-1788 they have looked at several receptors other than benzodiazepine and found nothing, so it is not any other known receptor. But CGS 8216 does have actions on adenosine.

DR. S. IVERSEN: I have first a rather specific question. It seemed that your anxiogenic effect to Ro 15-1788 varied in the two experiments. In the experiment in which you looked at the interaction with CGS 8216 the Ro 15-1788 seemed to be having more of an anxiogenic effect. Was that significant? Clearly it was not in the $\beta$-carboline experiment.

A general question is, would you comment on the anxiogenic effects of these compounds as they have been reported in man so far?

DR. FILE: First of all, when we looked at Ro 15-1788 on its own we got a significant anxiogenic effect. When we looked at it in the interaction study with β-carbolines, the reason its effect was not significant was we were also giving propylene glycol ethanol vehicle, and that was counteracting significantly the anxiogenic effect of Ro 15-1788. The reason it worked again in the interaction study with CGS 8216 is we were using different vehicles. So it is entirely the fault of propylene glycol.

The βCCE has not been given to man. There is a study from Germany on four men where they gave FG 7412, which is the methyl amide of βCCE, which had a very pronounced effect and produced marked panic attacks which apparently came in waves. The subjects were extremely anxious, and then less anxious, and then it came back without further administration of the drug. It was a completely open study on volunteers who knew what they were doing to the extent of going and asking for intravenous diazepam because they could not stand it. This is highly consistent with the animal data.

DR. GRAY: I was struck by the fact that you sometimes get a synergism and sometimes opposition. I wonder whether that may be because the effects you are getting are sometimes related to the different populations of GABA receptors, because we have found a similar variability. We showed a synergism between muscimol and baclofen. The synergism was in the behavioural task of punishment, but in our electrophysiological experiments we found that the effect of muscimol is apparently counteracted by baclofen. So we are similarly getting very variable effects.

DR. FILE: And it is in the same animal and the same test at the same moment. We just look at different behaviours. So it cannot be pharmacokinetic; it cannot be dose response.

I was very interested in what you were saying on baclofen because the GABA receptors that are linked in the complex of benzodiazepine receptors are known not to be the baclofen type.

DR. GRAY: is that now established?

DR. FILE: I think Dr. Iversen will know.

DR. L. IVERSEN: I do not want to be categorical about that. There is no interaction in the peripheral GABA-β receptors that you find on sympathetic nerve endings; that is, benzodiazepines do not enhance the effects of GABA on inhibiting noradrenaline release in the periphery. I do not know if it has been examined centrally.

THE CHAIRMAN: You described the German experiments with the βCCE analogue or the derivative. The waves of anxiety in the German experiment are much more typical of LSD administration than they are of any direct anxiogenic substance.

Benzodiazepines Divided
Edited by M. R. Trimble


# 11

# Benzodiazepines: Studies on a Possible Endogenous Ligand

MERTON SANDLER*

All the normal human urine samples we have examined contain some inhibitor of benzodiazepine (BDZ) receptor binding (Clow, Glover, Armando, Reynolds and Sandler, in preparation), apparently different from other putative endogenous ligands appearing in the literature (Braestrup *et al.*, 1980; Davis and Cohen, 1980; Rommelspacher *et al.*, 1980a; Kenessey *et al.*, 1981; Kuhn *et al.*, 1981; Möhler, 1981; Nagy *et al.*, 1981; Skolnick and Paul, 1981; Woolf and Nixon, 1981). Such samples also contain an endogenous inhibitor(s) of the enzyme monoamine oxidase (MAO) (Glover *et al.*, 1980) and as no extraction procedure or chromatographic system yet employed has separated these activities it is possible that the two actions may be caused by the same molecule (Glover *et al.*, 1981; Sandler, 1982). The output of endogenous MAO inhibitor has now been examined in a number of different conditions. It is greatly increased in rats stressed by cold restraint, an increase significantly attenuated by benzodiazepines (Glover *et al.*, 1981). In man, its excretion is raised after withdrawal from benzodiazepines (Petursson *et al.*, 1982) or alcohol (Petursson *et al.*, 1981; Bhattacharya *et al.*, 1982). The urinary inhibitor of BDZ receptor binding, like the MAO inhibitor, can be extracted into ethyl acetate at pH 1. When a group of urine samples from 16 normal subjects were so extracted, evaporated to dryness, and reconstituted, they brought about a mean inhibition of $^{3}$H-flunitrazepam binding to human cerebellar membranes in a standard test system (Braestrup *et al.*, 1980) of 13.5 ± 8.4% (s.d.).

The only clinical situation we have so far scrutinized both for urinary inhibition of BDZ receptor binding and MAO inhibitor is a group of neurological patients, including a subset of epileptics free from all BDZ drugs

*In collaboration with J. D. Elsworth, Angela Clow, Vivette Glover, R. D. C. Elwes, and E. H. Reynolds.

(Elwes, Clow, Glover, Reynolds and Sandler, in preparation). We decided to examine urine samples from epileptic subjects because the potent (if artefactual) benzodiazepine receptor ligand isolated by Braestrup *et al.* (1980) from human urine possesses the ability to lower the seizure threshold in experimental animals (Oakley and Jones, 1980; Cowen *et al.*, 1981). If our own endogenously generated compound or compounds, which we have called 'tribulin' had a similar action, one might predict that its increased production may be a convulsion-predisposing factor in some epileptic patients. The results are shown in Figures 1 and 2. The output of each factor was significantly increased both in epileptics and the complementary group of neurological patients with a miscellaneous collection of diagnoses, compared with controls. This raised output did not correlate with any of the drugs the patients were taking; it was also apparent to a significant degree, in a group of seven of the epileptic patients who were drug-free ($P<0.001$ for inhibition of BDZ binding; $P<0.005$ for inhibition of MAO activity; two-tailed Student's *t*-test). Further studies to determine the degree to which an increased output is linked with

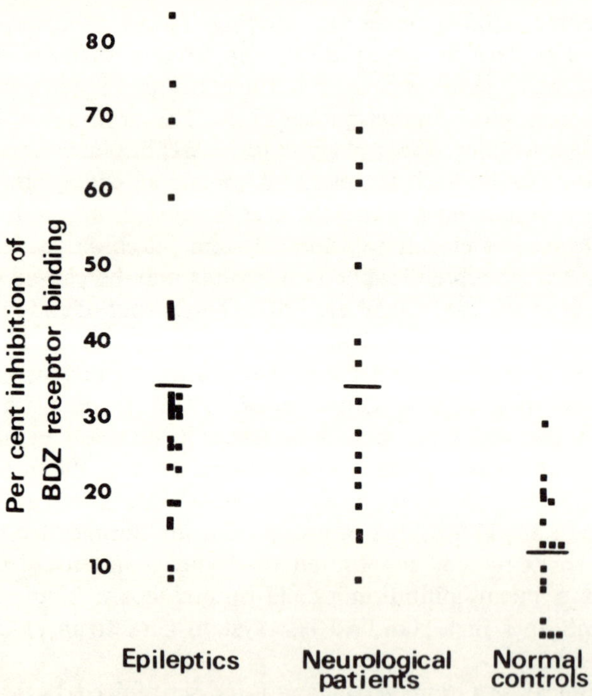


Figure 1 Output of urinary benzodiazepine (BDZ) receptor binding inhibitor in normal control subjects, in epileptics, and in a group of neurological patients of mixed aetiology. All 24-h urine samples were diluted to a concentration of 30 $\mu$g creatinine/100$\mu$l. Output in both groups are greater than controls ($P<0.0001$). (Two-tailed Student's *t*-test)

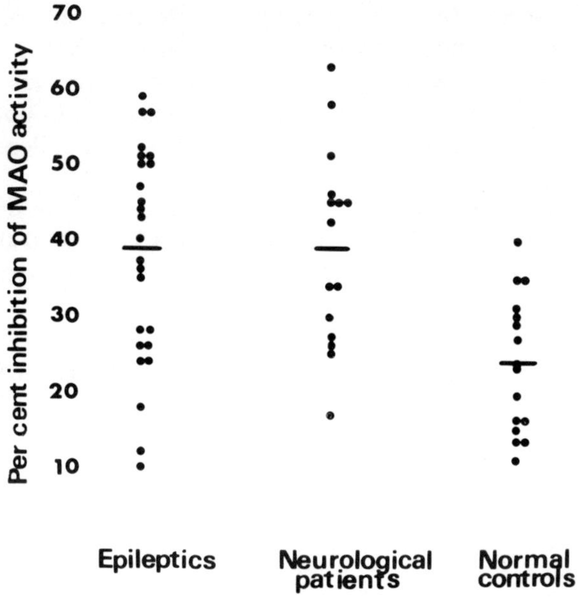


Figure 2 Output of monoamine oxidase (MAO) inhibitor in the same urine samples as in Figure 1. Output in both patient groups are greater than controls ($P<0.0001$). (Two-tailed Student's $t$-test)

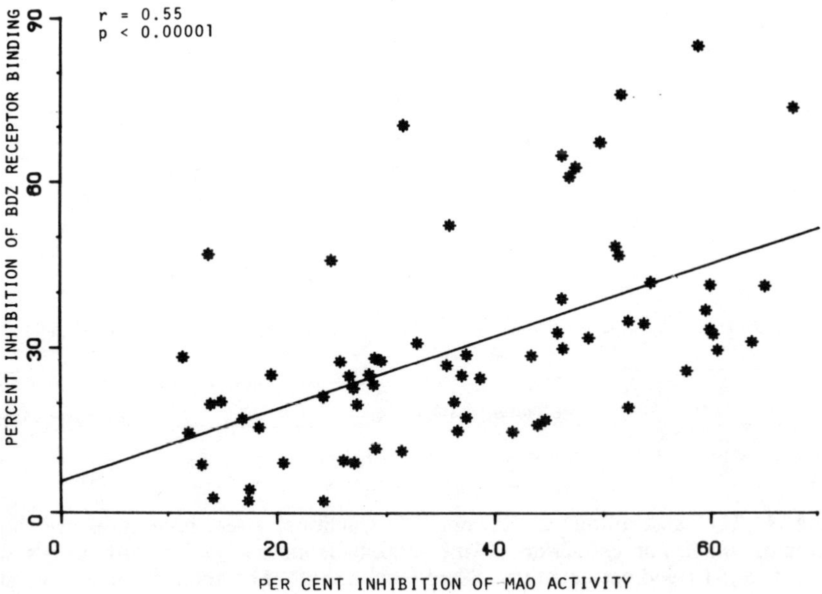


Figure 3 Correlation between the output of inhibitor of benzodiazepine (BDZ) receptor binding and monoamine oxidase (MAO) inhibitor in the urine samples shown in Figure 1

epilepsy are obviously necessary. It is of interest that seizures tend to be controlled by benzodiazepines. These results, as far as they go, show that the mean output of urinary BDZ receptor binding inhibitor was increased in epileptics but no more than in other neurological patients; in both, there was considerable overlap with controls. No specific link with epilepsy has so far emerged.

The output of BDZ receptor binding inhibitor and MAO inhibitor in these urine samples was highly significantly correlated ($r=0.55$, $P<0.0001$) (Figure 3), lending support to our working assumption that both actions derive from the

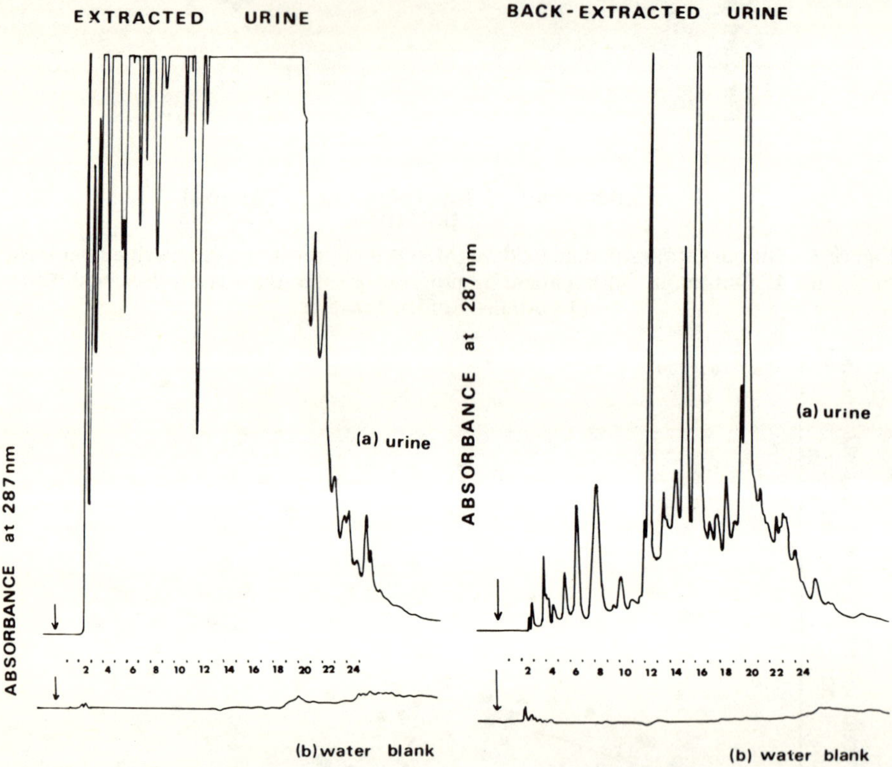


Figure 4 UV absorption at 287 nm of fractions after high pressure liquid chromatography. For extraction, 40 ml aliquots from six pooled 24-h urines were acidified to pH 1 and extracted into 80 ml ethyl acetate. For back extraction the ethyl acetate was washed with 20 ml of 1 M NaOH. Ethyl acetate was dried, reconstituted, and injected onto the column; 1 ml fractions were collected for subsequent assay. (a) Urine samples. (b) Water blank in which the procedure was repeated with water instead of urine

same molecule. This possibility has been further investigated by the purification of both types of activity by high pressure liquid chromatography (HPLC). Pooled ethyl acetate extracts from normal human acidified urine samples were run on a reverse phase column with a gradient of 10–90% methanol in water. Both MAO inhibitor and BDZ receptor binding inhibitory activity were present in more than one peak. Large amounts of UV absorbing material (287 nm) were eluted early in the run, before tube 19 (Figure 4), but the major peak both for MAO inhibitor and BDZ receptor binding inhibition eluted after this, being maximally present in tubes 19–21 (Figure 5). The elution pattern for both activities was similar, the correlation coefficient between them being 0.69 ($P<0.001$). The late emergence of these activities on this HPLC system suggests that the material is relatively non-polar.

The ethyl acetate extracts have been further purified by back extraction into 1 M NaOH. This manoeuvre should remove the more acidic components, leaving the more neutral ones in organic solution. Figure 4 also shows the trace

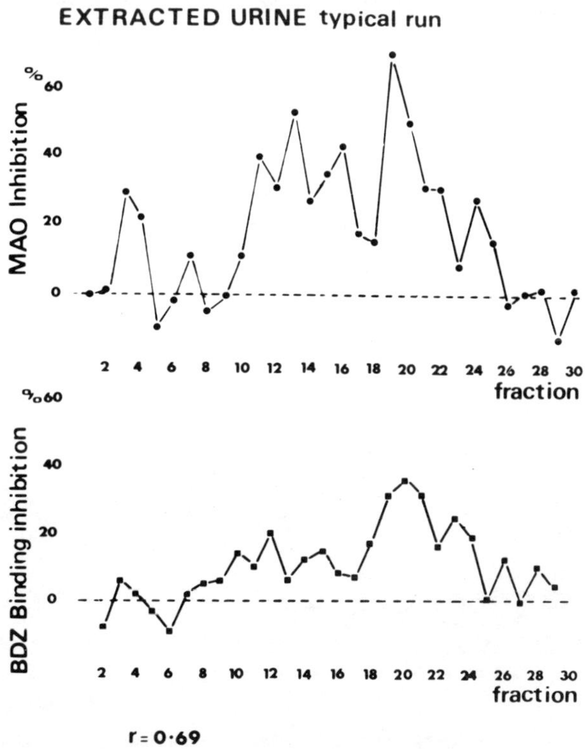


Figure 5 Monoamine oxidase (MAO) inhibition and inhibition of benzodiazepine (BDZ) receptor binding produced by urine extracted and separated by high pressure liquid chromatography as in Figure 4

after HPLC of an ethyl acetate extract which had been treated in this way. The UV trace shows the sample to have been considerably purified, with much less material absorbing at 287 nm than in the original extract. However, a substantial quantity of MAO inhibitor and some BDZ receptor binding inhibitor remained (Figure 6). Further analysis of the NaOH fraction (acidic compounds) by reverse phase HPLC using a different solvent gradient showed that a considerable amount of MAO inhibitor and most of the BDZ receptor binding inhibitor were present in this phase (Figure 7), and that the maxima of the two activities eluted in the same region. This indicates that MAO inhibition in urine is composed of at least two fractions, but that one of these may share identity with the BDZ receptor binding inhibitor, although full proof must await isolation and chemical characterization.

In the meantime, the nature of these molecules remains unknown. It seems unlikely that the urinary BDZ receptor binding inhibitor we are studying is identical with any of the endogenous BDZ receptor ligands previously proposed. Two β-carbolines which are potent BDZ receptor ligands have been isolated from urine. One is harmane (Rommelspacher *et al.*, 1980b). This is

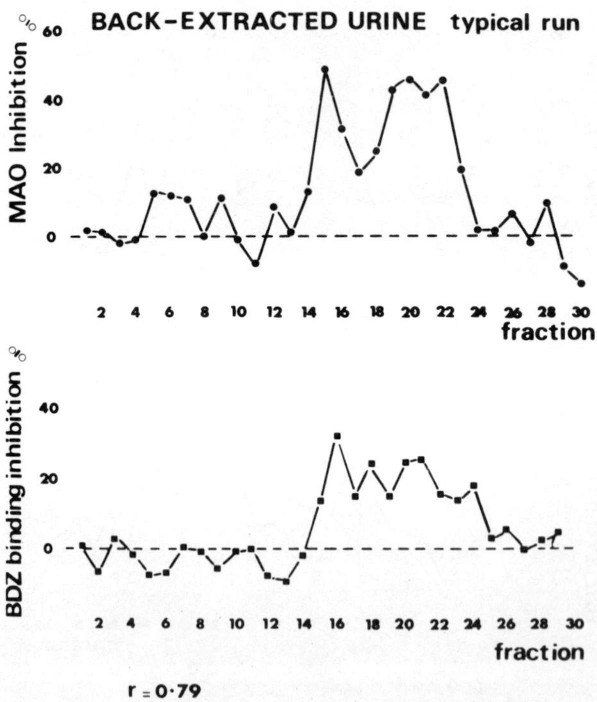


Figure 6 Monoamine oxidase (MAO) inhibition and inhibition of benzodiazepine (BDZ) receptor binding produced by urines back-extracted and separated by high pressure liquid chromatography as in Figure 4

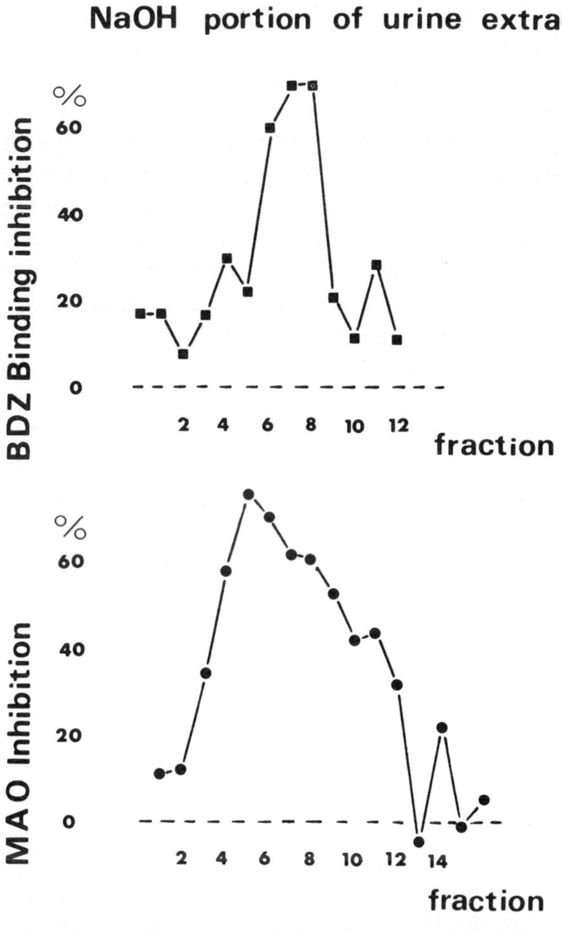


Figure 7 Monoamine oxidase (MAO) inhibition and inhibition of benzodiazepine (BDZ) receptor binding produced by the NaOH phase from the urine extraction procedure described in Figure 4. Urine (100 ml) from the same pool as in Figure 4 was extracted at pH 1 into 200 ml ethyl acetate. The organic phase was back-extracted into 25 ml NaOH which was adjusted to pH 1 and re-extracted into 125 ml ethyl acetate. This fraction was dried, reconstituted, and injected on the HPLC system described in the text. Fractions 18–23 were collected and dried, then reinjected on the same column, but with a 60–80% methanol in water gradient at 5% per min. Fractions (1 ml) were collected for assay

interesting because this compound is also a potent MAO inhibitor (Glover *et al.*, 1982); however harmane does not extract well into ethyl acetate at pH 1 (Clow, Glover, Armando, Reynolds and Sandler, in preparation) and its selective inhibition of MAO is different from that of the urinary inhibitor (Glover *et al.*, 1982). It remains possible, however, that what we are studying is closely related to harmane. The other ligand isolated from urine is β-carboline-3-carboxylic acid ethyl ester (βCEE), an artefact purified from human urine by Braestrup *et al.* (1980) and referred to above. Its parent acid is a much less potent ligand (Braestrup *et al.*, 1980). In our system, βCCE migrates to a different position on an HPLC run from any of the other BDZ receptor inhibiting peaks present in human urine. Both it and its parent acid are very poor MAO inhibitors and both are poorly extracted into ethyl acetate at pH 1. The other putative ligands, inosine, hypoxanthine and nicotinamide do not extract well into ethyl acetate at pH 1. The molecular weight of the urinary MAO inhibitor, at least, is too low, below 300 (Glover *et al.*, 1980) to be accounted for by large polypeptides or proteins.

We suspect that we are dealing with some new BDZ receptor ligand. If, indeed, it also turns out to be the endogenous MAO inhibitor, then its output is likely to be increased in stress, anxiety, and alcohol withdrawal (Sandler, 1982). Evidence is beginning to emerge that anxiety and panic can be generated pharmacologically and countered by benzodiazepines (Dorow, 1982). Whether tribulin, the biochemical system we are monitoring, is responsible for their spontaneous appearance is a question of outstanding importance.

## ACKNOWLEDGEMENTS

A.C. is supported by the Wellcome Trust. J.D.E. is supported by the Medical Research Council.

## REFERENCES

Bhattacharya, S. K., Glover, V., Sandler, M., Clow, A., Topham, A., Bernadt, M., and Murray, R. (1982). Raised endogenous monoamine oxidase inhibitor output in postwithdrawal alcoholics: effects of L-dopa and ethanol. *Biol. Psychiat.*, **17**, 829–836.

Braestrup, C., Nielsen, M. and Olsen, C-E. (1980). Urinary and brain β-carboline-3-carboxylates as potent inhibitors of brain benzodiazepine receptors. *Proc. Natl Acad. Sci., USA*, **77**, 2288–2292.

Cowen, P. J., Green, A. T., Nutt, D. J. and Martin, I. L. (1981). Ethyl β-carboline carboxylate lowers seizure threshold and antagonizes flurazepam-induced sedation in rats. *Nature, Lond.*, **290**, 54–55.

Davis, L. G. and Cohen, R. K. (1980). Identification of an endogenous peptide-ligand for the benzodiazepine receptor. *Biochem. Biophys. Res. Commun.*, **92**, 141–148.

Dorow, R. (1982). β-Carboline monomethylamide causes anxiety in man. *Abstr.* **I.** 13th C.I.N.P. Congress, Jerusalem, June, 1982.

Glover, V., Bhattacharya, S. K., Sandler, M. and File, S. E. (1981). Benzodiazepines reduce stress-augmented increase in rat urine monoamine oxidase inhibitor. *Nature, Lond.*, **292**, 347–349.

Glover, V., Liebowitz, J., Armando, I. and Sandler, M. (1982). β-Carbolines as selective monoamine oxidase inhibitors: *in vivo* implications. *J. Neural Transmiss.*, **54**, 209–218.

Glover, V., Reveley, M. A. and Sandler, M. (1980). A monoamine oxidase inhibitor in human urine. *Biochem. Pharmac.*, **29**, 467–470.

Kenessey, A., Lang, T. and Graf, L. (1981). Demonstration of an endogenous, highly potent, noncompetitive protein inhibitor(s) of $^{3}$H-diazepam binding in bovine brain. *Int. J. Peptide Protein Res.*, **18**, 103–106.

Kuhn, W., Neuser, D. and Przuntek, H. (1981). ($^{3}$H)Diazepam displacing activity in human cerebrospinal fluid. *J. Neurochem.*, **37**, 1045–1047.

Möhler, H. (1981). Benzodiazepine receptors: are there endogenous ligands in the brain? *Trends Pharmac. Sci.*, **2**, 116–119.

Nagy, J., Karcos, J., Maksay, G. and Simonyi, M. (1981). An endogenous substance from porcine brain antagonizes the anticonvulsant effect of diazepam. *Neuropharmacology*, **20**, 529–533.

Oakley, N. R. and Jones, B. J. (1980). The proconvulsant and diazepam-reversing effects of ethyl-β-carboline-3-carboxylate. *Eur. J. Pharmac.*, **68**, 381–382.

Petursson, H., Bhattacharya, S. K., Glover, V., Sandler, M. and Lader, M. H. (1982). Urinary monoamine oxidase inhibitor and benzodiazepine withdrawal. *Brit. J. Psychiat.*, **140**, 7–10.

Petursson, H., Reveley, M. A., Glover, V. and Sandler, M. (1981). Urinary MAO inhibitor in psychiatric illness. *Psychiat. Res.*, **5**, 335–340.

Rommelspacher, H., Nanz, C., Borbe, H. O., Fehske, K. J., Müller, W. E. and Wollert, U. (1980a). 1-Methyl-β-carboline (harmane), a potent endogenous inhibitor of benzodiazepine receptor binding. *Naunyn-Schmiedeberg's Arch. Pharmac.*, **314**, 97–100.

Rommelspacher, H., Strauss, S. and Lindemann, J. (1980b). Excretion of tetrahydroharmane and harmane into the urine of man and rat after a load of ethanol. *FEBS Letts.*, **109**, 209–212.

Sandler, M. (1982). The emergence of tribulin. *Trends Pharmac. Sci.* (in press).

Skolnick, P. and Paul, S. M. (1981). The mechanism(s) of the action of the benzodiazepines. *Med. Res. Rev.*, **1**, 3–22.

Woolf, J. H. and Nixon, J. C. (1981). Endogenous effector of the benzodiazepine binding site: purification and characterization. *Biochemistry*, **20**, 4263–4269.

## DISCUSSION

## CHAIRMAN: DR MICHAEL TRIMBLE

DR. FILE: I should like to clarify the question of whether the compound is a β-carboline and I would like to repeat that the β-carbolines will not extract out at pH 1. So we know that what you looked at is not a β-carboline.

PROFESSOR SANDLER: I would not agree; some β-carbolines might extract.

DR. LASCELLES: Can I ask more about the patients with epilepsy and the neurological controls? They were different from healthy subjects, is that right?

PROFESSOR SANDLER: They were largely hospitalized patients.

DR. LASCELLES: They were in hospital; they were not outpatients?

PROFESSOR SANDLER: Some were outpatients actually, but most were in hospital. So there is no pattern there.

DR. LASCELLES: Nothing to do with drugs, or diet, or anything like that?

PROFESSOR SANDLER: No. Some epileptics were quite drug-free. No patients were on benzodiazepines, of course, at the time, but a subset of the epileptics were drug-free and they had significantly high values compared with the controls.

DR. FILE: Do you know when they last had a seizure?

PROFESSOR SANDLER: We looked at some across an epileptic attack, and yet others who were seizure free. It did not make any difference.

Benzodiazepines Divided
Edited by M. R. Trimble


# 12

# Benzodiazepines, GABA, and Epilepsy —the Animal Evidence

MARKUS SCHMUTZ

## INTRODUCTION

Benzodiazepines exert potent anticonvulsant effects on a variety of experimentally induced seizures in animals. In man, however, their therapeutic use is limited, mainly because of unwanted effects, development of tolerance, and of rebound seizures after the withdrawal of treatment. There is evidence that the anticonvulsant activity of the benzodiazepines may be mediated primarily by an enhancement of GABA-ergic synaptic transmission. This is thought to be initiated by interactions with the benzodiazepine receptors. No direct link, however, has been demonstrated between the anticonvulsant effect, benzodiazepine receptors, and GABA-ergic transmission. Recently discovered benzodiazepine antagonists such as CGS 8216 and Ro 15-1788 provide the first direct evidence that the anticonvulsant activity of the benzodiazepines is mediated by interaction with their identified receptors. In addition, involvement of GABA is further suggested by the fact that CGS 8216 completely inhibited the decrease in the GABA turnover rate induced by diazepam.

## ANTICONVULSANT PROPERTIES OF BENZODIAZEPINES IN ANIMAL MODELS

One of the most interesting aspects of the benzodiazepines is their striking anticonvulsant properties in a variety of experimental models of epilepsy. Drugs such as clonazepam and diazepam are extremely effective in pentylenetetrazol-induced seizures (Koella *et al.*, 1976; Figure 1), oestrogen-induced spike-wave discharges (Julien *et al.*, 1975) or electrically induced spike-wave afterdischarges (Schmutz *et al.*, 1980), i.e. animal models indicative of drug

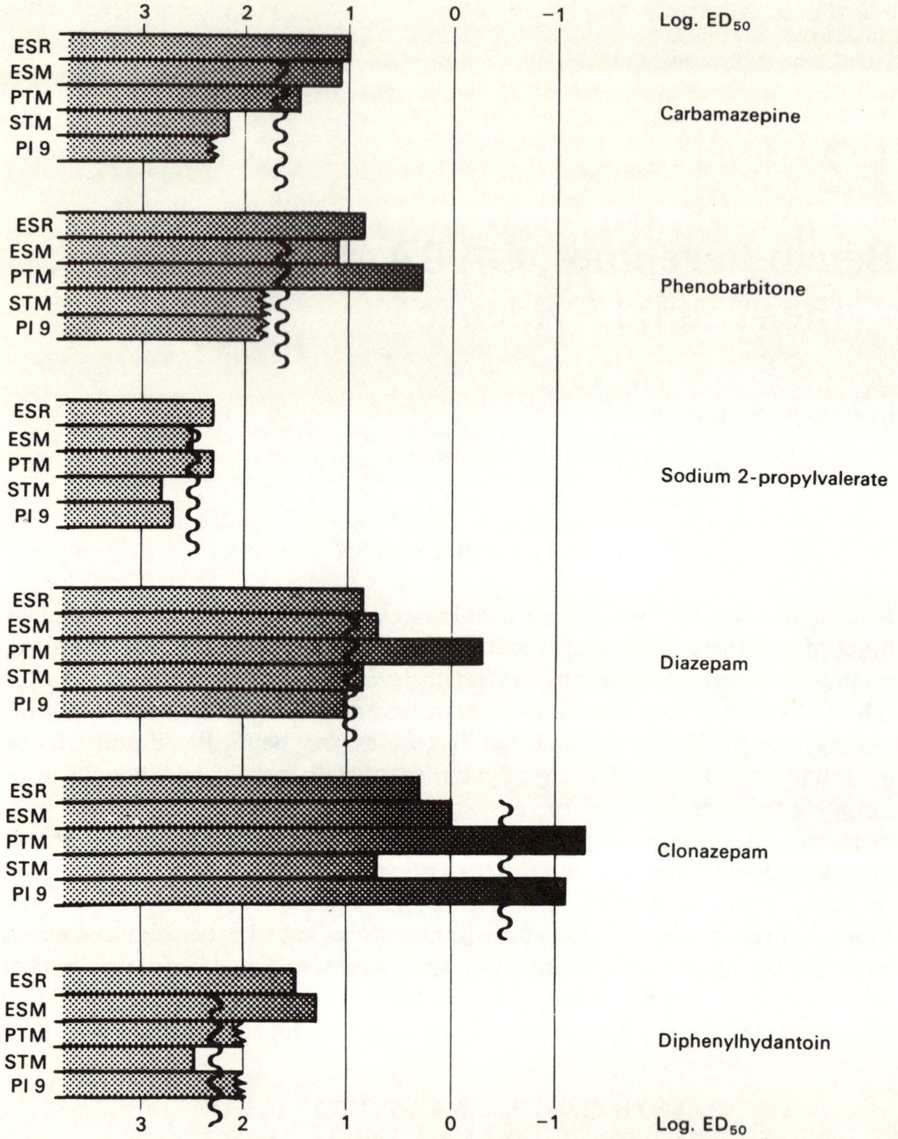


Figure 1 Oral 'potency' profiles ($ED_{50}$ values) of various antiepileptic drugs in 5 test situations. ESR = electroshock, rat; ESM = electroshock, mouse; PTM = pentylenetetrazole test, mouse; STM = strychnine test, mouse; PI9 = picrotoxin test, mouse (9 mg/kg picrotoxin i.p.). Abscissa: log $ED_{50}$ values (= log $1/ED_{50}$) as a measure of potency. The dose inducing sedation in the mouse is indicated in each instance by a vertical wavy line. Reproduced by permission of Hans Huber Publishers, Bern, from *Epileptic Seizures—Behaviour—Pain* (ed. W. Birkmayer) 1976

activity in human absence-type epilepsy. Also in one of the most widely employed tests related to generalized epilepsy with tonic–clonic convulsions, the electroshock test, the benzodiazepines exert considerable anticonvulsant potency (Koella *et al.*, 1976; Figure 1). In addition, they antagonize seizures in animal models for epilepsies with simple or complex partial seizures, e.g. in cats stimulated electrically in the hippocampus (Schmutz *et al.*, 1981; Figure 2). Furthermore, the benzodiazepines also suppress photic seizures in *Papio papio* (Killam, 1976), convulsions produced by antagonists of GABA and glycine (Koella *et al.*, 1976; Figure 1) and they delay the development and generalization of epileptogenic phenomena in the kindling experiment (Wise and Chinerman, 1974; Baltzer *et al.*, 1981). The above data suggest that the benzodiazepines clinically would show a broader spectrum of activity in the treatment of the epilepsies than most other antiepileptics. This turns out to be true to some extent for clonazepam, whereas drugs such as diazepam, nitrazepam, or chlordiazepoxide have a more limited therapeutic use (Browne and Penry, 1973; Vassella, 1980; Trimble, chapter 20, this edition).

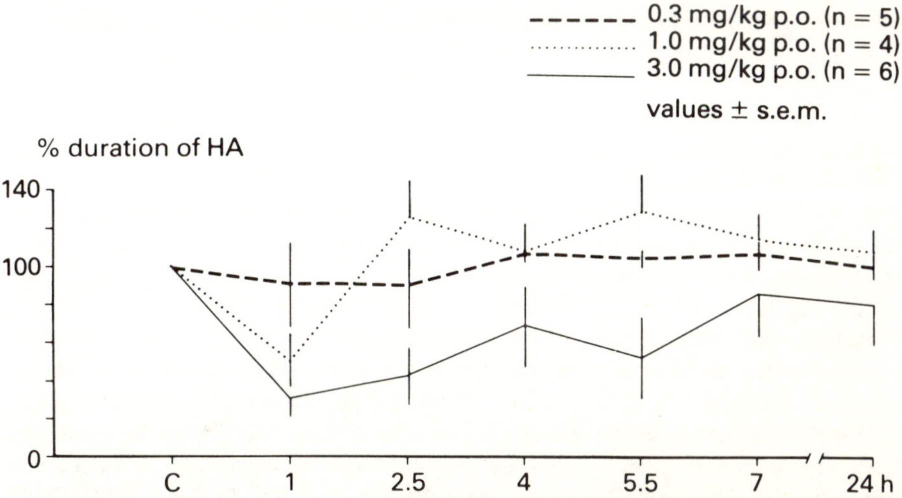


Figure 2 Time course of the effect of diazepam on the electrically induced hippocampal after-discharge (HA) in the cat. Ordinate: duration of HA expressed in per cent of the control value: Abscissa: time after drug administration in hours (C = control value before drug administration). Reproduced, with permission, from Schmutz *et al.* (1980), published by Raven Press, New York

Besides antagonizing convulsions of various kinds, the benzodiazepines on the one hand also exert clear-cut sedation, ataxia, and muscular hypotonia in rodents (Koella *et al.*, 1976), cats (Schmutz *et al.*, 1981), and monkeys (David and Grewal, 1982). On the other hand, signs of tolerance and rebound seizures in animals treated chronically with diazepam or clonazepam have been reported by Baltzer *et al.* (1980), David and Grewal (1982), and Killam *et al.* (1973). These above-mentioned effects, and in addition the occurrence of psychomotor impairment have also been observed in epileptic patients treated with benzodiazepines (Browne and Penry, 1973; Browne, 1976; Vassella, 1980). These drawbacks are responsible for the fact that the clinical value of benzodiazepines in the treatment of the epilepsies is not as great as might be expected from their spectrum of activity in acute animal models. In this respect also the most prominent 'newcomer', the 1,5-benzodiazepine clobazam, may not be a true innovation (Wolf *et al.*, 1981). Nevertheless, further research in this field is justified considering the broad spectrum activity and the high efficacy of this class of compounds in experimental models of the epilepsies.

## THE ROLE OF GABA IN THE ANTICONVULSANT ACTION OF THE BENZODIAZEPINES

There exist several hypotheses about the origin and the development of epileptogenic phenomena. It is certainly not too speculative to assume that an imbalance between excitatory and inhibitory neurotransmitter systems may be one cause of epileptogenesis. Generally speaking, more central excitation or less inhibition than usual will consequently lead to neuronal hyperactivity, that under chronic conditions can be the trigger for the development of an epileptic focus.

GABA is a powerful inhibitory neurotransmitter in the central nervous system. There are two main reasons to implicate GABA with the epilepsies: on the one hand, drugs such as bicuculline or picrotoxin that antagonize GABA-ergic inhibition at various levels are known to act as convulsant agents; on the other hand, drugs such as valproate sodium (see Kerwin *et al.*, 1980), diazepam, or clonazepam enhance GABA-ergic inhibition while being anticonvulsant agents. For the latter drugs, one, or even *the* anticonvulsant mode of action is thought to be the result of their interactions with the GABA system.

Within the past years numerous reports have been published that point to the fact that benzodiazepines enhance GABA-ergic transmission in most areas of the mammalian central nervous system (for review see Haefely, 1982): it has been shown that benzodiazepines enhance presynaptic inhibition in the spinal cord (Schmidt *et al.*, 1967) and the cuneate nucleus of the cat (Polc and Haefely, 1976). Also GABA-mediated postsynaptic inhibition is enhanced in the cuneate nucleus (Polc and Haefely, 1976), the substantia nigra (Schaffner and Haefely, 1975) and in the cortex (Raabe and Gumnit, 1977). Increased GABA-ergic activity following administration of benzodiazepines has also been reported to occur in the limbic system (Jahnsen and Laursen, 1981; Wolf and Haas, 1977) and cerebellar cortex (Pieri and Haefely, 1976). Furthermore benzodiazepines influence other neurotransmitters such as noradrenaline in the locus coeruleus (Grant *et al.*, 1980) or serotonin in the raphé nuclei

(Polc *et al.*, 1981); these latter effects are thought to be secondary and mediated also by interactions of the benzodiazepines with GABA.

Of special interest for the anticonvulsant mode of action of benzodiazepines is the fact that compounds such as diazepam and clonazepam antagonize convulsions elicited by drugs which reduce the activity of GABA, e.g. bicuculline, picrotoxin, isoniazid or 3-mercaptopropionic acid (Koella *et al.*, 1976; Stone and Javid, 1978; Shenoy *et al.*, 1982). In addition, biochemical investigations revealed that benzodiazepines reduce the turnover rate of GABA, yet were without effect on either GAD, GABA-T, GABA levels, GABA uptake, or GABA release (Bernasconi *et al.*, 1982a,b; Figures 3,4). It is interesting to note that in parallel to pharmacological and clinical findings here also tolerance develops, in that after chronic treatment with diazepam the GABA turnover rate is much less reduced than under acute conditions (Figure 3).

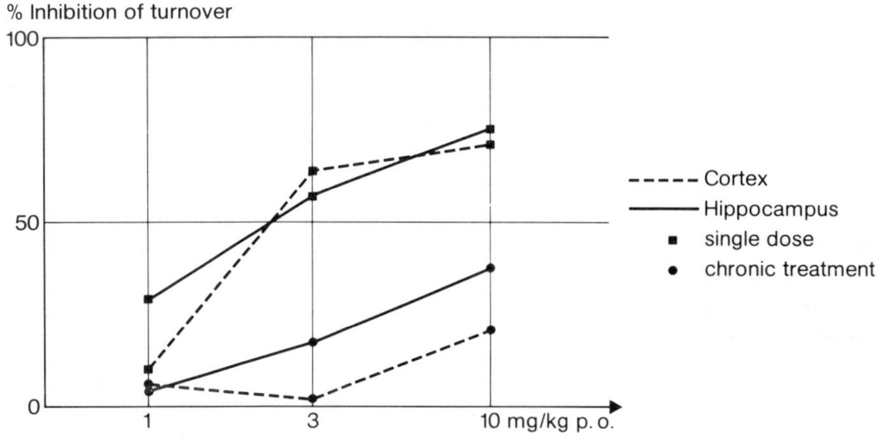


Figure 3 Reduction of GABA turnover induced by diazepam after acute and chronic treatment (4 weeks). Ordinate: inhibition of turnover in per cent. Abscissa: doses of diazepam in mg/kg p.o. The difference in the effect of the diazepam after acute and chronic treatment is indicative of tolerance

The pharmacological and biochemical evidence of benzodiazepine–GABA interactions presented in this chapter can be explained by the fact that GABA- and benzodiazepine-receptors seem to be functionally linked together to form a GABA–benzodiazepine receptor complex. Although benzodiazepines fail to displace labelled GABA from high affinity receptor sites, there is evidence that in the presence of benzodiazepines the binding of GABA is modified. As modification, an increase in the number of high affinity GABA binding sites is suggested. Interestingly enough, also the reverse has been reported: GABA itself seems to modulate the affinity of benzodiazepine binding sites and to

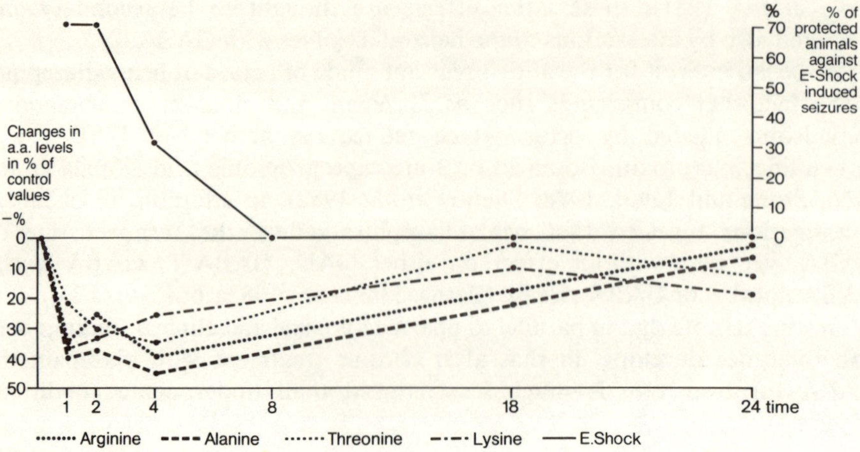


Figure 4 Effects of diazepam (10 mg/kg p.o.) on electroshock induced convulsions in mice and on the amino acid levels in the mouse cortex. Ordinate at left: changes in amino acid levels in per cent of the respective control values. Ordinate at right: per cent of protected mice against electroshock induced seizures. Abscissa: time after drug administration in hours

enhance the binding of benzodiazepines to their receptors (e.g. Möhler and Okada, 1977; Müller, 1981; Costa and Guidotti, 1982). Further evidence for the role of GABA in the mode of action of benzodiazepines is indicated by the fact that benzodiazepine receptors have been found at GABA-ergic synapses (Möhler *et al.*, 1981).

## THE ROLE OF BENZODIAZEPINE RECEPTORS IN THE ANTICONVULSANT ACTION OF THE BENZODIAZEPINES

Although the existence of benzodiazepine receptors and the importance of GABA for the effects of benzodiazepines are hardly questioned, up to now only very few direct links have been demonstrated between these receptors, GABA-ergic transmission, and the anticonvulsant activity of the benzodiazepines.

First, several research groups have shown that the anticonvulsant activity of diazepam can be antagonized by so-called benzodiazepine antagonists, i.e. drugs such as CGS 8216 (Figure 5; e.g. Czernik *et al.*, 1982) or Ro 15-1788 (Figure 6; e.g. Hunkeler *et al.*, 1981); both are neither convulsants nor anticonvulsants but have high affinity for benzodiazepine receptors. In an extended study, first presented at the Epilepsy International Symposium in London (Schmutz, 1982), our group presented data on pharmacological

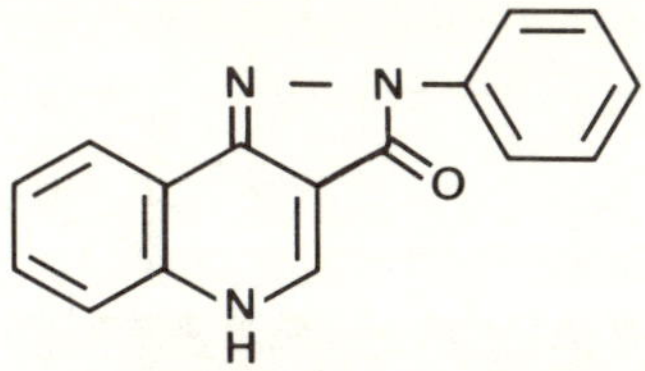


**CGS 8216**

Figure 5 Structural formula of CGS 8216

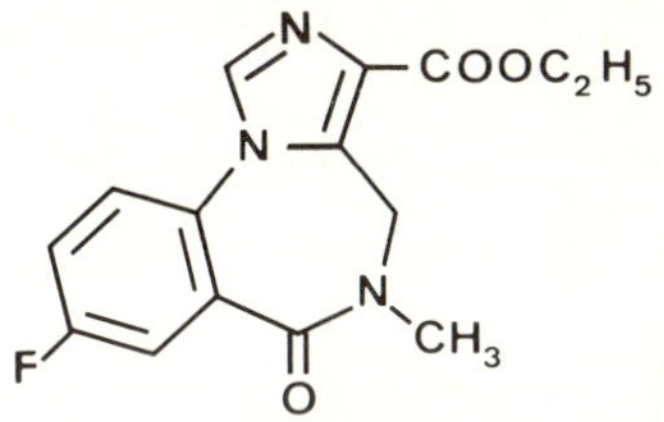


**Ro 15-1788**

Figure 6 Structural formula of Ro 15-1788

interaction studies of all major antiepileptic drugs in clinical use against CGS 8216 and Ro 15-1788.

**Methods**

In the electroshock test in mice, tonic convulsions of the hind extremities were induced by passing an alternating electrical current of 50 Hz and 16 mA for 0.2 seconds through corneal electrodes. Anticonvulsants and CGS 8216 were administered orally one hour, and Ro 15-1788 half an hour, before seizure induction. Ten animals per dose and dose-combination were used; one group served as control. The number of animals protected from tonic hind limb extension seizures was determined. For representation of the results a latin square design was chosen.

In the pentylenetetrazole test in mice, the same procedure as above was used with the exception that clonic seizures were induced by the intraperitoneal injection of 70 mg/kg pentylenetetrazol. The number of animals protected from clonic seizures was determined. The following drugs were used: CGS 8216, Ro 15-1788, diazepam, clonazepam, clobazam, carbamazepine, oxcarbazepine (Baltzer and Schmutz, 1978; Rai *et al.*, 1982), phenytoin, phenobarbitone, valproate sodium, and acetazolamide.

**Results**

CGS 8216 and Ro 15-1788 had neither convulsant nor anticonvulsant effects in the electroshock test and the pentylenetetrazole test.

| | DIAZEPAM | | | | | |
|---|---|---|---|---|---|---|
| | DOSES | 0 | 1 | 3 | 10 | 30 |
| CGS 8216 | 0 | 0 | 0 | 20 | 70 | 100 |
| | 1 | 0 | 0 | - | 40 | 100 |
| | 3 | 0 | 0 | - | 30 | 100 |
| | 10 | 0 | 0 | 0 | 0 | 100 |
| | 30 | 0 | 0 | 0 | 0 | 40 |

Figure 7 Influence of CGS 8216 on the anticonvulsant activity of diazepam in the electroshock test on mice ($n = 10$ per dose). Unshaded area: doses in mg/kg p.o. Figures in the shaded areas indicate percentage of animals protected against seizures. The lightly shaded area shows the effects of both drugs given together; the darkly shaded area shows the effects of each drug given alone. –: no value for the respective dose combination

The anticonvulsant activity of diazepam was diminished by both antagonists in the electroshock test and in the pentylenetetrazole test (Figures 7, 8). The most pronounced reduction in anticonvulsant activity was observed at those doses of diazepam which were too low to protect 100% of the animals from seizures.

Qualitatively similar results were obtained with clonazepam and clobazam (electroshock test, CGS 8216), indicating no major differences between 1,4- and 1,5-benzodiazepines in this respect.

The anticonvulsant activity of phenytoin (Figure 9), phenobarbitone, valproate sodium, and acetazolamide was not or only marginally diminished by CGS 8216 and/or Ro 15-1788 over the whole dose range.

The results with carbamazepine were somewhat unexpected: whereas both antagonists exerted similar effects when combined with the beforementioned antiepileptics, this did not seem to turn out to be true for carbamazepine

DIAZEPAM

RO 15 - 1788

| DOSES | 0 | 3 | 10 | 30 |
|---|---|---|---|---|
| 0 | 0 | 0 | 60 | 100 |
| 1 | 0 | 0 | 20 | 90 |
| 3 | 0 | 0 | 20 | 90 |
| 10 | 0 | 0 | 0 | 50 |
| 30 | 0 | 0 | 0 | 80 |

Figure 8 Influence of Ro 15-1788 on the anticonvulsant activity of diazepam in the electroshock test on mice ($n = 10$ per dose). Unshaded area: doses in mg/kg p.o. Figures in the shaded areas indicate percentage of animals protected against seizures. The lightly shaded area shows the effects of both drugs given together; the darkly shaded area shows the effects of each drug given alone

(Figures 10–12). In the electroshock and the pentylenetetrazol test, Ro 15-1788 did not reduce the anticonvulsant effect of carbamazepine; however, CGS 8216 diminished the anticonvulsant effect of carbamazepine in both tests. This antagonistic effect was somewhat less than with diazepam, yet clearly stronger than with phenytoin, phenobarbitone, valproate sodium, and acetazolamide. With oxcarbazepine similar results to those with carbamazepine were obtained.

In general, both antagonists exerted qualitatively similar effects on the anticonvulsant activity of the antiepileptic drugs tested with regard to the electroshock test and the pentylenetetrazol test.

PHENYTOIN

| RO 15 - 1788 DOSES | 0 | 3 | 10 | 30 |
|---|---|---|---|---|
| 0 | 0 | 10 | 40 | 100 |
| 1 | 0 | 0 | 40 | 100 |
| 3 | 0 | 0 | 30 | 90 |
| 10 | 0 | 0 | 50 | 100 |
| 30 | 0 | 0 | 70 | 100 |

Figure 9 Influence of Ro 15-1788 on the anticonvulsant activity of phenytoin in the electroshock test on mice ($n = 10$ per dose). Unshaded area: doses in mg/kg p.o. Figures in the shaded areas indicate percentage of animals protected against seizures. The lightly shaded area shows the effects of both drugs given together; the darkly shaded area shows the effects of each drug given alone

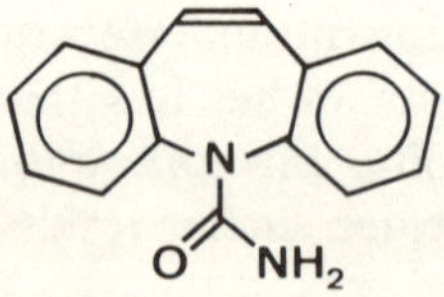


**Carbamazepine**

Figure 10 Structural formula of carbamazepine

CARBAMAZEPINE

RO 15 - 1788

| DOSES | 0 | 10 | 20 | 30 |
|---|---|---|---|---|
| 0 | 0 | 0 | 50 | 100 |
| 1 | 0 | 0 | 50 | 100 |
| 3 | 0 | 0 | 60 | 100 |
| 10 | 0 | 0 | 40 | 100 |
| 30 | 0 | 0 | 100 | 100 |

Figure 11 Influence of Ro 15-1788 on the anticonvulsant activity of carbamazepine in the electroshock test on mice ($n = 10$ per dose). Unshaded area: doses in mg/kg p.o. Figures in the shaded area indicate percentage of animals protected against seizures. The lightly shaded area shows the effects of both drugs given together; the darkly shaded area shows the effects of each drug given alone

## Discussion

According to these results, the anticonvulsant effect of the 1,4- and 1,5-benzodiazepines is mediated by benzodiazepine receptors as it was antagonized by CGS 8216 and/or Ro 15-1788. The anticonvulsant activity of valproate sodium, phenytoin, phenobarbitone and acetazolamide was at best only marginally diminished by these antagonists, indicating that there is no direct correlation of the anticonvulsant mode of action of these drugs with benzodiazepine receptors. The reduction of the anticonvulsant activity of carbamazepine and oxcarbazepine by CGS 8216 may on the one hand be mediated by benzodiazepine receptors; in this context it is interesting to note that at high doses

CARBAMAZEPINE

CGS 8216

| DOSES | 0 | 5 | 10 | 10* | 20 |
|---|---|---|---|---|---|
| 0 | 0 | 0 | 20 | 40 | 100 |
| 1 | 0 | 0 | 0 | 0 | 80 |
| 3 | 0 | 0 | 0 | 0 | 90 |
| 10 | 0 | 0 | 0 | 0 | 80 |
| 30 | 0 | 0 | 0 | - | 70 |

Figure 12 Influence of CGS 8216 on the anticonvulsant activity of carbamazepine in the electroshock test on mice ($n = 10$ per dose). Unshaded area: doses in mg/kg p.o. Figures in the shaded area indicate percentage of animals protected against seizures. The lightly shaded area shows the effects of both drugs given together; the darkly shaded area shows the effects of each drug given alone. -: no value for the respective dose combination. *: two different experiments with the dose of 10 mg/kg p.o. of carbamazepine

both antiepileptics also reduce the GABA turnover rate in mice (Bernasconi *et al.*, 1982a). In this case CGS 8216 would be a more 'complete' benzodiazepine antagonist than Ro 15-1788 as far as its effects on GABA are concerned. On the other hand, CGS 8216 also interacts with adenosine receptors (Czernik *et al.*, 1982); it may well be that this effect is responsible for the reduction of the anticonvulsant activity of carbamazepine and oxcarbazepine. This interpretation is strengthened by the fact that carbamazepine has been described to inhibit the binding of $^3$H-phenylisopropyladenosine to adenosine receptors on rat brain membranes in 'therapeutic' concentrations (Skerritt *et al.*, 1982).

Besides this approach some other data related to the anticonvulsant effect of benzodiazepines and benzodiazepine receptors are of interest: it has been reported that the displacing potencies of benzodiazepines for $^3$H-diazepam binding sites correlate significantly with their antagonism against pentylenetetrazol-induced convulsions in mice (Möhler and Okada, 1977). And Paul *et al.* (1979) have shown an excellent correlation between benzodiazepine receptor occupancy by diazepam and the protection against pentylenetetrazol-induced seizures. They further demonstrated that only a small fraction of benzodiazepine receptors needs to be occupied to produce complete protection against this type of seizure.

Finally, an involvement of GABA in the receptor-mediated activity of benzodiazepines could be demonstrated by Bernasconi (1983): CGS 8216 in mice completely inhibited the decrease in the GABA turnover rate induced by diazepam.

## OUTLOOK

It is unquestionable that the benzodiazepines exert potent anticonvulsant effects on a variety of experimentally induced seizures in animals. Strong pharmacological and biochemical evidence indicates that the principal effects of benzodiazepines on the central nervous system may be mediated primarily by an enhancement of GABA-ergic synaptic transmission. These effects are thought to be initiated by interactions with the benzodiazepine receptors which seem to be localized in part at GABA-ergic synapses. In experimental epilepsy, benzodiazepines that bind to their receptors in general have been shown also to possess anticonvulsant potency. With benzodiazepine antagonists such as CGS 8216 or Ro 15-1788 direct evidence is provided that the anticonvulsant activity of the benzodiazepines is indeed mediated by interaction with their identified receptors. In addition, involvement of GABA is further suggested by the fact that CGS 8216 completely inhibited the decrease in the GABA turnover rate induced by diazepam.

However, it remains to be convincingly demonstrated that this is the only mechanism mediating the anticonvulsant activity of benzodiazepines; various neurotransmitters besides GABA are influenced by benzodiazepines and it seems worthwhile to raise the question whether the following interactions are all primarily mediated by GABA: benzodiazepines decreasing the turnover rates of dopamine, noradrenaline (Corrodi *et al.*, 1967; Dolce and Kaemmerer, 1967), acetylcholine (Zsilla *et al.*, 1976), and serotonin (Wise *et al.*, 1972); benzodiazepines decreasing the cortical levels of alanine, arginine, lysine, and threonine (Bernasconi *et al.*, 1982b; Figure 4); benzodiazepines inhibiting the uptake of adenosine and binding to glycine receptors (Snyder and Enna, 1975). The same question of benzodiazepine effects being mediated by GABA alone can be raised in the chemically induced seizure models: that is, benzodiazepines block pentylenetetrazol-induced seizures more potently than seizures induced by antagonists of GABA-ergic effects such as bicuculline or picrotoxin (Koella *et al.*, 1976; Stone and Javid, 1978; Shenoy *et al.*, 1982). In addition, studies with benzodiazepine antagonists must be interpreted carefully, since these compounds may also bind to other types of receptors (see results of the combination of CGS 8216 and carbamazepine). In this context the reverse situation also is possible, since U 43,465 F, a benzodiazepine, is known to have 'antidepressant' effects in mice that are not mediated by benzodiazepine receptors. These effects can be reversed by propranolol but not by Ro 15-1788; the anxiolytic effects of this compound are, however, mediated by benzodiazepine receptors since they can be antagonized by Ro 15-1788 (Thiebot *et al.*, 1982).

Finally, the existence of GABA-independent benzodiazepine receptors associated to a chloride ionophore (Le Fur *et al.*, 1981) and of micromolar benzodiazepine receptors, to which also phenytoin binds (Bowling and De Lorenzo, 1982), has been claimed recently. Thus, the precise mechanism of action of the benzodiazepines is not yet fully understood, and we certainly need further clarification of the molecular mechanisms mediating the (anticonvulsant) effects of this class of compounds. Nevertheless, this paper and the data reviewed provide convincing evidence that enhancement of GABA-ergic transmission is of great importance for the anticonvulsant activity of the benzodiazepines and that this activity is initiated by interactions with receptors to which benzodiazepines bind with high affinity.

## ACKNOWLEDGEMENTS

The author gratefully acknowledges the help of Dr. Raymond Bernasconi and Dr. Helmut Bittiger in preparing this manuscript.

## REFERENCES

Baltzer, V., Baud, J., Degen, P. and Koella, W. P. (1980). A procedure to detect development of tolerance ('Escape') to antiepileptic drugs: first results. In: *Advances in Epileptology: The 10th Epilepsy International Symposium*, pp.310–320 (Eds. Wada, J. A. and Penry, J. K.), Raven Press, New York.

Baltzer, V., Klebs, K. and Schmutz, M. (1981). Effects of oxcarbazepine, a compound related to carbamazepine, and of GP 47 779, its main metabolite in man, on the evaluation of amygdaloid-kindled seizures in the rat. In: *13th Epilepsy International Symposium, Kyoto*, Abstracts, p.151.

Baltzer, V. and Schmutz, M. (1978). Experimental anticonvulsive properties of GP 47 680 and of GP 47 779, its main human metabolite. In: *Advances in Epileptology 1977*, pp.295–299 (Eds Meinardi, H. and Rowan, A. J.), Swets and Zeitlinger BV, Amsterdam.

Bernasconi, R. (1983). L'hypothèse GABAergique du méchanisme d'action des anti-épileptiques. *J. Pharmac. (Paris)*, in press.

Bernasconi, R., Klein, M., Martin, P. and Schmutz, M. (1982a). The influence of anti-convulsant drugs on GABA-turnover. In: *Basic and Clinical aspects of Molecular Neurobiology*, p.394 (Eds. Giuffrida Stella, A. M. *et al.*), Fondazione Internazionale Menarini, Milano.

Bernasconi, R., Martin, P. and Schmutz, M. (1982b). Effects of antiepileptic drugs on amino acid concentrations in mouse brain as a function of time: correlation with anticonvulsant activity. In: *IBRO Congress Lausanne*, Abstracts, p.24.

Bowling, A. C. and De Lorenzo, R. J. (1982). Micromolar affinity benzodiazepine receptors: identification and characterization in central nervous system. *Science*, **216**, 1247–1250.

Browne, T. R. (1976). Clonazepam, a review of a new anticonvulsant drug. *Arch. Neurol.*, **33**, 326–332.

Browne, T. R. and Penry, J. K. (1973). Benzodiazepines in the treatment of epilepsy. A review. *Epilepsia*, **14**, 277–310.

Corrodi, H., Fuxe, K. and Hokfelt, T. (1967). The effect of some psychoactive drugs on central monoamine neurons. *Eur. J. Pharmac.*, **1**, 363–368.

Costa, E. and Guidotti, A. (1982). Molecular mechanisms whereby benzodiazepines interact with gamma-amino-butyric acid recognition sites. In: *Brain Peptides and Hormones*, pp.107–114 (Eds. Collu, R. *et al.*), Raven Press, New York.

Czernik, A. J., Petrack, B., Kalinsky, H. J., Psychoyos, S., Cash, W., Tsai, C., Rinehart, R. K., Granat, F. R., Lovell, R. A., Brundish, D. E. and Wade, R. (1982). CGS 8216: receptor binding characteristics of a potent benzodiazepine antagonist. *Life Sci.*, **30**, 363–372.

David, J. C. and Grewal, R. S. (1982). Unpublished results. CIBA-GEIGY Research Centre, Goregaon East, Bombay, India.

Dolce, G. and Kaemmerer, E. (1967). Neurophysiological studies with 7-chlor-1,3-dihydro-3-hydroxy-5-phenyl-2H-1,4-benzodiazepin-2-one in animal experiments. *Arzneim. Forsch.*, **17**, 1057–1060.

Grant, S. J., Huang, Y. H. and Redmond, D. E. (1980). Benzodiazepines attenuate single unit activity in the locus coeruleus. *Life Sci.*, **27**, 2231–2236.

Haefely, W. (1982). Behavioural and neuropharmacological aspects of benzodiazepines. In: *Brain Peptides and Hormones*, pp.81–91 (Eds. Collu, R. *et al.*), Raven Press, New York.

Hunkeler, W., Möhler, H., Pieri, L., Polc, P., Bonetti, E. P., Cumin, R., Schaffner, R. and Haefely, W. (1981). Selective antagonists of benzodiazepines. *Nature*, **290**, 514–516.

Jahnsen, H. and Laursen, A. M. (1981). The effects of a benzodiazepine on the hyperpolarizing and the depolarizing responses of hippocampal cells to GABA. *Brain Res.*, **207**, 214–217.

Julien, R. M., Fowler, G. W. and Danielson, M. G. (1975). The effects of antiepileptic drugs on estrogen-induced electrographic spike-wave discharge. *J. Pharmac. exp. Ther.*, **193**, 647–656.

Killam, E. K. (1976). Measurement of anticonvulsant activity in the Papio papio model of epilepsy. *Fed. Proc.*, **35**, 2264–2269.

Killam, E. K., Matsuzaki, M. and Killam, K. F. (1973). Studies of anticonvulsant compounds in the Papio papio model of epilepsy. In: *Chemical Modulation of Brain Function*, pp.161–171 (Ed. Sabelli, M. C.), Raven Press, New York.

Kerwin, R. W., Olpe, H. R. and Schmutz, M. (1980). The effect of sodium-n-dipropyl acetate on GABA dependent inhibition in the rat cortex and substantia nigra in relation to its anticonvulsant activity. *Brit. J. Pharmac.*, **71**, 545–551.

Koella, W. P., Levin, P. and Baltzer, V. (1976). The pharmacology of carbamazepine and some other antiepileptic drugs. In: *Epileptic Seizures-Behaviour-Pain*, pp.23–48 (Ed. Birkmayer, W.), Huber, Bern Stuttgart Vienna.

Le Fur, G. Mizoule, J., Burgevin, M. C., Ferris, O., Heaulme, M., Gauthier, A., Guérémy, C. and Uzan, A. (1981). Multiple benzodiazepine receptors: evidence of a dissociation between anticonflict and anticonvulsant properties by PK 8165 and PK 9084 (two quinoline derivatives). *Life Sci.*, **28**, 1439–1448.

Möhler, H. and Okada, T. (1977). Benzodiazepine receptor: demonstration in the central nervous system. *Science*, **198**, 849–851.

Möhler, H., Richards, J. G. and Wu, J. Y. (1981). Autoradiographic localization of benzodiazepine receptors in immunocytochemically identified gamma-aminobutyrergic synapses. *Proc. Natl Acad. Sci. USA*, **78**, 1935–1938.

Müller, W. E. (1981). The benzodiazepine receptor, an update. *Pharmacology*, **22**, 153–161.

Paul, S. M., Syapin, P. J., Paugh, B. A., Moncada, V. and Skolnick, P. (1979). Correlation between benzodiazepine receptor occupation and anticonvulsant effects of diazepam. *Nature*, **281**, 688–689.

Pieri, L. and Haefely, W. (1976). The effect of diphenylhydantoin, diazepam and clonazepam on the activity of Purkinje cells in the rat cerebellum. *Naunyn-Schmiedeberg's Arch. Pharmac.*, **296**, 1–4.

Polc, P. and Haefely, W. (1976). Effects of two benzodiazepines, phenobarbitone and baclofen on synaptic transmission in the cat cuneate nucleus. *Naunyn-Schmiedeberg's Arch. Pharmac.*, **294**, 121–131.

Polc, P., Laurent, J. P., Scherschlicht, R. and Haefely, W. (1981). Electrophysiological studies on the specific benzodiazepine antagonist Ro 15-1788. *Naunyn-Schmiedeberg's Arch. Pharmac.*, **316**, 317–325.

Raabe, W. and Gumnit, R. J. (1977). Anticonvulsant action of diazepam: Increase of cortical postsynaptic inhibition. *Epilepsia*, **18**, 117–120.

Rai, P. V., Egli, M. and Wad, N. (1982). Report of a 6 years clinical evaluation on a new antiepileptic drug, oxcarbazepine. In: *14th Epilepsy International Symposium, London, Abstracts*, pp.56–57.

Schaffner, R. and Haefely, W. (1975). The effects of diazepam and bicuculline on the strio-nigral evoked potential. *Experientia*, **31**, 732.

Schmidt, R. F., Vogel, E. and Zimmermann, M. (1967). Die Wirkung von Diazepam auf die präsynaptische Hemmung und andere Rückenmarksreflexe. *Naunyn-Schmiedeberg's Arch. Pharmak. exp. Path.*, **258**, 69–82.

Schmutz, M. (1982). Inhibition of the anticonvulsant activity of benzodiazepines and other anticonvulsants by CGS 8216: pharmacological interaction studies as a tool to detect correlations between anticonvulsant drug effect and benzodiazepine receptor binding. In: *14th Epilepsy International Symposium, London*, Abstracts, p.149.

Schmutz, M., Bürki, H. and Koella, W. P. (1981). Electrically induced hippocampal afterdischarge in the freely moving cat: an animal model of focal (possibly temporal lobe) epilepsy. In: *Advances in Epileptology: The 12th Epilepsy International Symposium*, pp.59–65 (Eds. Dam, M. *et al.*), Raven Press, New York.

Schmutz, M., Klebs, K. and Koella, W. P. (1980). A chronic petit mal model. In: *Advances in Epileptology: The 10th Epilepsy International Symposium*, pp.311–314 (Eds. Wada, J. A. and Penry, J. K.), Raven Press, New York.

Shenoy, A. K., Miyahara, J. T., Swinyard, E. A. and Kupferberg, H. J. (1982). Comparative anticonvulsant activity and neurotoxicity of clobazam, diazepam, phenobarbital and valproate in mice and rats. *Epilepsia*, **23**, 399–408.

Skerritt, H., Davies, L. P. and Johnston, G. A. R. (1982). A purinergic component in the anticonvulsant action of carbamazepine? *Eur. J. Pharmac.*, **82**, 195–197.

Snyder, S. H. and Enna, S. J. (1975). The role of central glycine receptors in the pharmacologic actions of benzodiazepines. *Adv. Biochem. Psychopharmac.*, **14**, 81–91.

Stone, W. E. and Javid, M. J. (1978). Benzodiazepines and phenobarbital as antagonists of dissimilar chemical convulsants. *Epilepsia*, **19**, 361–368.

Thiebot, M. H., Doare, L., Puech, A. J. and Simon, P. (1982). U 43,465 F: a benzodiazepine with antidepressant activity? Interaction with Ro 15-1788 and *d,l*-propranolol. *Eur. J. Pharmac.*, **84**, 103–106.

Vassella, F. (1980). Benzodiazepine in der Behandlung der Epilepsien. *Schweiz. Rundschau Med. (PRAXIS)*, **69**, 827–834.
Wise, C. D., Berger, B. D. and Stein, L. (1972). Benzodiazepines: anxiety-reducing activity by reduction of serotonin turnover in the brain. *Science*, **177**, 180–183.
Wise, R. A. and Chinerman, J. (1974). Effects of diazepam and phenobarbital on electrically-induced amygdaloid seizures and seizure development. *Exp. Neurol.*, **45**, 355–363.
Wolf, P., Beck-Mannagetta, G., Knorz, A., Meencke, J., Röder, U. U. and Schmidt, D. (1981). How useful is clobazam as an antiepileptic drug? In: *13th Epilepsy International Symposium, Kyoto*, Abstracts, p.166.
Wolf, P. and Haas, H. L. (1977). Effects of diazepines and barbiturates on hippocampal recurrent inhibition. *Naunyn-Schmiedeberg's Arch. Pharmac.*, **299**, 211–218.
Zsilla, G., Cheney, D. L. and Costa, E. (1976). Regional changes in the rate of turnover of acetylcholine in rat brain following diazepam or muscimol. *Naunyn-Schmiedeberg's Arch. Pharmac.*, **294**, 251–255.

## DISCUSSION

## CHAIRMAN: PROFESSOR MALCOLM LADER

DR. GRAY: I am not skilled at translating oral to intraperitoneal doses, but is my impression correct that the doses of your, for example, diazepam that are effective in controlling seizures are very much higher than those that would be effective in a typical behavioural test? For antianxiety action, for example, diazepam 1 mg/kg intraperitoneally would be ample.

DR. SCHMUTZ: That is in part correct, in part not. It depends on the type of seizures. With electric shock induced convulsions the $ED_{50}$ of diazepam is about 6 mg/kg per os. When you have a look at the pentylenetetrazol-induced seizures, the $ED_{50}$ of diazepam is below 1 mg/kg.

DR. TRIMBLE: Clinically, if tolerance did not develop to the effect of these compounds, they would be extremely effective anticonvulsants. We do not seem to see tolerance to their anxiolytic effects. Do we know anything about the biochemical changes related to tolerance?

DR. SCHMUTZ: Tolerance has been reported to occur with chronic treatment in electric shock induced seizures, and also in seizures induced by aluminium hydroxide. There is some evidence that in pentylenetetrazol-induced seizures, no tolerance develops. Some people claim that pentylenetetrazol-induced seizures are more related to anxiety, where tolerance with benzodiazepines is much less seen than in epilepsy. The biochemical publications dealing with receptors and chronic treatment with benzodiazepines provide only equivocal data.

DR. GRAY: Can I just comment that the animal behavioural studies confirm what Dr. Trimble just said, namely that you do not get tolerance to the anxiolytic effects of benzodiazepines; at least, I have not seen them and I have not seen them reported.

DR. FILE: We reported in 1979 tolerance to the anxiolytic effects.

DR. GRAY: Over what sort of timing?

DR. FILE: This is the interesting thing and it is not really in conflict with what Dr. Trimble says: you get tolerance to the sedative effects in 3–5 days, you get tolerance to the antipentylenetetrazol effects in from 5 to 10 days, to the antistress effects as measured by corticosterone rises in about 10 days, and to the anxiolytic effects in 15–21 days.

DR. GRAY: Those figures are in a sense in agreement with our data, in that we have looked up to about 20 days. You have evidently gone on longer than we did.

PROFESSOR I. OSWALD: May I remind us that there is a very powerful circadian rhythm, and such things as measures of $ED_{50}$, and of the ease with which convulsions can be induced in rodents vary enormously with the time or the phase or the circadian cycle. It would follow, I would have supposed, that anticonvulsant effects would also vary, as would antagonism to anticonvulsant effects.

Benzodiazepines Divided
Edited by M. R. Trimble


# 13

# Where in the Brain do Benzodiazepines Act?

SUSAN IVERSEN

## INTRODUCTION

The benzodiazepines have a selective psychopharmacological profile in animals. They release responding which has been suppressed by the presentation of a noxious stimulus; a procedure described as punishment. As we have seen (chapter 8), this is usually achieved by initially establishing a baseline of responding for food reward and then introducing an aversive stimulus, such as shock, so that in order to obtain reward the animal must simultaneously accept electric shock. The consequence of this interaction is described as conflict, and is considered to generate anxiety and disrupt responding. Benzodiazepines are thought to influence this emotional state and the result is observed as higher levels of responding during the periods of conflict. It can be demonstrated that non-specific stimulatory or sedative effects of these drugs, although they exist to some extent, do not account for their profound anxiolytic action. They are also devoid of significant analgesic action. Barbiturates and muscle relaxants, such as meprobamate also share these properties and are also effective anxiolytic compounds; however, in these cases it is more difficult to separate the sedative and anxiolytic actions.

The selectivity of the action of the benzodiazepines on conflict has encouraged us to believe that an equally selective site of action in the CNS is likely to account for this effect. I believe this to be misguided, first on behavioural grounds. It is clear as we saw earlier that although we arbitrarily monitor anxiety with an operant response, this is only a tiny part of the response profile. If we confine our attention to the conflict procedure we may provide an explanation of the effects of benzodiazepines on the response suppression mechanism, which may indeed involve a discrete brain structure and its immediate circuitry. However, the full behavioural expression of anxiety is likely to involve substrates extending from cortex to brain stem. We should be looking not for a site of action, but sites of action and trying to build up a circuit mediating the complex of respondent, operant, and cognitive responses which constitute an emotional state. Second, recent advances in our understanding of the CNS pharmacology of benzodiazepines reinforce this view. A growing list of neurotransmitters and their receptor types are implicated in the action of benzodiazepines and barbiturates.

Having said this, although it is clear that the research strategy is inadequate to the problem, the correlation of structure and function remains one of the few approaches which we can actually use. Thus, the majority of experiments to be discussed consider the involvement of a given structure or pathway in relation to anxiety. In a piecemeal fashion one can then begin to fit the picture together.

## THE BRAIN SUBSTRATES INVOLVED IN EMOTIONAL BEHAVIOUR — WITH SPECIAL REFERENCE TO ANXIETY

Bolles and Fanselow (1980) have proposed a theory of fear and anxiety based on principles of conditioning. Fear is considered a motivational state activated by painful aversive events, novelty, and significant species-specific stimuli, which signal danger and which the animal does not have to learn about. Fear motivation once activated induces arousal and three classes of events:

1. autonomic changes;
2. defensive behaviour (freezing or activity);
3. perceptual changes.

Fear is also claimed to inhibit the overt response to pain which is seen to be recuperative (Figure 1). Classical conditioning forms the basis for generation of fear motivation which brings the theory closely in line with classical two-process models of learning. After conditioning, neutral stimuli (CS) presented with the aversive event (US) come to elicit the expectancy of an unpleasant experience (E[US]). The anticipation of the pain generates fear and mobilizes defensive behaviour (SSDR) and activates the endogeneous opiate system which inhibits the response to pain.

In a more physiologically oriented theory, Gray (1982) has identified four classes of stimuli which generate the behavioural state of anxiety (Figure 2), and result in changes in operant behaviour. Suppression of behaviour is most commonly used as a reflection of anxiety but it is important to note that the presentation of aversive stimuli may lead to increases in behavioural output associated, Gray suggests, with enhanced levels of arousal and attention. It is notable that Gray's own model behavioural system, the partial reinforcement effect, results in behavioural invigoration as a response to anxiety rather than

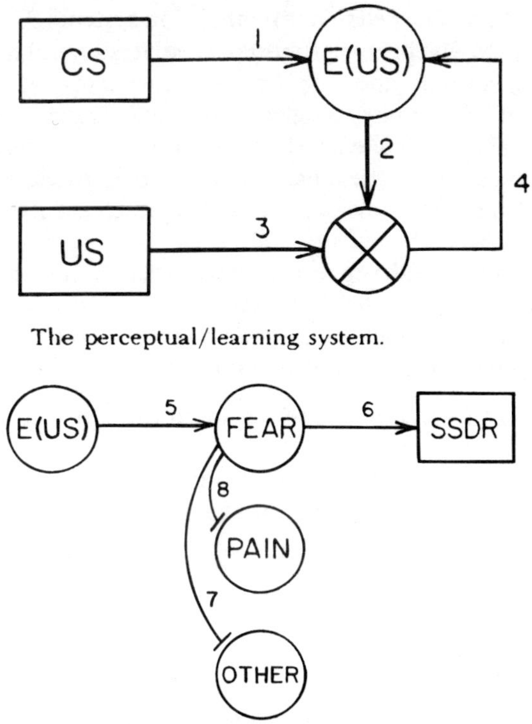


Figure 1 Schematic diagrams reproduced from Bolles and Fanselow (1980) illustrating the conditioning phase (above) and fear eliciting mechanism (below) proposed in their model of fear and pain

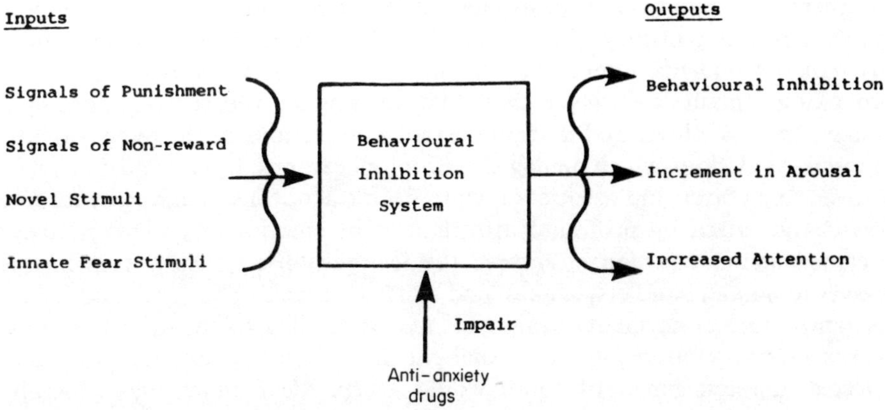


Figure 2 The behavioural inhibition system as proposed by Gray (1982). This responds to any of its adequate inputs with all of its outputs, and comprises the hypothetical substrate on which the antianxiety drugs act to reduce anxiety

behavioural inhibition. The behavioural inhibition system (BIS) is invoked as a theoretical construct, which, it is proposed, mediates the relationship between anxiety-provoking stimuli and the operant correlates of anxiety. In an extensive series of electrophysiological, pharmacological, and anatomical studies Gray and his colleagues have provided evidence that the septohippocampal circuit of the limbic system is the critical neuroanatomical substrate of the BIS system (reviewed admirably in Gray, 1982 and chapter 9, this edition).

While not wishing to undermine the importance of the septohippocampal circuit it is proposed that we should accept that the brain systems involved in anxiety are more extensive than proposed in Gray's original theory.

Three kinds of evidence are complementary:

1. What do we know in anatomical terms about the substrates involved in the expression of anxiety?
2. What do we know about the neurotransmitters operating in these structures?
3. What do we know about the pharmacological properties of the benzodiazepines?

**The substrates involved**

The limbic system includes structures and extensive anatomical projections at a number of levels in the CNS (Nauta, 1982; Iversen, 1983). There are many reasons to believe that structures and circuits removed from, but nevertheless anatomically closely related to, the septohippocampal system are also essential for the generation and expression of emotional behaviour. This is as true of anxiety as of other emotional states. The amygdala, for example, which together with hippocampus constitutes the forebrain contribution of the limbic system has a long history of involvement with emotion. Indeed, many would say that the evidence implicating the amygdala in the response to emotion-provoking stimuli is stronger than that relating to the septohippocampal system. In 1939 Kluver and Bucy made radical resections of the temporal lobe in monkeys, lesions which damaged both hippocampus and amygdala as well as overlying cortex and associated white fibre tracts. The resulting syndrome was characterized by profound disturbances of emotionality. The monkeys became tame and no longer showed the fear response typically seen in this species to human handlers, snakes, and stuffed animals. They could no longer recognize objects normally meaningful and rewarding to them, for example offensive, or preferred foods or sexual partners. Consequently they no longer selected amongst bowls of food, would accept meat which was generally rejected by monkeys, attempted to mate with their own sex or indeed inanimate objects. This profile was considered to reflect blunting of the normal response to meaningful stimuli in the environment, and it was noted that the changed responses to aversive stimuli were particularly dramatic. In subsequent studies, where more restricted lesions were made, it became clear that damage to the amygdala rather than the hippocampus produced these changes. In rats, lesions to the basolateral amygdala also produce dramatic changes in the response to meaningful stimuli, particularly in novel stimulus situations (Rolls and Rolls, 1973).

If we turn to the literature describing the effects of electrical stimulation of brain on emotional behaviour, it is again clear that an extensive substrate related to the limbic system is involved in the generation of emotional patterns of behaviour. Since this is an extensive area of research, we shall consider only studies in which brain stimulation induces responding consonant with general activation of defensive behaviour.

The use of electrical stimulation for defining brain substrates involved in motivational behaviour has a long history. The evidence relating to defensive behaviour has been reviewed recently by Graeff (1981). In both cat and rat it has been shown that stimulation of the midbrain periaqueductal grey matter (PAG) induces defensive behaviour. As illustrated in Figure 3 the PAG has extensive anatomical relationships anteriorly with hypothalamus and amygdala and posteriorly with pons and medulla, and at all these sites defensive behaviour, including profound autonomic changes, may be elicited.

Rats, cats, and monkeys if stimulated in the PAG will learn new responses to turn off the aversive stimuli, indicating that this substrate is a crucial focus for fear-motivated behaviour as well as defensive actions. Close by are sites where stimulation is rewarding or induces analgesia suggesting that in the PAG the substrates mediating the response to reward, punishment, and pain are closely intermingled, a physiological fact which mirrors the behavioural interactions seen in conditioning experiments.

Graeff (1981) uses the term 'brain aversive system' (BAS) to encompass this complex brain stem substrate which influences a wide range of possible responses to aversive events. It seems likely that conditions under which the BAS is activated determine the involvement of a number of different circuits. For example, the evidence from lesion and drug studies indicates that behavioural suppression induced by central stimulation of BAS is subserved to some extent by different substrates than suppression induced with peripheral shock. Equally stimulation of BAS, given in conditions where escape is or is not possible, has different consequences.

## The neurotransmitters

Even the most cursory consideration of this question makes us realize that many of the earlier formulations of a neuropharmacological theory of anxiety must be at best incomplete and at most incorrect. Our knowledge of the classical transmitter pathways of the brain has advanced dramatically in the

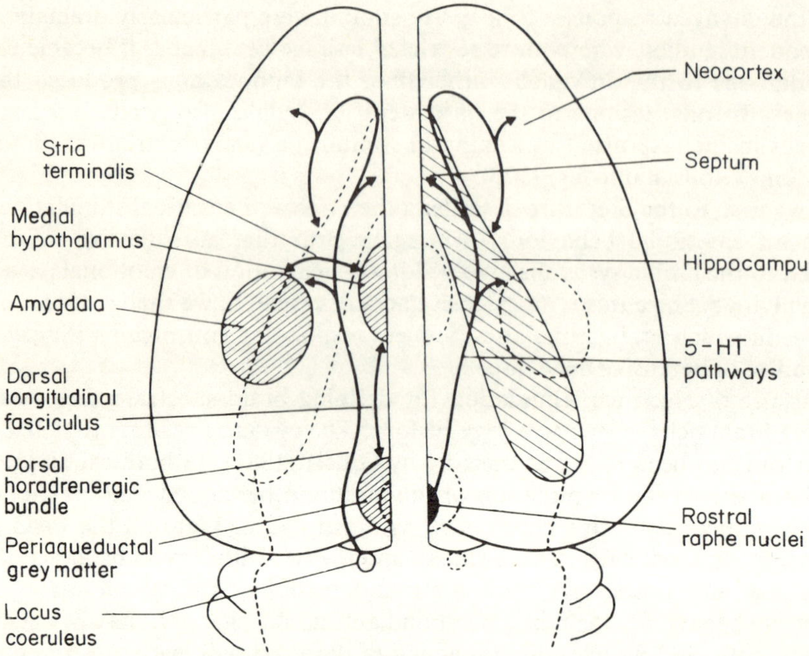


Figure 3 Schematic representation in rat brain of neuron systems integrating defensive behaviours. Superimposed are the trajectories of the noradrenaline (left) and serotonin (5HT) neurons arising in brain stem and innervating limbic structures. (Reproduced from Graeff, 1981)

past decade. First the number of transmitters increases year by year. In addition to the monoaminergic transmitters, adrenaline (A), noradrenaline (NA), dopamine (DA), serotonin (5HT), and acetylcholine (ACH), inhibitory GABA, and excitatory amino acids, must be added a large number of peptides of varying importance in the CNS. In many cases, these neurotransmitters have been shown to exist in specific pathways and structures. Particularly striking in relation to the limbic structures implicated in emotional behaviour are the distributions of NA and 5HT (Figure 3).

It is notable also that DA provides a minor innervation to the classical limbic areas. What is interesting, however, is that the structures which receive a rich innervation from A10 DA neurons of the mesencephalon (nucleus accumbens, ventral striatum) are classified anatomically as 'limbic orientated' structures, which according to Nauta provide a link between the core limbic nuclei and the motor output systems of the brain. Thus it has been suggested that DA may serve an enabling function by which highly integrated information in limbic systems and cortex gains access to response mechanisms (Iversen, 1983).

### Pharmacological properties

It is perhaps in the domain of pharmacology that recent advances have posed problems to the neuropsychologist attempting to provide a general theory of anxiety. It has been known for decades that benzodiazepines influenced NA and 5HT transmission in brain. The NA responses were shown to adapt rapidly and in parallel with the tolerance to the sedative effects. The 5HT response on the other hand did not show tolerance and appeared to correlate with the maintained anxiolytic action of the drugs.

With the discovery of the benzodiazepine receptor in brain, attention has switched from the monamines. The benzodiazepine receptor is widely distributed in brain but not in any obvious or exclusive relationship to other transmitters. There are some striking covariances such as the high density of 5HT and benzodiazepine receptors in amygdala, which may be of importance, but some equally puzzling facts at first sight, such as the very high density of benzodiazepine receptors in cortex. Furthermore, it is not clear how the benzodiazepine receptor relates to the other transmitter receptors either in terms of localization or function. It is now clear that the benzodiazepine receptor (and the barbiturate receptor) is part of a larger receptor complex involving GABA, and it is this larger receptor element which must be viewed in relation to other transmitter systems. Perhaps the benzodiazepine receptor complex regulates the release of other transmitters at critical sites. Evidence for such interactions is still lacking. However, an involvement of GABA in benzodiazepine action must be taken seriously, and already there is preliminary evidence that manipulation of functional levels of GABA in brain may mimic or block benzodiazepine action.

Thus we have many new facts to accommodate in formulating a neuropsychological theory of anxiety and future experiments must attempt to take these into account using new experimental tools as they become available. To illustrate this approach the remaining sections will review evidence implicating anatomically defined neurotransmitter pathways in the expression of anxiety. Particular attention will be given to behavioural suppression as a correlate of anxiety states.

## INVOLVEMENT OF SEROTONIN (5HT) PATHWAYS ORIGINATING IN PAG IN PUNISHMENT-INDUCED BEHAVIOURAL SUPPRESSION

The 5HT innervation of forebrain has been extensively reviewed by Azmitia (1978) and arises mainly from raphé nuclei of the rostral brain stem which are embedded in the PAG located in the ventral tegmentum. The dorsal raphé nucleus innervates neocortex, amygdala, and basal ganglia, whereas the median raphé nucleus innervates the medial septum and hippocampus. Midline thalamus and hypothalamus receive input from both sources.

The clearest evidence exists for an involvement of 5HT in suppression of behaviour induced with foot shock. The earlier evidence on this point has been reviewed (Iversen, 1979) and attention will focus largely on new developments in this area of research.

Tye *et al.* (1977) reported that lesions of the 5HT fibre pathways at the level of the medial forebrain bundle prevented the acquisition of behavioural suppression on a conflict schedule. Subsequently Tye (unpublished findings) found that the same lesion abolished previously acquired behavioural suppression, and resulted in a release of punished behaviour equivalent to that seen after systemic administration of benzodiazepines. Chlordiazepoxide was not able to increase further the rate of responding during conflict in the lesioned animals, presumably because the maximum level of release had already been recorded (Figure 4). The implication of these findings is that reduced 5HT levels result in release of punished responding or in other words impair the response to anxiety provoking stimuli. In support of this hypothesis it has been found that 5HT antagonists, such as cyproheptadine and methysergide, release behavioural inhibition, while increased 5HT transmission enhances suppression. Since benzodiazepines reduce the turnover of 5HT, it is likely that these anxiolytic compounds, probably acting at a number of levels in CNS and perhaps acting indirectly by involving other transmitters, involve 5HT neurons in their mode of action.

More recent attempts have been made to manipulate the cell body and terminal innervations of the raphé 5HT system. The dorsal raphé appears to be the significant cell body site. Thiébot *et al.* (1980) describe an 'on-baseline' CER procedure in which rats are trained to press a lever for food on a continuous reinforcement (CRF) schedule. Subsequently they received 7 days of training on a conflict schedule: lights on 5 min CRF—lights off 5 min CRF plus 50% responses for food punished with electric shock—lights on 3 min CRF—lights off 5 min punishment—lights on 2 min CRF. After such training responding is largely restricted to the lights-on phase. Chlordiazepoxide injected into the dorsal raphé ($5 \times 10^{-5}$M) or given systemically, released responding in the punished lights-off phase (Figure 5). Lesions to raphé 5HT system induced with 5,7-dihydroxytryptamine prevent the releasing effect of chlordiazepoxide on this punishment schedule (Thiébot *et al.*, 1982). The exact mode of action of benzodiazepines on the 5HT neurons remains obscure (Thiébot *et al.*, 1980, 1982). Benzodiazepines release 5HT from neurons and thus in the raphé, 5HT release could act directly on 5HT autoreceptors. Since both peripherally administered benzodiazepines, and 5HT iontophoretically applied to raphé inhibits the firing of 5HT neurons (Haigler and Aghajanian, 1977), such an action would be consistent with our hypothesis. However benzodiazepine/5HT/GABA interactions have been described in the raphé, and equally benzodiazepines could act by enhancing GABA transmission onto the raphé neurons. GABA accumulating cells have been found in the dorsal

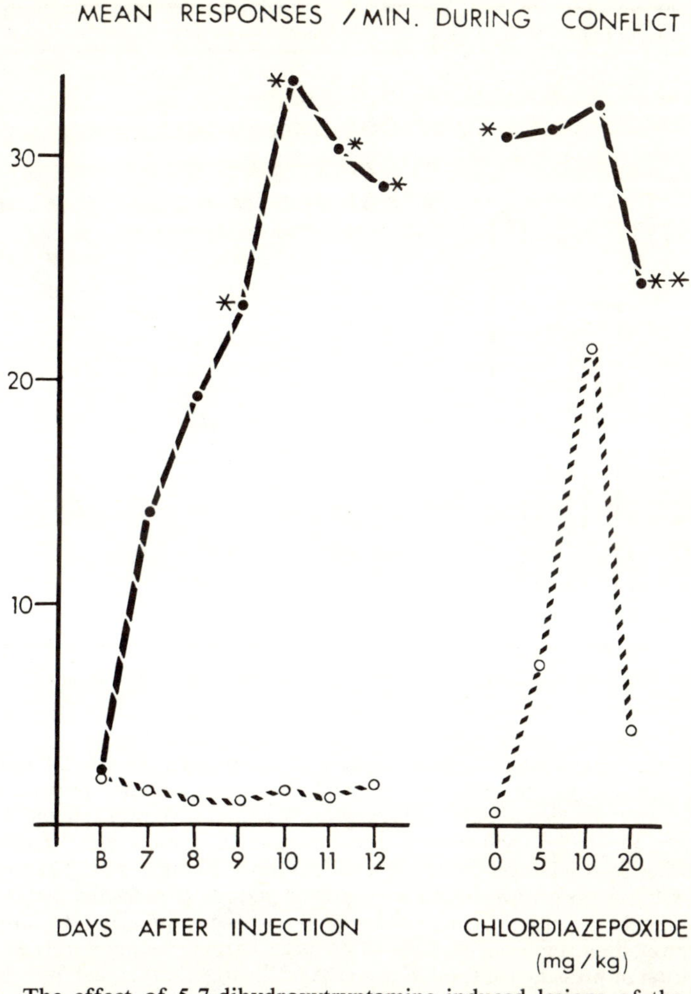


Figure 4 The effect of 5,7-dihydroxytryptamine induced lesions of the brain 5HT pathway on a conflict schedule learned before the lesion. Filled circles: 5HT lesion group. Open circles: control lesion group. The schedule involved three components: (Variable interval) VI reward–time out–VI reward + punishment of every rewarded response. Responding during the conflict phase is illustrated above. B = baseline suppression after training and before surgery performed. Left: lesion results in release of suppression when tested 7 days after surgery. Right: chlordiazepoxide (10 mg/kg) released suppression in control rats but caused no further release in lesioned rats

raphé, and GABA is reported to exert an inhibitory control upon 5HT neurons. Since benzodiazepines facilitate GABA transmission (Costa *et al.*, 1978), the inhibition of 5HT neurons by benzodiazepines could be achieved in this way. Electrophysiological studies also suggest that there is a potentiation

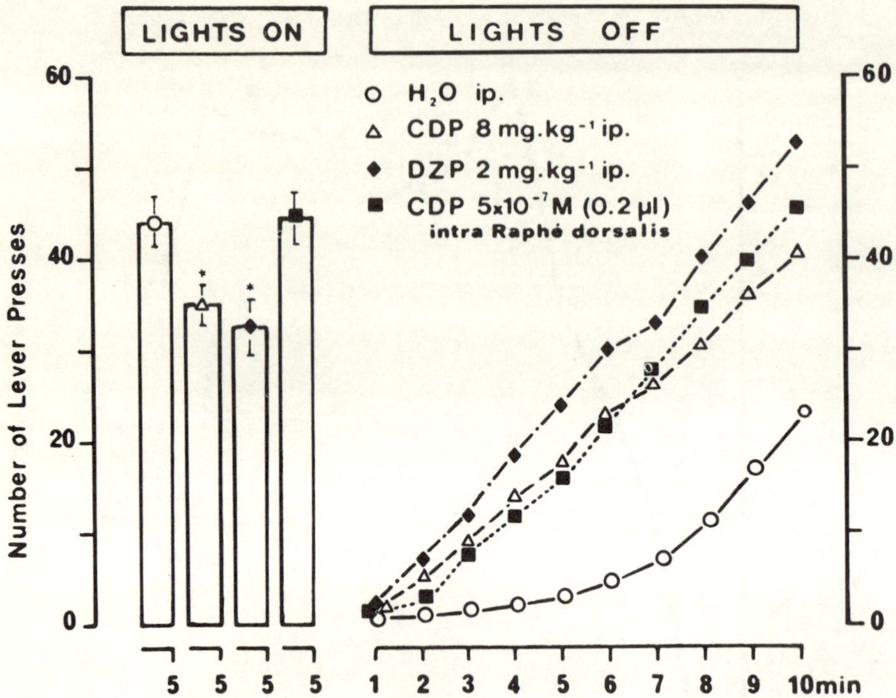


Figure 5 Effects of parenteral administration of chlordiazepoxide (CDP), diazepam (DZP), and of microinjection of CDP into the dorsal raphé, on lever pressing for food during the delivery of a signal (lights-off) previously paired with punishment. Rats were trained to press a lever for food reward according to a continuous reinforced schedule (CRF = 1 pellet for each lever press), in an illuminated Skinner box. They were then subjected to CRF sessions with alternating signalled periods of punished (lights-off, one electric foot shock, 1.5 mA, 45 ms, following every second press) and non-punished (lights-on) responding for food. At the end of these learning sessions, rats exhibited a strong inhibition of pressing for food in presence of the lights-off signal (4 ± 1 presses/10 min, as compared to 70 ± 5 presses during the 10 min non-punished periods). On the test day, rats were given either CEP infused (0.2 $\mu$l in 3 min into the raphé dorsalis via a chronically implanted cannula (stereotaxic coordinates according to Konig and Klippel, 1963; A = 0.16; L = 0; H = –0.8) or CDP or DZP i.p. They were subjected to the experimental session which started with a 5 min (lights-on) non-punished period followed by a continuous 10 min lights-off period during which *responding was no longer punished* (conditioned conflictual response). The values are the mean ± s.e.m. of the presses effected by separate groups of rats ($n$ = 7–12) during the initial 5 min lights-on period and the mean of the presses per minute during the subsequent 10 min lights-off period. *$P<0.05$ as compared to controls (Student's $t$-test). During the lights-off period the three groups of treated rats did not differ from each other ($F(2, 367) = 2.047$, NS) but differ significantly from the control group ($F(1, 367) = 43.315$:$P<0.01$) as calculated by two-way (time and subjects) analysis of variance. (Reproduced from Thiébot *et al.*, 1983)

between GABA and benzodiazepines; the latter enhances the inhibitory control exerted by GABA or GABA agonists on the firing rate of 5HT cells in the dorsal raphé. Consequently, microinjections of GABA into the raphé would be expected to release behavioural suppression induced by punishment and indeed this is the case (Thiébot *et al.*, 1980). Although there are some equivocal results in the literature (Thiébot *et al.*, 1980), the GABA agonist muscimol has been reported on systemic injection and on intra-amygdaloid infusion (Petersen *et al.*, 1982) to release punished responding. Benzodiazepines also appear to act via an enhancement of GABA transmission to reverse the escape from aversive brain stimulation (Brandào *et al.*, 1982) despite the fact that the 5HT substrates of raphé are not apparently as directly involved in this escape response as in the response to peripheral foot shock (Graeff, 1981).

The raphé 5HT neurons innervate widely in forebrain but, as indicated earlier, the rich 5HT innnervation of cortical and basolateral nuclei of amygdala deserves attention with respect to anxiety. Benzodiazepine receptors are found in dense concentration in these areas of amygdala as indicated with radioautographic techniques (Young and Kuhar, 1980) and benzodiazepine receptor binding assays (Thomas, unpublished findings). Wang and Aghajanian (1977) made an electrophysiological study of this 5HT pathway to the amygdala and report that the dorsal raphé nucleus exerts an inhibitory influence on amygdala neurone, which can also be inhibited by direct iontophoretic application of 5HT. Lesions of the 5HT pathway or treatment with 5HT antagonists abolished the effect of raphé stimulation. It is tempting to conclude that the induction of behavioural suppression in brain stem sites, and its abolition by selective 5HT lesions, involve this pathway to the amygdala.

The test of this hypothesis would be the abolition or induction of suppression by means of direct manipulation of 5HT levels in amygdala or by direct application of benzodiazepines or GABA manipulations to the amygdala. We have begun such experiments using the conditioned emotional response task of Thiébot. We have validated the systemic benzodiazepines release behaviour suppressed by a signal previously associated with shock, thus enlarging the list of positive studies involving benzodiazepines and the CER paradigm (Cicala and Hartley, 1967; Miczek, 1973; Leslie and Garrud, 1976). In further experiments (Thomas and Iversen, unpublished) chlordiazepoxide was injected bilaterally into the lateral amygdala of the behaving rat. Significant release of behavioural suppression was observed (Figure 6). Further experiments are required to evaluate dosage, site, and drug specificity. However, similar results are reported by Petersen *et al.* (1982) using punished drinking as the behavioural measure. Bilateral infusions of the benzodiazepine midazolam into the lateral nuclei of amygdala released suppressed drinking, and this effect was reversed by the simultaneous administration of the

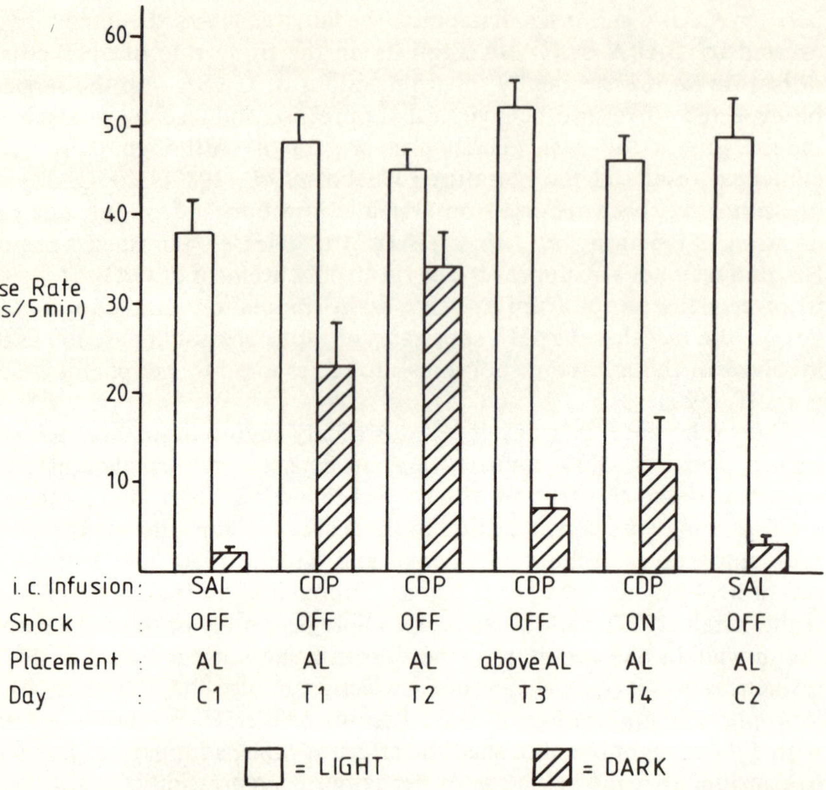


Figure 6 Effect of intra-amygdala infusion of chlordiazepoxide on suppression induced by signal previously associated with shock. On all test days except T4 the shock was not presented during the lights-off phase of the schedule. Under control conditions (CI) suppression was virtually complete during the dark phase. Effects of identical infusions of chlordiazepoxide (10 $\mu$g in 1 $\mu$l at a rate of 0.5 $\mu$l/min) on conditioned suppression (expressed as group mean, $n = 11$) tested in the absence of shock (second and third tests) and in the presence of shock (fifth test), compared with infusions of the saline vehicle at same volume and rate (first and last tests) and a control placement above the amygdaloid complex (fourth test). Response rates are shown separately for 'shock' (shaded) and 'no-shock' (plain bars) periods for each session; note that these figures are calculated for 5 minute bins. Compared with saline controls, CDP significantly increased 'shock period' response rates in the presence and absence of shock (both $P<0.005$, Wilcoxon test); the control placement had no significant effect, and non-shock response rates were also unaffected (all NS, Wilcoxon test). (Thomas, unpublished results)

GABA antagonist bicuculline methiodide. Shibata *et al.* (1982) also reported that in rats, infusions of diazepam, chlordiazepoxide, and midazolam into the amygdala released responding suppressed on a Geller Seifter conflict schedule.

## THE ROLE OF NA IN ANXIETY

If one considers the behavioural suppression seen in conflict situations as a measure of anxiety, it has been shown in my laboratory that bilateral lesions to the dorsal noradrenaline bundle arising in locus coeruleus, and providing the NA innervation to cortex and hippocampus, do not release punished responding or impair the acquisition of behavioural suppression. This stands in marked contrast to the massive release of suppression seen after 5HT lesions.

However, there is reason to believe that NA does play a role in certain forms of behaviour associated with anxiety. In particular in Gray's laboratory, where the behavioural test used involves partial reinforcement and results in enhancement of arousal associated with the anxiety, impairment of the response to partial reinforcement has been found after NA lesions and other manipulations which reduce NA transmission. Redmond and Huang (1979) support the view that the locus coeruleus has a role in anxiety. Electrolytic lesions of the locus coeruleus in the monkey produce placid animals who do not respond to threats, and electrical stimulation of this nucleus elicits species specific responses associated with fear. Drugs which are known to reduce the activity of locus coeruleus neurons, including benzodiazepines, tricyclic antidepressants, barbiturates, opiates, and the $\beta$-adrenergic antagonist propranolol have anxiolytic properties, whereas piperoxane and yohimbine, which increase locus coeruleus activity, cause anxiety in man, as does electrical stimulation of this part of the brain (Redmond *et al.*, 1977).

We also know from numerable instances that transmitter systems in brain interact with each other as well as influencing their areas of terminal innervation. In regard to our present topic, it is interesting to note that the locus coeruleus influences the 5HT raphé neurone at the level of the brain stem. Clonidine, a noradrenergic $\alpha_2$-agonist inhibits locus coeruleus neurone by acting on $\alpha_2$-autoreceptors and indirectly, via this effect on locus coeruleus, is thought to inhibit serotonergic neurons of the dorsal raphé nucleus. In turn 5HT neurone influence the DA neurone of the substantia nigra. Bunney and De Riemer (1982) have reported that the firing rate of DA neurone is depressed by DA agonists, an effect which can be reversed by clonidine. A general theory of dorsal bundle NA function has been proposed (Mason and Iversen, 1979) which suggests that cortical and hippocampal NA is involved in aspects of attentional behaviour. If, in a test situation devised to induce anxiety, demands are placed on the ability to attend to crucial environmental events, then we predict that dorsal bundle lesions would impair the anxiety response. If, however, the task does not involve high levels of attention, then the dorsal bundle lesion would not be predicted to have an effect. In this way we can reconcile the positive findings with NA lesions of Gray using partial reinforcement paradigms (attention and arousal), with the negative findings using conflict paradigms (behavioural suppression). In commenting on Redmond's results, Mason (1981) notes that the stimuli used 'were of a cognitive nature in their induction of fear of snakes, human experimenters, lights, and tones paired with punishment; primary negative reinforcers like footshock were not used. Thus it is possible that the attentional functions of the dorsal bundle in interpreting and sampling stimuli of cognitive importance were being tapped, rather than any primary role in fear'. This is an interesting suggestion which would predict that in anxiety states, where attentional/cognitive processing is strongly involved, anxiolytic drugs blocking noradrenergic function would be of therapeutic use. It is interesting to note that benzodiazepines lower NA turnover and inhibit locus coeruleus activity. The latter effect may well involve GABA as the intermediating transmitter in parallel with what we saw in the 5HT system. There are GABA receptors on the locus coeruleus which inhibits its firing.

## THE ROLE OF DA IN ANXIETY

When painful aversive stimuli are presented to an animal irrespective of its behaviour, it is said to be stressed. Clearly in the paradigm discussed in relation to anxiety, the levels of overt stress vary considerably. We know that under conditions of unavoidable stress, (e.g. repeated application of electric shock, immobilization, placing in cold water) in addition to the overt behavioural responses observed, various neurotransmitter pathways of brain (5HT, NA, and DA) respond by changing their level of activity.

Stress in a specific environment leads to subsequent behavioural suppression and immobility in that environment. Dantzer (1983) has demonstrated the environment specificity in experiments where rats were shocked in an environment and returned to it 24 hours later to show markedly reduced activity. Treatment with benzodiazepines before the initial shock experience significantly reduced the behavioural suppression seen on the subsequent test session.

Using a very similar test paradigm, but it must be stressed using much less severe but highly unpredictable shocks, Reinhard *et al.* (1982) have reported that DA turnover in frontal cortex (and to a lesser degree in nucleus accumbens), but not in striatum, is increased by the stress. Pretreatment with benzodiazepines before the initial shock stress significantly attenuates the increase in DA turnover (Figure 7). Since the frontal DA system appears to mediate an inhibitory hold over lower motor output systems, stress would be likely to enhance inhibition and decrease motor output, the behavioural consequence observed by Dantzer. It is therefore possible that the frontal DA system plays a significant role in the behavioural inhibition associated with certain anxiety states.

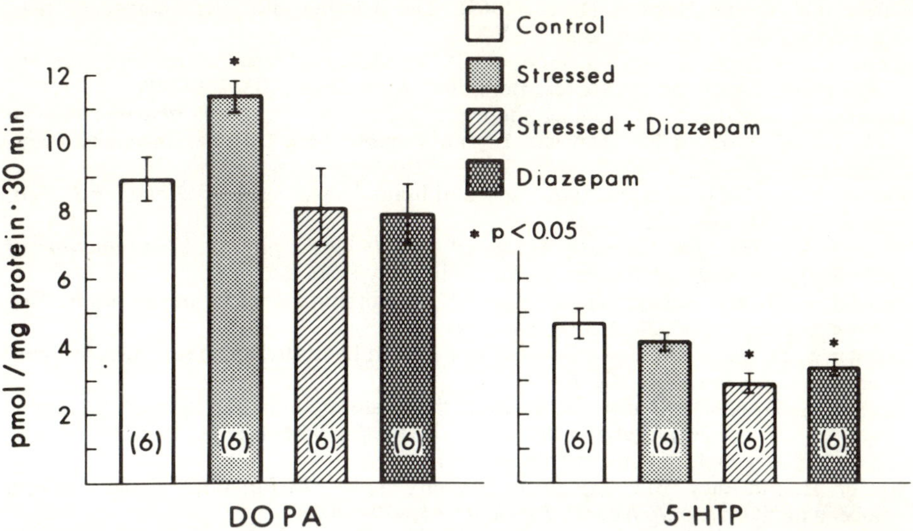


Figure 7 The effect of stress, diazepam or their combination on catechol and indole synthesis in frontal cortex. Rats received unavoidable mild foot shock; 30 minutes later brain levels of DA and 5HT were assayed. Stress significantly increased DOPA levels in frontal cortex, an effect reversed by pretreatment with diazepam. (Reproduced from Reinhard *et al.*, 1982)

## CONCLUDING STATEMENT

Benzodiazepines appear to act at different levels in the CNS and influence a range of neurotransmitter substrates. A GABA-mediated interaction on raphé 5HT systems appears to mediate the behavioural suppression associated with punishment. However, the neurotransmitter systems of the limbic brain operate not in isolation but in concert, and NA and DA clearly are involved in some aspects of the expression of anxiety.

## REFERENCES

Azmitia, E. C. (1978). The serotonin-producing neurons of the midbrain median and dorsal raphé nuclei. In: *Handbook of Psychopharmacology*, Vol. 9, pp.233–314 (Eds. Iversen, L. L., Iversen, S. D. and Snyder, S. H.).

Bolles, R. C. and Fanselow, M. S. (1980). A perceptual-defensive recuperative model of fear and pain. *Behav. Brain Sci.*, **3**, 291–323.

Brandào, M. L., Aguiar, J. C. de and Graeff, F. G. (1982). GABA mediation of the anti-aversive action of minor tranquilisers. *Pharmac. Biochem. Behav.*, **16**, 397–402.

Bunney, B. J. and De Riemer, S. (1982). Effect of clonidine on dopaminergic neurone activity in the substantia nigra: possible indirect mediation by noradrenergic regulation of the serotonergic raphé system. In: *Gilles de la Tourette Syndrome* (Eds. Friedhoft, A. J. and Chase, T. N.) *Adv. in Neurology* **35**, 99–104, Raven Press, New York.

Cicala, G. A. and Hartley, D. L. (1967). The learning and performance of fear. *J. comp. Physiol. Psychol.*, **64**, 175–178.

Costa, E., Guidotti, A. and Tofftano, G. (1978). Molecular mechanisms mediating the action of diazepam on GABA receptors. *Brit. J. Psychiat.*, **133**, 239–248.

Dantzer, R. (1983) Benzodiazepines and the limbic system. In: *Psychopharmacology of the Limbic System* (Eds. Zarifian, E. and Trimble, M.), Oxford University Press, Oxford.

Graeff, F. G. (1981). Minor tranquilizers and brain defense systems. *Brazilian J. med. biol. Res.*, **14**, 239–265.

Gray, J. A. (1982). *The Neuropsychology of Anxiety: an Enquiry into the Functions of the Septo-hippocampal System*, Oxford University Press, Oxford.

Haigler, H. J. and Aghajanian, G. K. (1977). Serotonin receptors in the brain. *Fed. Proc. Soc. exp. Biol.*, **36**, 2159–2164.

Iversen, S. D. (1979). Animal models of anxiety and benzodiazepine actions. *Arzniem-Forsch. (Drug Res.)*, **30**, 862–868.

Iversen, S. D. (1983). Recent advances in the anatomy and chemistry of the limbic system. In: *The Psychopharmacology of the Limbic System* (Eds. Zarifian, E. and Trimble, M.), Oxford University Press, Oxford.

Kluver, H. and Bucy, P. C. (1939). Preliminary analysis of functions of the temporal lobe in monkeys. *Arch. Neurol. Psychiat.*, **42**, 979–1000.

König, J. F. and Klippel, R. A. (1963). *The Rat Brain: A Stereotaxic Atlas of the Forebrain and Lower Parts of the Brain Stem.* Williams and Wilkins, Baltimore.

Leslie, J. C. and Garrud, P. (1976). Conditioned suppression of a positively reinforced shuttle response. *Animal Learning and Behav.*, **4**, 99–104.

Mason, S. T. (1981). Noradrenaline in the brain: progress in theories of behavioural function. *Progress in Neurobiology*, **16**, 263–303.

Mason, S. T. and Iversen, S. D. (1979). Theories of the dorsal bundle extinction effect. *Brain Res. Rev.*, **1**, 107–137.

Miczek, K. A. (1973). Effects of scopolamine, amphetamine and benzodiazepines on conditioned suppression. *Pharmac. Biochem. Behav.*, **1**, 401–411.

Nauta, J. (1982). Neural associations of the limbic system. In: *The Neural Basis of Behaviour*, pp.175–206. (Ed. Beckman, A.), Spectrum Publications Inc., New York.

Petersen, E. N., Braestrup, C. and Scheel-Kruger, J. (1982). Intraamygdaloid application of benzodiazepines exert anticonflict effect by a GABA-ergic mechanism. Presented at *OHOLO Conference on Behavioural Models and the Analysis of Drug Action.* Israel Institute for Biological Research.

Redmond, D. E. and Huang, Y. H. (1979). New evidence for a locus coeruleus-norepinephrine connection with anxiety. *Life Sci.*, **25**, 2149–2162.

Redmond, D. E., Maas, J. W., Huang, Y. H., Snyder, D. R. and Baulu, J. (1977). *Anxiety: the Locus Coeruleus Connection*, American Psychiatric Association, Toronto.

Reinhard, J. F., Bannon, M. J. and Roth, R. H. (1982). Acceleration by stress of dopamine synthesis and metabolism in prefrontal cortex: antagonism by diazepam. *N-S Arch. Pharmac.*, **318**, 374–377.

Rolls, B. J. and Rolls, E. T. (1973). Altered food preferences after lesions in the basolateral region of the amygdala in the rat. *J. Comp. Physiol. Psychol.*, **83**, 248–259.

Shibata, K., Kataoka, Y., Gomita, Y. and Ueki, J. (1982). Localization of the site of the anticonflict action of benzodiazepines in the amygdaloid nucleus of rats. *Brain Res.*, **234**, 442–446.

Thiébot, M. H., Hamon, M. and Soubrie, P. (1982). Attenuation of induced anxiety in rats by chlordiazepoxide: role of raphé dorsalis benzodiazepine binding sites and serotonergic neurones. *Neuroscience*, **7**, 2287–2294.

Thiébot, M. H., Hamon, M. and Soubrie, P. (1983). Serotonergic neurons and anxiety related behaviour in rats. In: *Psychopharmacology of the Limbic System* (Eds. Zarifian, E. and Trimble, M.), Oxford University Press, Oxford.

Thiébot, M. H., Jebert, A. and Soubrie, P. (1980). Chlordiazepoxide and GABA injected into raphé dorsalis release the conditioned behavioural suppression induced in rats by a conflict procedure without nociceptive component. *Neuropharmacology*, **19**, 633–641.

Tye, N. C., Everett, B. J. and Iversen, S. D. (1977). 5-hydroxytryptamine and punishment. *Nature*, **268**, 741–743.

Wang, R. Y. and Aghajanian, G. K. (1977). Inhibition of neurones in the amygdala by dorsal raphé stimulation: mediation through a direct serotonergic pathway. *Brain Res.*, **120**, 85–102.

Young, W. S. and Kuhar, M. J. (1980). Radiohistochemical localization of benzodiazepine receptors in rat brain. *J. Pharmac. exp. Ther.*, **212**, 337–346.

## DISCUSSION

## CHAIRMAN: PROFESSOR M. LADER

DR. J. GRAY: I entirely agree with Dr. Iversen's conclusions. One could attempt to put the pieces together a little. I agree that the 5HT pathways are very likely involved in the behavioural inhibition component of anxiety, and, very probably, that the ascending noradrenergic fibres are more involved in arousal and/or cognitive changes. I do not think that one should think of these, however, as acting quite separately. They would normally go together in different proportions. I also agree about the possibility that the interactions are taking place in the brain stem rather than upstream.

Adding one point, you mentioned the increased dopamine turnover in the prefrontal cortex—that is almost the only place, as far as I am aware, in which increased dopamine turnover has been reported, under stress conditions. Indeed, in other parts of the brain, if anything, there has been a tendency for dopamine turnover to be reduced. The other area for which I have seen an equivalent report is the cingulate cortex. Both of those regions (prefrontal and cingulate cortices) receive their dopamine innervation from A10 in the ventral tegmental area. There is evidence for a locus coeruleus projection to the A10 cell bodies. It is conceivable that the particular involvement of those dopamine pathways is secondary to increased action in the locus coeruleus cell bodies. That would account also for the fact that you have the selectivity of the benzodiazepine and other antianxiety drug action on that increased turnover. In other words, the change produced by the benzodiazepine in the prefrontal cortex may be secondary to an action on the noradrenergic innervation of the ventral tegmental area.

Similarly, the cell bodies of the locus coeruleus and the raphé nuclei, I think, have reciprocal connections. There are plenty of possibilities for integration at that end. You have also plenty of possibilities for integration in the forebrain. I was very struck by what was said about the locus within the amygdala of the intracerebral drug effects. I was told recently (Crow, T.) that there is evidence for a direct projection in rat from the nucleus centralis of the amygdala—which I believe is the one in which you achieved your greatest effects—to the hippocampus. Although there has been evidence before in primates for some kind of an amygdala-hippocampal projection, it has never been very clear, and this is the first evidence I have heard of a direct projection from amygdala to hippocampus. That would make sense.

The prefrontal cortex, in which you get the increased dopamine turnover, also projects back into the septohippocampal system. So many different parts are involved but they function as a unity.

What is the specific locus of action of these drugs when they reduce anxiety? In a sense we have heard evidence which would cause us to reject the biochemical answer to that question. That is, it does not look as though it is a special kind of receptor that is involved in the antianxiety effects of the benzodiazepines, whether a special type of GABA receptor or a benzodiazepine receptor.

I suggest the following: the suggestion originally comes from Heafely that the specificity of action of the benzodiazepines turns not upon what the drug is doing at particular receptors, but rather upon what the animal is doing and what the animal's brain is doing under particular circumstances when you give the drug. If these drugs are acting by facilitating GABA, we know that a lot of GABA neurons form part of recurrent inhibitory circuits—sometimes very small, local circuits, sometimes very much longer circuits involving many points of the brain. The characteristic feature of a recurrent inhibitory circuit is that the GABA synapse that is involved is only going to be active at those parts in the brain where the principal cells are active and causing the recurrent inhibitory loop to start functioning. If the benzodiazepines work by facilitating the action of GABA, then the selectivity will depend upon which GABA synapses are active at a particular moment. That, in turn, will depend upon what the animal's brain is doing at a particular moment. So we may have to go for our selectivity rather in the behaviour or the environment that is acting upon the animal and what the animal is doing at the time we give them our drugs.

DR. FILE: May I take up the point Dr. Iversen made, that possibly the different tests are tapping different aspects of anxiety and therefore the neural substrates may differ? Dr. Herbert noted that in some of these condition paradigms the animal knows specifically what to fear and probably what appropriate response to make; whereas, when we have to put him in an unfamiliar situation, such as I do, he does not know what to be frightened of and certainly does not know what response is appropriate.

For that reason, we were very interested to try to repeat your kind of data on lesions in the social-interaction test. We went a long way to completely agreeing with you, because when we made specific lesions of the dorsal raphé nucleus we got an anxiolytic profile. If we lesion the median raphé nucleus we do not. We then turned to the central nucleus of the amygdala, because we had already found when we injected with morphine into that site, but not adjacent nuclei, we got an anxiolytic profile. When we made specific 57DHT lesions, however, all we got was very marked sedation. No anxiolytic profile was seen. The animals were so hypoactive, they did less of anything we cared to measure. This seems to be a recurring problem in our laboratory: every time we do a bigger depletion of 5HT we tip over from the antianxiety effect into sedation.

DR. S. IVERSEN: Surgical lesions to the amygdala have yielded equivocal results. However, they may not be specific since there are any number of neuropeptides and neurotransmitters within the central and lateral nuclei of the amygdala, and presumably they are contributing to the kinds of lesion effects that we see. Serotonergic lesions in the amygdala might not be expected to release anxiety since a number of other 5HT projections to forebrain may be involved. If, on the other hand, you are using a specific toxin focused on a particular cell group, the chances of a specific lesion in the terminal region is that much greater.

DR. FILE: We used a specific toxin, but it was injected in the cell body area, in the terminal region. In fact, we get an anxiolytic profile when we place 57DHT in the lateral septum, whereas we did not in the amygdala.

DR. S. IVERSEN: I was not trying in any way to exclude the septohippocampal system; I was really focusing on other parts of the circuitry. I believe Dr. Gray would probably now agree that we have to take into account the amygdala in these forebrain circuits, certainly with respect to the involvement of cognitive anxiety behaviour.

DR. GRAY: In my recent book I did not include much about the amygdala. There are two reasons for that. The first is that, if you look at the overall behavioural profile of lesions to the amygdala—and I am talking about large lesions since it is a complex structure which has so far been rather recalcitrant to the attempts of psychologists and physiologists to perform small, discrete lesions within it—you do not get anything at all resembling the effects of antianxiety drugs. In contrast, you do, as I said, get such a resemblance after lesions to either the septal area or the hippocampus. While you get the release of punished behaviour after amygdala lesions you also get a lot of other changes which are in no way like the antianxiety profile, whereas in the septohippocampal system you get a closely resembling profile.

The other reason I ignored the amygdala was because I could not see any close anatomical relationship yet between the amygdala and the septohippocampal system, in spite of everybody always saying over the years that such a relationship exists. I certainly do not wish to suggest that there is any opposition between the notion of a septohippocampal system involved in anxiety and the amygdala. The key things are the ascending monoamine pathways; it is upon them that the antianxiety drugs act. What critical role is played by the forebrain targets of these ascending monoamine pathways depends upon the behavioural task, with different effects such as behavioural inhibition, arousal, increased attention (depending on the different tasks) all being dealt with by different brain structures. So that the particular role played by the particular forebrain target is going to vary from task to task.

Benzodiazepines Divided
Edited by M. R. Trimble


# 14

# Clinical Pharmacokinetics of Benzodiazepines

ALAN RICHENS*

## INTRODUCTION

All 1,4-benzodiazepines have broadly the same profile of pharmacological activity, including antianxiety, sedative/hypnotic, anticonvulsant, and muscle relaxing actions, although the relative balance of these effects may differ to some extent between individual compounds. The 1,5-benzodiazepine, clobazam, has been claimed to display a wider separation of tranquillizing properties from impairment of motor coordination and this is associated with a relative lack of muscle relaxant activity.

Pharmacokinetically, however, there are major differences between the benzodiazepine drugs in clinical use, particularly in their lipid solubility (which influences rate of absorption and distribution), the route of metabolism and the presence or absence of active metabolites, and the duration of the plasma half-life of the active component. These characteristics are paramount in determining their clinical applications.

## ABSORPTION AND DISTRIBUTION

All benzodiazepines are well absorbed following oral administration. Peak concentrations are usually reached within 30–240 minutes. However, not all the parent compounds are themselves active; clorazepate and prazepam are prodrugs, both being activated by conversion to *N*-desmethyldiazepam. *In vitro*, the hydrolysis of clorazepate is dependent on pH; the lower the pH the faster the hydrolysis. Consequently, *in vivo* it would seem likely that hydrolysis takes place in the stomach and that concurrent administration of antacid preparations might affect the availability of active drug (Shader *et al.*,

*In collaboration with A. Griffiths.

1978). However, there is evidence that the conversion to desmethyldiazepam also takes place in the gut wall, and the presystemic circulation or the systemic circulation (Ochs *et al.*, 1979; Shader *et al.*, 1982). Prazepam, the other prodrug, is converted to desmethyldiazepam by dealkylation in the liver (Greenblatt and Shader, 1978). The rate of appearance of desmethyldiazepam in the blood following administration of these prodrugs differs; prazepam produces desmethyldiazepam more slowly than does clorazepate. This makes prazepam useful for patients who are prone to drug misuse or abuse (Shader and Greenblatt, 1979).

The presence of food in the stomach also affects benzodiazepine absorption. It has been reported that there is a 26% increase in bioavailability (AUC to 48 hours) in subjects taking 5 mg diazepam after a meal as compared with the same dose on an empty stomach (Greenblatt *et al.*, 1978a). The time to peak plasma concentration, however, is longer following a meal.

Intramuscular administration of chlordiazepoxide (Greenblatt *et al.*, 1978b) and diazepam (Mandelli *et al.*, 1978) results in a slow and erratic absorption that yields lower peak plasma concentrations than after oral administration; crystallization at the injection site has been suggested as one possible reason. Intramuscular injection of lorazepam on the other hand yields peak plasma levels at 1.5 hours (Bellantuono *et al.*, 1980), a rapid and complete absorption. Lorazepam is less lipid soluble than diazepam and hence may avoid concentrating in adipose tissue. Flunitrazepam has also been shown to be well absorbed following intramuscular administration resulting in 'effective' plasma levels at 10–20 minutes; the authors did not, however, define what they mean by 'effective' (Mattila and Larni, 1980).

Rectal administration of diazepam solution has been reported by many workers to be effective (Moolenaar *et al.*, 1980), particularly in children (Knudsen, 1977, 1979). This route of administration is a useful alternative to intravenous administration when the latter is impractical or impossible. Pharmacokinetic studies in children have shown rapid absorption from the rectum achieving peak serum levels within 10–20 minutes. Intermittent rectal administration of diazepam solution in children is clinically effective as an acute treatment of seizures and is of value in preventing recurrent febrile convulsions (Knudsen and Westermark, 1978; Knudsen, 1979). A liquid formulation (Stesolid, Weddel) is now available in the UK for rectal use. Wax-based diazepam suppositories, which are currently marketed in the UK by Roche, while being more convenient do not release the drug as quickly as do solutions and they produce lower plasma levels. This preparation is not satisfactory for the urgent control of seizures, but an experimental solid solution suppository has a much more satisfactory plasma concentration profile and may be as effective and more convenient an alternative to liquid formulations (Dhillon *et al.*, 1982). In adults, absorption of diazepam from the rectum varies considerably between subjects. Nevertheless rectal administration is significantly better than placebo in preventing serial seizures in adult patients prone to fits in clusters (Milligan, 1982).

Despite rectal diazepam being a potential alternative to intravenous diazepam, the latter remains the treatment of first choice for status epilepticus, being effective in 93% of cases of absence status, 88% of tonic-clonic status, and 75% of complex partial status (Browne and Penry, 1973). The rate of onset of action of intravenous diazepam is fast, usually within 3 minutes. Tedeschi *et al.* (1983) have compared the rate of entry of two benzodiazepines into the CNS following intravenous administration. Diazepam and lorazepam were compared using a saccadic eye movement method (Bittencourt *et al.*, 1981; Smith *et al.*, 1981) that provides an index of neuronal depression in a specific area of the brain stem. Their results (Figure 1, Table 1) show that diazepam produces its peak most rapidly, while lorazepam is relatively slow

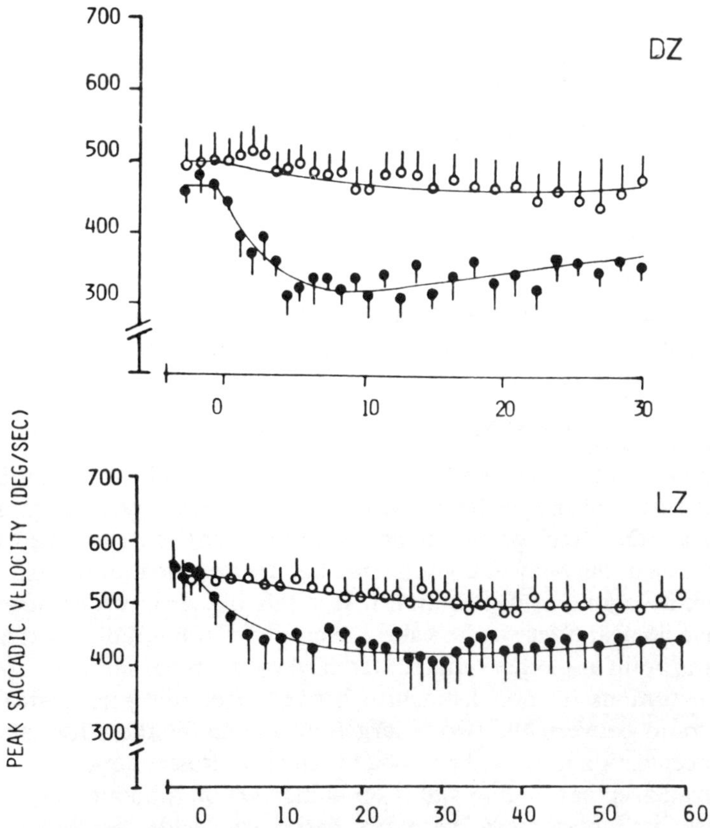


Figure 1 Peak saccadic velocity (degrees/second) against time (min) for 2 mg intravenous lorazepam (LZ) and 5 mg intravenous diazepam (DZ). In both cases • is the active treatment and ○ is placebo

Table 1 Time (min) to achieve maximum effect ($T_{max}$) on peak saccadic velocity (PSV), saccade duration (SD) and saccade reaction time (SRT) after diazepam 5 mg and lorazepam 2 mg (see Figure 1)

| | | Diazepam | Lorazepam |
|---|---|---|---|
| PSV | $T_{max}$ | 8.2 | 23.3 |
| SD | $T_{max}$ | 10.3 | 31.9 |
| SRT | $T_{max}$ | 11.6 | 30.9 |

Table 2 Lipid solubility of benzodiazepines. Octanol: buffer partition coefficient

| | |
|---|---|
| Diazepam | 309 |
| Chlordiazepoxide | 171 |
| Temazepam | 62 |
| Desmethyldiazepam | 54 |
| Oxazepam | 97 |
| Lorazepam | 73 |
| Clobazam | 9 |
| Alprazolam | 19 |

*In vitro* fat solubility: octanol: buffer partitioning at pH 7.4 (after Arendt, R. M. *et al.*, 1982).

in onset. This rapidity of onset of effect is the same as the order of lipid solubility of these drugs (Table 2). Diazepam, being the most lipid soluble, crosses the blood–brain barrier more quickly than lorazepam.

## PLASMA PROTEIN BINDING

Many benzodiazepine drugs bind extensively to plasma and tissue proteins and this characteristic influences their distribution. The concentration of drug in plasma water (the 'free' or 'unbound' concentration) is determined by the amount of drug in the body at a given time, and by the extent of its distribution (the 'apparent volume of distribution'). It is this free drug which determines the pharmacological effect and creates the concentration gradient driving the drug into the brain and other tissues. Standard methods for measuring plasma drug concentrations do not distinguish between free and bound drug, and where the ratio between the two is largely in favour of the latter, the total plasma concentration may not be a good measure of drug action.

The benzodiazepines bind to site II on human serum albumin; site II drugs are, besides benzodiazepines, generally carboxylic acids (Sjolholm *et al.*, 1979). Diazepam is frequently used as a model drug for the examination of drug displacements, because of its large apparent volume of distribution ($V_d$) and the extent of its binding to plasma proteins (96.8–98.5% bound;

Table 3 Pharmacokinetic data for selected benzodiazepines

| | $t_{½}$ (hours) | Volume of distribution (ℓ/kg) | % bound to plasma proteins |
|---|---|---|---|
| Chlordiazepoxide | 6–28 | 0.26–0.58 | 94–97 |
| Clobazam | 9–30 | NA | 87–90 |
| Clorazepate | 24–60 | NA | 82 |
| Demoxepam | 14–95 | NA | NA |
| Diazepam | 20–70 | 0.95–2 | 96.8–98.6 |
| *N*-Desmethyldiazepam | 48–57 | 0.93–1.27 | 97.6 |
| *N*-Desalkylflurazepam | 51–100 | NA | NA |
| Flurazepam | Very short | NA | NA |
| Lorazepam | 9–22 | 0.7–1 | 85 |
| Medazepam | 1–2 | NA | 98.7–99.5 |
| Midazolam | 1.3–3.1 | 50.2 | NA |
| Nitrazepam | 18–31 | 1.5–2.76 | 86–87 |
| Oxazepam | 4–13 | 0.6 | 87–90 |
| Temazepam | 7.8–8.3 | NA | NA |
| Triazolam | 2.2 | NA | NA |

References: Breimer, 1979; Whelpton, 1979; Bellantuono *et al.*, 1980; Breimer *et al.*, 1980; Heizmann *et al.*, 1983.

Bellantuono *et al.*, 1980). The degree of binding of other benzodiazepines is summarized in Table 3.

The displacement of a benzodiazepine from plasma protein binding sites is not generally of much clinical significance because the displaced drug distributes extensively and because the therapeutic ratio is relatively large. However, it is likely that displacement by drug interaction may often be accompanied by displacement of drug from tissue binding sites and by some degree of inhibition of metabolism, and under these circumstances an enhanced drug effect might be expected.

Liver dysfunction not only affects the metabolism of drugs, but also produces alterations in free fraction due to quantitative and qualitative changes in plasma albumin. *In vitro* studies with plasma from cirrhotic patients shows reduced binding of diazepam (Klotz *et al.*, 1975; Thiessen *et al.*, 1976), chlordiazepoxide (Roberts *et al.*, 1978), and lorazepam (Kraus *et al.*, 1978) when compared with normal plasma. *In vivo*, this increased unbound fraction compensates for the decrease in intrinsic hepatic clearance and so the decrease in clearance calculated from the total drug concentrations is an underestimate of hepatic dysfunction (Wilkinson, 1980). Also when $V_d$ is calculated from total drug concentration an increase is seen, but when determined from free concentration no change is observed provided that $V_d$ is reasonably large and that tissue binding is not altered.

Binding interactions due to the presence of other drugs, e.g. valproic acid

(Dhillon and Richens, 1982a,b) or antirheumatic agents (Sjolholm *et al.*, 1979), or endogenous compounds, e.g. free fatty acids (Tsutsumi *et al.*, 1975; Sjodin, 1977; Colburn and Gibaldi, 1978; Wong and Sellers, 1979) do occur although in themselves are of little clinical importance. The transient rise in free drug concentrations produced acutely by these interactions will lead to a temporary increase in systemic clearance of total drug, but once the displaced drug is cleared the free concentration will return to normal. However, as mentioned earlier, binding interactions are seldom clear-cut; if we examine the 'interaction' between valproic acid and diazepam it will be seen that there are two opposing processes at work. The first is the displacement of diazepam from plasma protein binding sites and the second is the reduction of unbound valproic acid clearance due to metabolic inhibition in the liver. The former effect would be expected to increase the free fraction and reduce the total plasma concentration (because the displaced drug redistributes), while the second effect would tend to reverse the latter. Consequently the overall effect depends on the balance of these two trends.

If routine monitoring of benzodiazepine serum levels becomes justified by future studies, these effects may have to be taken into account in interpreting laboratory results, but in the meantime it is the clinical pharmacologist who will be mostly concerned with the details of effects on drug binding.

## METABOLISM AND ELIMINATION

The metabolic pathways of selected benzodiazepines are shown in Figures 2(a) and (b). The difference between short (Figure 2(a)) and long (Figure 2(b))

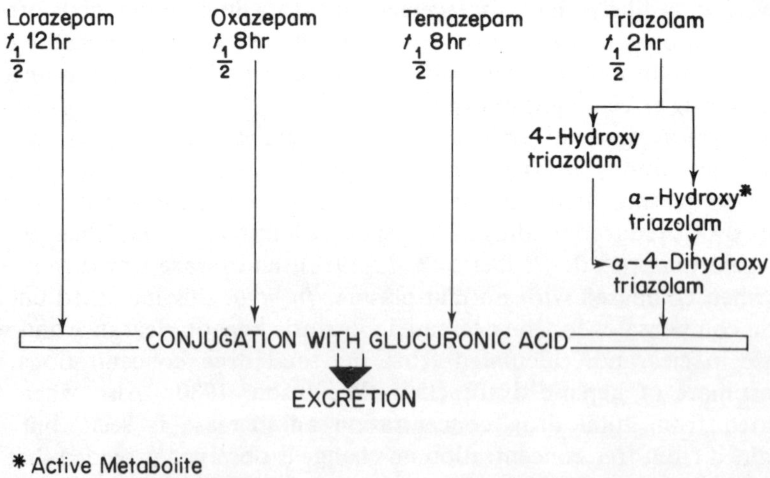


Figure 2(a) Metabolic pathways of selected short elimination half-life benzodiazepines

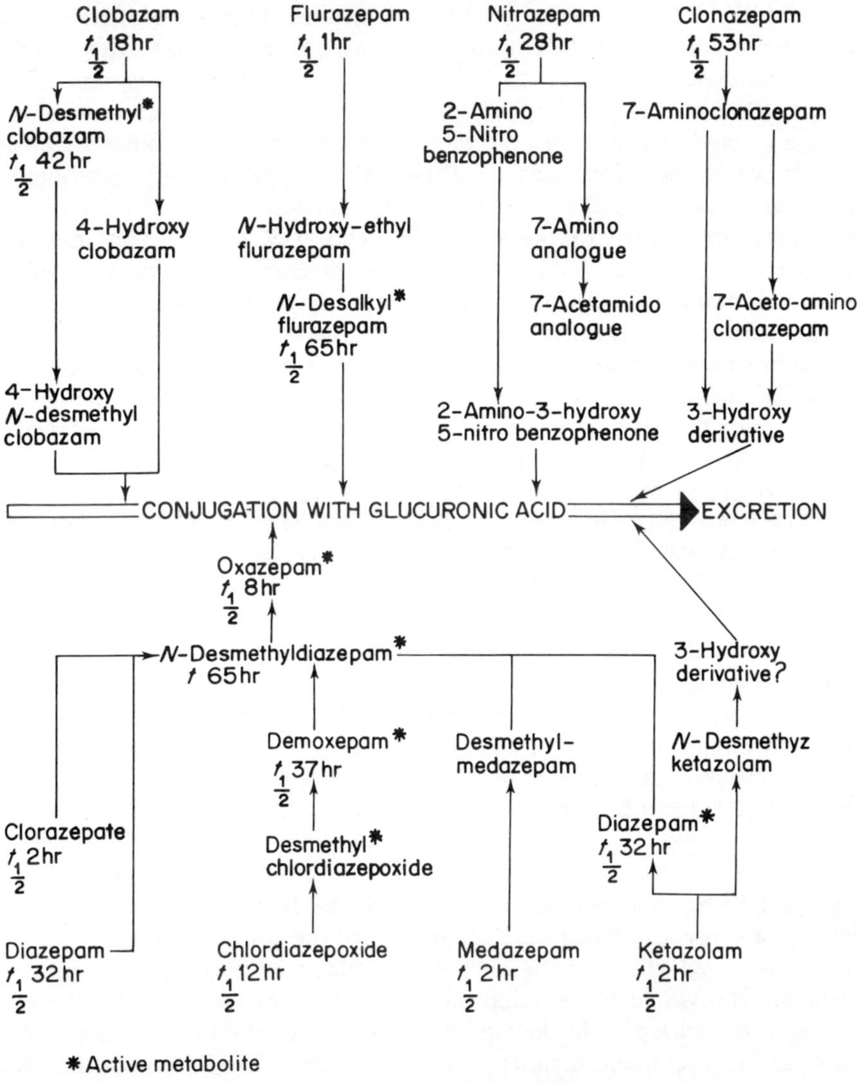


Figure 2(b) Metabolic pathways of selected long-acting benzodiazepines

acting benzodiazepines lies in the half-lives of the drugs or metabolites. Many of the long-acting benzodiazepines have desmethyldiazepam as an active metabolite; the half-life of this compound is 48–57 hours (Klotz *et al.*, 1977) and consequently it extends the activity of the parent benzodiazepine. For the various uses of benzodiazepines this difference of half-lives is of fundamental importance.

Interindividual variation of benzodiazepine pharmacokinetics is of profound importance in the clinical use of this group of drugs often requiring substantial dose adjustments in order to obtain an optimal response from a patient (Breimer *et al.*, 1980). Table 3 reveals the large variation in pharmacokinetic parameters; the data are gathered from studies of healthy subjects where the differences are attributable to genetic and environmental factors as well as age and sex. A pharmacogenetic difference between orientals and caucasians has been reported by Ghoneim *et al.* (1981). They describe a decrease in $V_d$ at steady state and decrease clearance of diazepam with an increase in desmethyldiazepam serum levels in orientals and they also suggest that chronic dosing may produce more profound CNS depression in orientals.

Drug metabolism and distribution can be further perturbed by disease. The type of biotransformation reaction by which a benzodiazepine is metabolized can be predictive of the effect of age or liver dysfunction on metabolism. Benzodiazepines that are primarily oxidized tend to have longer half-lives in the elderly due to an increased $V_d$ and lowered metabolic clearance (Roberts *et al.*, 1978; Klotz and Muller-Seyditz, 1979; Divoll Allen *et al.*, 1980; Greenblatt *et al.*, 1981). Sex may also have an influence; it has been shown that desmethyldiazepam and desalkylflurazepam, both of which are hydroxylated, have reduced clearance particularly among elderly males (Greenblatt and Shader, 1980; Greenblatt *et al.*, 1982). In contrast, benzodiazepines which are primarily conjugated with either glucuronide or sulphate are virtually unaffected by ageing; disposition may be affected, however (Kraus *et al.*, 1978; Greenblatt *et al.*, 1979; Divoll *et al.*, 1981). Liver disease has a similar effect on metabolism; oxidation may be markedly reduced whereas conjugation is little affected. (Schull *et al.*, 1976; Kraus *et al.*, 1978; Roberts *et al.*, 1978; Sellers *et al.*, 1979).

Nitrazepam, which has a nitro-reduction as its primary metabolic step, appears to be half way between these two groups. Jochemsen *et al.* (1983) have reported an absence of ageing effect on intrinsic clearance of nitrazepam while there was a reduction of metabolizing capacity in patients with alcoholic cirrhosis. This would suggest that the reported increased incidence of adverse reactions to nitrazepam in the elderly (Castleden *et al.*, 1977; Greenblatt and Allen, 1978) is as much a function of the increased sensitivity of the ageing brain to benzodiazepines as it is to pharmacokinetic change.

Benzodiazepine metabolism can also be affected by other drugs given concurrently. Cimetidine is known to inhibit oxidative metabolism (Desmond *et al.*, 1980; Klotz and Reimann, 1980, 1981; Patwardhan *et al.*, 1980) which would be expected to increase the half-lives of such benzodiazepines as desmethyldiazepam and desalkylflurazepam while leaving the benzodiazepines which are primarily conjugated unaffected. A similar effect is seen with disulfiram. Sellers *et al.* (1980) demonstrated that disulfiram and ethanol exhibit independent inhibitory effects of variable magnitudes on both

*N*-desmethylation and *C*-hydroxylation by hepatic mixed function oxidases. They therefore infer that oxazepam or lorazepam would be preferable for chronic alcoholics requiring therapy with benzodiazepines. Smoking also affects benzodiazepine metabolism. Norman *et al.* (1981) reported on the pharmacokinetics of desmethyldiazepam after a single oral dose of clorazepate and recorded a shortened half-life ($t_{½\beta}$) and lowered peak serum concentrations in smokers. Abernethy *et al.* (1982) reported an impairment of diazepam total metabolic clearance with low dose oral contraceptive steroid therapy, which could lead to an enhanced clinical effect during chronic therapy.

Enzyme induction due to chronic antiepileptic drugs administration increases the rate of diazepam metabolism to the desmethyl derivative (Viala *et al.*, 1971; Dhillon, 1981) (see Table 4). However, evidence for the effects of enzyme induction on other benzodiazepines is scanty.

Table 4 Diazepam pharmacokinetics in enzyme-induced patients

| | Enzyme-induced patients ($n=6$) | Normal volunteers ($n=6$) | |
|---|---|---|---|
| $AUC_{0-\infty}$ ($\mu g \cdot \ell^{-1} h$) | 3551 ± 1231 | 9059 ± 3018 | ($P<0.01$) |
| $t_{½\alpha}$ (h) | 0.15 ± 0.07 | 0.24 ± 0.11 | (NS) |
| $t_{½\beta}$ (h) | 13.1 ± 4.3 | 34.0 ± 14.0 | ($P<0.01$) |
| $V_d$ ($\ell \cdot kg^{-1}$) | 0.86 ± 0.29 | 0.80 ± 0.33 | (NS) |
| $C\ell$ ($\ell \cdot h^{-1}$) | 3.10 ± 1.00 | 1.20 ± 0.35 | ($P<0.01$) |

Elimination half-lives of diazepam are shorter when used acutely as compared with chronically (Klotz and Reimann, 1981). These authors have shown that this, in part, can be attributed to product inhibition of diazepam elimination by desmethyldiazepam (Klotz and Reimann, 1982). More generally benzodiazepines have been shown not to induce their own metabolism (Lackner and Hunt, 1968; Breckenridge and Orme, 1971; Orme *et al.*, 1972; Robinson and Amidon, 1973).

## CLINICAL USE AND PLASMA LEVEL PROFILES

Benzodiazepines used chronically as anxiolytics and anticonvulsants require a constant non-sedative effect while for hypnotic use, drug action needs to be intermittent. Although benzodiazepines have broadly similar pharmacological profiles, the marked pharmacokinetic differences between individual compounds make some more suitable for the first indication whereas others are better for short duration hypnotic effects.

The rate of onset of drug action depends on the lipid solubility of the compound and on the pharmaceutical formulation used. Hypnotics are usually required to produce a fast onset of action, i.e. to induce sleep quickly. In this respect nitrazepam and flurazepam are satisfactory hypnotics despite their long elimination half-lives. Oxazepam and lorazepam are more suitable for use as anxiolytics as their rate of absorption is too slow for hypnotic use, in spite of oxazepam and lorazepam having short elimination half-lives, a quality which is desirable for a drug used as an hypnotic. None the less the elimination half-life is an important factor in determining duration of drug action; for instance clonazepam, with an elimination half-life of 53 hours is a conveniently long-acting anticonvulsant drug and diazepam which is metabolized to *N*-desmethyldiazepam, with an elimination half-life of up to 100 hours, is a widely used antianxiety drug. On the other hand triazolam and temazepam have much shorter half-lives and have been promoted as short-acting hypnotics which produce minimal hangover effects. On this basis nitrazepam and flurazepam would be unsatisfactory as hypnotics. Figure 3 shows the effect of different elimination half-lives on accumulation after chronic administration. Clearly the compound with an 8 hour half-life is preferable to the compound with a 24 hour half-life as an hypnotic, whereas for an anxiolytic or anticonvulsant the reverse is true. The duration of action and likelihood of accumulation of a benzodiazepine is dependent on elimination half-life of both parent compound and any active metabolite present.

However, this is not the whole story. Benzodiazepine pharmacokinetics are generally held to be best represented by a two compartment model, although on occasion a single or three compartment model has been used. Figure 4 represents an idealized two compartment system after oral dosing. One must

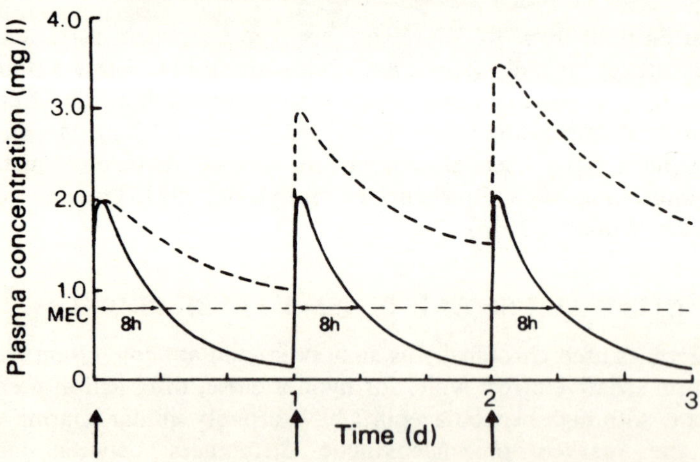


Figure 3 Theoretical plasma concentration profile of two hypnotics with different elimination half-lives: solid line 6 h; dotted line 24 h during nightly administration. MEC refers to the minimal effective concentration; in hypnotic therapy the drug effect should last 8 h or less. $D$ = 100 mg; $\Delta_t$ = 24 h; $V_d$ = 50 l. (Taken from Breimer (1979) with permission)

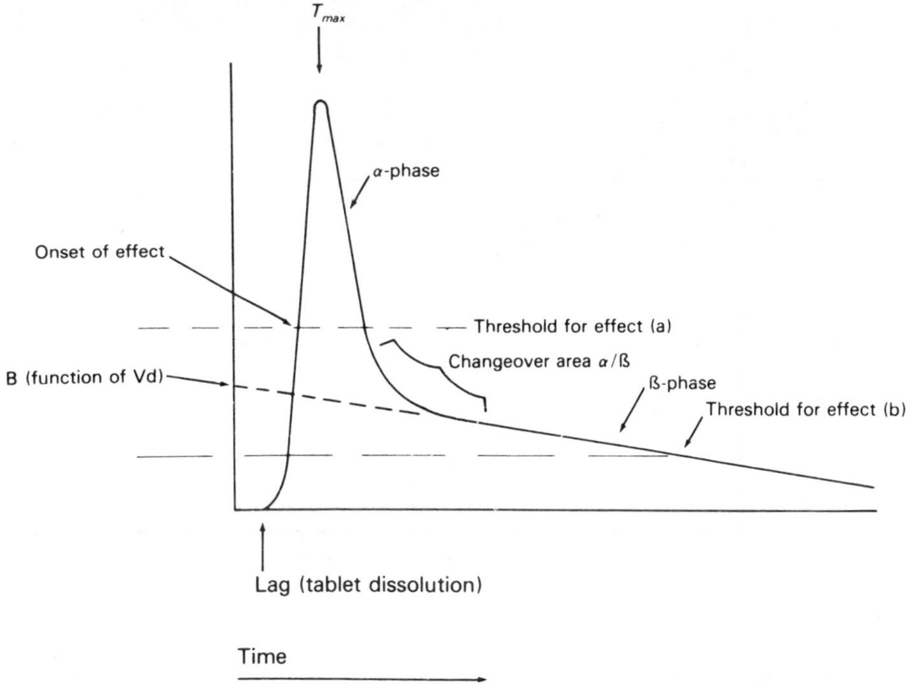


Figure 4 Annotated model plasma concentration graph (semi-log plot) for a two compartment system and oral dosing. (Taken from Curry and Whelpton (1979) with permission)

assume that drug effects last for the time the concentration is above the threshold for effect. Curry and Whelpton (1979) pointed out that initially there is a delay before onset of action and that the effect may wear off either during the $\alpha$ phase (the distribution phase) or below the $\alpha/\beta$ inflexion (i.e. during the $\beta$ or elimination phase). The relative importance of the two phases may thus determine the duration of action and the degree to which they influence the latter is a function of the compartment sizes and of volume of distribution. The profound effect on serum levels of a difference in the ratio between volume of distribution in two phases despite identical absorption rates ($K_a$), $\alpha$ and $\beta$ is shown in Figure 5. This figure clearly shows that the traditional classification of benzodiazepines purely on $t_{1/2\beta}$ is unreliable and potentially misleading. Amrein *et al.* (1983) have suggested an alternative parameter 'residual fraction ($r_{12.1}$)' which is calculated from the plasma drug concentration 12 hours following drug intake and the maximum plasma drug concentration. This parameter is claimed to be a predictive guide of a benzodiazepine's therapeutic applications. Compounds with a small $r_{12.1}$ are suitable for hypnotic use, i.e. they are rapidly removed from the central

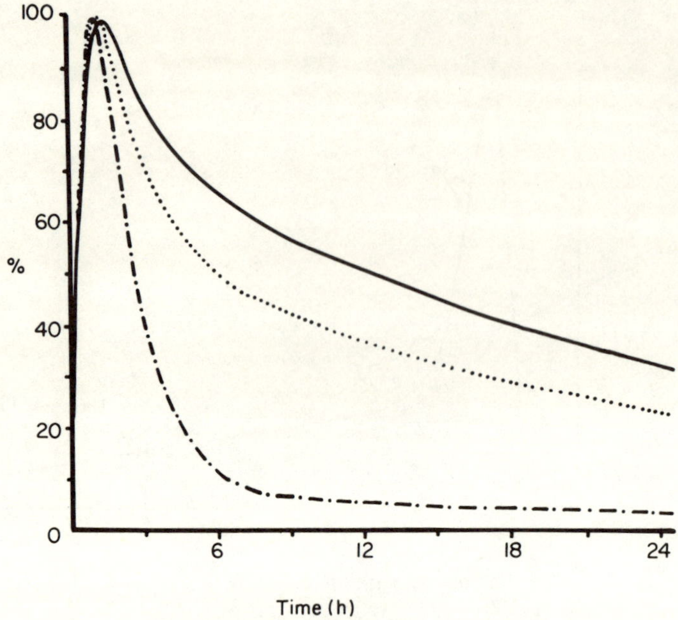


Figure 5 Three theoretical plasma concentration profiles (percentage of maximum concentration against time) for which the following are the same:

1. absorption rate $K_a = 2.0$ (= invasion $t_3$ of 20 min);
2. diffusion rate $\alpha = 0.693$ (= $t_{½\alpha} = 1$ h);
3. elimination rate $\beta = 0.0395$ (= $t_{½\beta} = 20$ h).

The differences amongst the curves are due solely to the differences in the ratio between volumes of distribution in each individual curve. ______ A:B = 2:3; ...... :B = 3:2; —·—·—. A:B = 19:1. (Taken from Amrein *et al.* (1983) with permission)

Table 5 Residual fraction ($r_{12.1}$) and half-life ($t_{½\beta}$) of several benzodiazepines

| | $r_{12.1}$ | $t_{½}$ (hours) |
|---|---|---|
| Midazolam | ≤0.01 | 2 |
| Triazolam | 0.16 | 2 |
| Flunitrazepam | 0.25 | 22 |
| Oxazepam | 0.40 | 8 |
| Temazepam | 0.42 | 8 |
| Nitrazepam | 0.70 | 25 |
| Desmethyldiazepam | 0.71 | 84 |

$r_{12.1}$ = quotient of plasma concentration at 12 hours after drug intake to plasma $C_{max}$.
Modified from Amrein *et al.* (1983).

compartment, while a large $r_{12.1}$ would suggest that the compound is best used as an anxiolytic; intermediate $r_{12.1}$ benzodiazepines are suggested to be hypnoanxiolytics (see Table 5). This new parameter is more helpful than elimination ($\beta$ phase) half-life but still has limitations in that it does not take accumulation of drug and tolerance to drug into account. These two factors are of major importance when benzodiazepines are used chronically.

Tolerance has the effect of gradually increasing the minimum effective concentration. The actual time course and extent of tolerance to benzodiazepines in man has not been clearly investigated. Our studies of nitrazepam have led us to believe that tolerance to the sedative effects of nitrazepam has appeared within 6 days. The therapeutic implications of this are not clear as nitrazepam has been reported to be effective as an hypnotic for up to 24 weeks (Oswald *et al.*, 1982 and chapter 19).

These principles are, of course, only a guideline, and other contributors to this book have expressed differing viewpoints. Interindividual differences in drug metabolism and elimination, as well as in the development of tolerance, will blur the distinction between the marketed benzodiazepines and therefore the choice of compound for a particular indication must remain flexible.

## SERUM LEVEL MONITORING

The routine measurement of plasma benzodiazepine drug concentrations cannot be justified at present because the therapeutic ranges for these compounds have not been defined and because a poor relationship appears to exist between serum level and effects with chronic dosing, probably partly as a result of the development of tolerance. Furthermore, their therapeutic ratios are relatively large and sedation is usually a satisfactory clinical indicator that the dose is excessive.

It has, on occasion, proved possible to relate plasma levels to effect in acute situations. Fink *et al.* (1976) demonstrated a linear correlation between the amount of EEG activity and serum diazepam concentration. Aschoff (1968) found a linear correlation between dosage of diazepam and the decrease of peak velocity of saccadic eye movements. Bittencourt *et al.* (1981) took this further and demonstrated a log-linear relationship between peak saccadic velocity and log concentration of temazepam, nitrazepam, and diazepam. It would seem that interindividual variation in benzodiazepine sensitivity may be the main reason why plasma level:effect relationships have so seldom been found even in an acute situation.

Also using eye movements, Griffiths *et al.* (1983) investigated the effects of chronic administration of nitrazepam (long $t_{1/2}$) and temazepam (short $t_{1/2}$) on normal subjects and showed that the residual performance impairment produced by nitrazepam on the first day of treatment had disappeared by day 6, despite much higher serum levels (see Figures 6 and 7). Temazepam on the

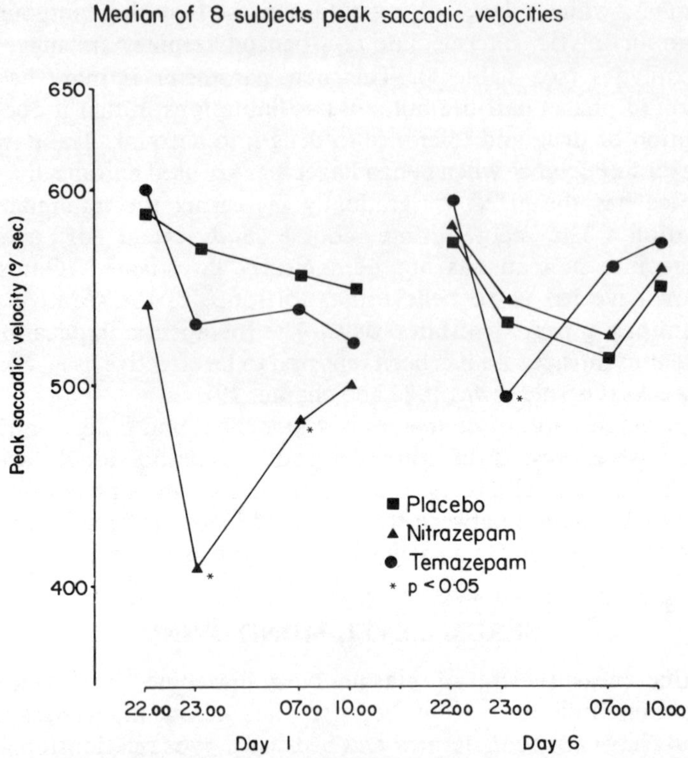


Figure 6 Nitrazepam (10 mg), temazepam (20 mg) and placebo were given nightly for 6 days. On the first the sixth night peak saccadic velocity was measured at 22.00 (time of drug intake), 23.00, 07.00 and 10.00. Significant performance impairment (between drug and placebo) occurred with nitrazepam on day 1 at 23.00 and 07.00 with temazepam on day 6 at 23.00 ($P<0.05$ in all cases). Eight subjects took part in the study

other hand produced no residual effects on day 1 but by day 6, with slightly higher serum levels, a significant performance impairment was seen. This would suggest that nitrazepam has produced tolerance to itself, possibly by desensitization of the benzodiazepine receptor, while temazepam had not. One explanation of this is that the receptors in the central nervous system are exposed for much longer periods to a high concentration of nitrazepam, but less so with temazepam. Desensitization to the effects of nitrazepam therefore predominates.

The reverse side of tolerance is withdrawal. Benzodiazepines do produce withdrawal symptoms, notably rebound insomnia and anxiety though this may in part be due to the removal of the pill taking ritual. The actual withdrawal effects may take some days to develop due to the long half-life of some of the metabolites, notably desmethyldiazepam. This gradual decrease of drug level

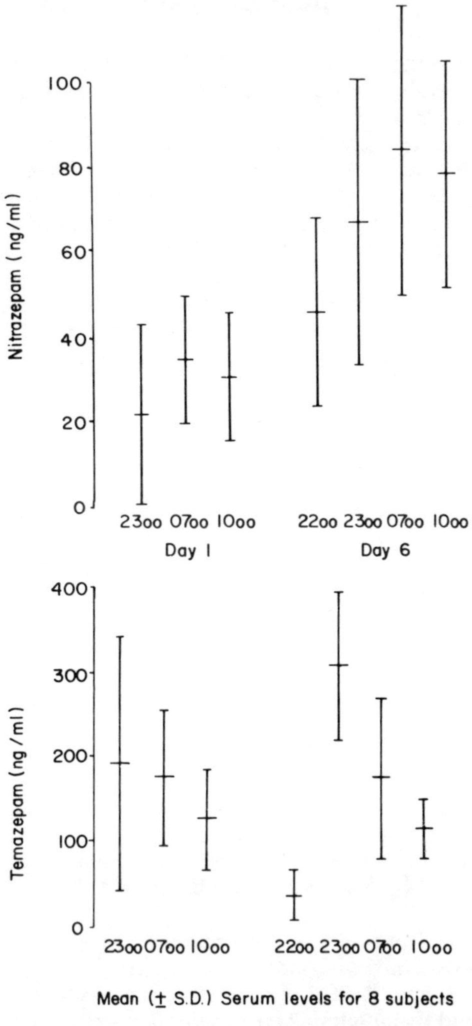


Figure 7 Serum level data for Figure 6. Nitrazepam can be seen to have accumulated over the 6 day period, while temazepam had not

may in some patients cushion the withdrawal. Short-acting benzodiazepines used in large doses can produce rebound anxiety the morning following night time administration for insomnia. Morgan and Oswald (1982 and page 265) have reported this effect for triazolam. If this is substantiated, there may be important implications for the future use and development of very short-acting drugs like triazolam and midazolam.

## REFERENCES


Abernethy, D. R., Greenblatt, D. J., Divoll, M. and Arendt, R. (1982). Impairment of diazepam clearance with low dose and oral contraceptive steroid therapy. *Clin. Pharmac. Ther.*, **31**, 198–199.

Amrein, R., Eckert, M., Haefely, H. and Leishman, B. (1983). Pharmacokinetic and clinical considerations in the choice of a hypnotic. *Brit. J. clin. Pharmac.* (In press).

Arendt, R. M., Greenblatt, D. J., Divoll, M., Abernethy, D. R., Giles, H. G. and Sellers, E. M. (1982). Predicting *in vivo* benzodiazepine distribution based on *in vitro* lipophilicity. *Clin. Pharmac. Ther.*, **31**, 200–201.

Aschoff, C. J. (1968). Verandenugen rascher blick bewegungen (Saccaden) beim menschen inter diazepam (valium). *Arch. Psychiat. Nervemb.*, **211**, 325–332.

Bellantuono, C., Reggi, V., Tognoni, G. and Garattini, S. (1980). Benzodiazepines: clinical pharmacology and therapeutic use. *Drugs*, **19**, 195–219.

Bittencourt, P. R. M., Wade, P., Smith, A. T. and Richens, A. (1981). The relationship between peak saccadic eye movements and serum benzodiazepine concentrations. *Brit. J. clin. Pharmac.*, **12**, 523–534.

Breckenridge, A. and Orme, M. (1971). Clinical implications of enzyme induction. *Ann. NY Acad. Sci.*, **179**, 421–431.

Breimer, D. D. (1979). Pharmacokinetics and metabolism of various benzodiazepines used as hypnotics. *Brit. J. clin. Pharmac.*, **8**, 7S–13S.

Breimer, D. D., Jochemsen, R. von and Albert, H. H. (1980). Pharmacokinetics of benzodiazepines—short acting vs. long acting. *Arzneim Forsch/Drug Res.*, **30(I)** Nr 5a, 875–882.

Browne, T. R. and Penry, J. K. (1973). Benzodiazepines in the treatment of epilepsy. *Epilepsia*, **14**, 277–310.

Castleden, C. M., George, C. F., Marcer, D. and Hallett, C. (1977). Increased sensitivity to nitrazepam in old age. *Brit. med. J.* **1**, 10–12.

Colburn, W. A. and Gibaldi, M. (1978). Plasma protein binding of diazepam after a single dose of sodium oleate. *J. Pharm. Sci.*, **67**, 891–892.

Curry, S. H. and Whelpton, R. (1979). Pharmacokinetics of closely related benzodiazepines. *Brit. J. clin. Pharmac.*, **8**, 155–215.

Desmond, P. V., Patwardham, R. V., Schenker, S. and Speeg, K. V. Jr. (1980). Cimetidine impairs the elimination of chlordiazepoxide in man. *Ann. intern. Med.*, **93**, 266–268.

Dhillon, S. (1981). Rectal absorption and pharmacokinetics of diazepam in epileptic patients. Ph.D. Thesis, Univ. of London.

Dhillon, S., Oxley, J. and Richens, A. (1982). Bioavailability of diazepam after intravenous, oral and rectal administration in adult epileptic patients. *Brit. J. clin. Pharmac.*, **13**, 427–432.

Dhillon, S. and Richens, A. (1982a). Serum protein binding of diazepam and its displacement by valproic acid in vitro. *Brit. J. clin. Pharmac.*, **12**, 591–592.

Dhillon, S. and Richens, A. (1982b). Valproic acid and diazepam interaction in vivo. *Brit. J. clin. Pharmac.*, **13**, 553–560.

Divoll Allen, M., Greenblatt, D. J., Harmatz, J. S. and Shader, R. I. (1980). Desmethyldiazepam kinetics in the elderly after oral prazepam. *Clin. Pharmac. Ther.*, **28**, 196–202.

Divoll, M., Greenblatt, D. J., Harmatz, J. S. and Shader, R. I. (1981). Effect of age and gender on disposition of temazepam. *J. Pharm. Sci.*, **70**, 1104–1108.

Fink, M., Irwin, P., Weinfeld, R. E., Schwartz, M. A. and Conney, A. H. (1976). Blood levels and EEG effects of diazepam and bromazepam. *Clin. Pharmac. Ther.*, **20**, 184–191.

Ghoneim, M. M., Korttilia, K., Chiang, C. K., Jacobs, L., Schoenwald, R. D., Mewalot, S. P. and Kayaba, K-O. (1981). Diazepam effects and kinetics in caucasians and orientals. *Clin. Pharmac. Ther.*, **29**, 749–756.

Greenblatt, D. J. and Allen, M. D. (1978). Toxicity of nitrazepam in the elderly. A report from the Boston collaborative drug surveillance program. *Brit. J. clin. Pharmac.*, **5**, 407–413.

Greenblatt, D. J., Divoll Allen M., Lochnisar, A., Harmatz, J. S. and Shader, R. I. (1979). Lorazepam kinetics in the elderly. *Clin. Pharmac. Ther.*, **26**, 103–113.

Greenblatt, D. J., Divoll Allen, M., MacLaughlin, D., Harmatz, J. S. and Shader, R. I. (1978a). Diazepam absorbtion: effects of antacids and food. *Clin. Pharmac. Ther.*, **24**, 600–609.

Greenblatt, D. J., Divoll, M., Abernathy, D. R., Harmatz, J. S. and Shader, R. I. (1982). Antipyrine kinetics in the elderly—prediction of age related changes in benzodiazepine oxidizing capacity. *J. Pharmac. exp. Ther.*, **200**, 120–126.

Greenblatt, D. J., Divoll, M., Harmatz, J. S., Maclaughlin, D. S. and Shader, R. I. (1981). Kinetics and clinical effects of flurazepam in young and elderly insomniacs. *Clin. Pharmac. Ther.*, **30**, 475–486.

Greenblatt, D. J. and Shader, R. I. (1978). Prazepam and lorazepam, two new benzodiazepines. *New Engl. J. Med.*, **299**, 1342–1344.

Greenblatt, D. J. and Shader, R. I. (1980). Effects of age and other drugs on benzodiazepine kinetics. *Arzneim Forsch/Drug Res.*, **30(1)**, Nr. 5a, 886–890.

Greenblatt, D. S., Shader, R. I., Macleod, S. M. and Sellers, E. M. (1978b). Clinical pharmacokinetics of chlordiazepoxide. *Clin. Pharmacokinet.*, **3**, 381–394.

Griffiths, A., Tedeschi, G., Smith, A. T. and Richens, A. (1983). The effects of repeated doses of temazepam and nitrazepam on human psychomotor performance. *Br. J. clin. Pharmac.* (In press)

Heizmann, P., Eckert, M. and Ziegler, W. (1983). Pharmacokinetics and bioavailability of midazolam in man. *Br. J. clin. Pharmac.* (in press).

Jochemsen, R., Van Bucsekom, B. R., Spoelstra, P., Janssens, A. R. and Breimer, D. D: (1983). Effect of age and liver cirrhosis on the pharmacokinetics of nitrazepam. *Br. J. clin. Pharmac.* (in press).

Klotz, U., Antonin, K. H., Burgel, H. and Breck, P. R. (1977). Disposition of diazepam and its major metabolite desmethyldiazepam in patients with liver disease. *Clin. Pharmac. Ther.*, **21**, 430.

Klotz, U., Avant, G. R., Moyumpa, A., Sclenker, S. and Wilkinson, G. R. (1975). The effects of age and liver disease on the disposition and elimination of diazepam in adult man. *J. clin. Invest.*, **55**, 347–359.

Klotz, U. and Muller-Seyditz, P. (1979). Altered elimination of desmethyldiazepam in the elderly. *Br. J. clin. Pharmac.*, **7**, 119–120.

Klotz, U. and Reimann, I. (1980). Influence of cimetidine on the pharmacokinetics of desmethyldiazepam and oxazepam. *Eur. J. clin. Pharmac.*, **18**, 517–520.

Klotz, U. and Reimann, I. (1981). Elevation of steady state diazepam levels by cimetidine. *Clin. Pharmac. Ther.*, **30**, 513–517.

Klotz, U. and Reimann, I. (1982). Clearance of diazepam can be impaired by its major metabolite desmethyldiazepam. *Eur. J. clin. Pharmac.*, **21**, 161–163.

Knudsen, F. U. (1977). Plasma diazepam in infants after rectal administration in solution and by suppository. *Acta paed. scand.*, **66**, 563–567.

Knudsen, F. U. (1979). Rectal administration of diazepam in solution in the acute treatment of convulsions in infants and children. *Archs Dis. Child.*, **54**, 855–857.

Knudsen, F. U. and Westermark, S. (1978). Prophylactic diazepam or phenobarbitone in febrile convulsions: a prospective controlled study. *Archs Dis. Child.*, **53**, 660–663.

Kraus, J. W., Desond, P. V., Marshall, J. P., Johnson, R. F., Schenker, S. and

Wilkinson, G. R. (1978). The effects of ageing and liver disease on disposition of lorazepam in man. *Clin. Pharmac. Ther.*, **24**, 411–419.

Lackner, M. and Hunt, V. E. (1968). The effect of Librium on hemostasis. *Am. J. med. Sci.*, **256**, 368–372.

Mandelli, M., Tognoni, M. and Garattini, S. (1978). Clinical pharmacokinetics of diazepam. *Clin. Pharmacokinet.*, **3**, 72–91.

Mattila, M. A. K. and Larni, H. M. (1980). Furnitrazepam: a review of its pharmacological properties and therapeutic use. *Drugs*, **20**, 353–374.

Milligan, N. (1982). Methods of assessment of antiepileptic drugs in man. M.D. Thesis, Univ. of Birmingham.

Moolenaar, F., Bakker, S., Visser, J. and Huizargen, T. (1980). Biopharmaceuticals of rectal administration of drugs in man IX. Comparative biopharmaceuticals of diazepam after single rectal, oral and intravenous administration in man. *Int. J. Pharmaceut.*, **5**, 127–137.

Morgan, K. and Oswald, I. (1982). Anxiety caused by a short life hypnotic. *Brit. med. J.*, **284**, 942.

Norman, T. R., Fulton, W., Burrows, G. D. and Maguire, K. P. (1981). Pharmacokinetics of desmethyldiazepam after a single oral dose of clorazepate. The effect of smoking. *Eur. J. clin. Pharmac.*, **21**, 229–233.

Ochs, H. R., Greenblatt, D. J., Allen, M. D., Harmatz, J. S., Shader, R. I. and Bodens, G. (1979). Effect of age and Billroth gastrectomy on absorption of desmethyldiazepam from clorazepate. *Clin. Pharmac. Ther.*, **26**, 449–456.

Orme, M., Breckenridge, A. and Brooks, R. V. (1972). Interactions of benzodiazepines with warfarin. *Brit. med. J.*, **3**, 611–614.

Oswald, I., French, C., Adam, K. and Gilham, J. (1982). Benzodiazepine hypnotics remain effective for 24 weeks. *Brit. Med. J.*, **284**, 860–863.

Patwardhan, R. V., Yarborough, G. W., Desmond, P. V., Johnson, R. F., Schenler, S. and Speeg, K. V. Jr. (1980). Cimetidine spares the glucuronidation of lorazapam and oxazepam. *Gastroenterology*, **79**, 912–916.

Roberts, R. K., Wilkinson, G. R., Branch, R. A. and Scherler, S. (1978). Effects of age and parenchymal liver disease on the disposition and elimination of chlordiazepoxide. *Gastroenterology*, **78**, 479–485.

Robinson, D. S. and Amidon, E. L. (1973). Interactions of benzodiazepines with warfarin in man. In: *The Benzodiazepines*, pp.641–646 (Eds. Garattini, S., Mussini, E. and Randall, L. O.), Raven Press, New York.

Schull, H. J. Jr., Wilkinson, G. R., Johnson, R. and Schenken, S. (1976). Normal disposition of oxazepam in acute viral hepatitis and cirrhosis. *Ann. intern. Med.*, **84**, 420–425.

Sellers, E. M., Giles, M. G., Greenblatt, D. J. and Naranjo, C. A. (1980). Differential effects on benzodiazepine disposition by disulfiram and ethanol. *Arzneim-Forsch/ Drug Res.*, **30 (1)** Nr 5a, 882–885.

Sellers, E. M., Greenblatt, D. J., Giles, M. G., Naranjo, C. A., Kaplan, H. and Macleod, S. M. (1979). Chlordiazepoxide and oxazepam disposition in cirrhosis. *Clin. Pharmac. Ther.*, **26**, 240–246.

Shader, R. I., Ciranlo, D. A., Greenblatt, D. J. and Harmatz, J. S. (1982). Steady state plasma desmethyldiazepam during long term clorazepate use. Effect of antacids. *Clin. Pharmac. Ther.*, **31**, 180–183.

Shader, R. I., Georgotas, A., Greenblatt, D. J., Harmatz, J. S. and Allen, M. D. (1978). Impaired absorbtion of desmethyldiazepam from clorazepate by magnesium aluminium hydroxide. *Clin. Pharmac. Ther.*, **24**, 308–315.

Shader, R. I. and Greenblatt, D. J. (1979). Benzodiazepines: some aspects of their clinical pharmacology. *Ciba Found. Symp.*, **(74)**, 141–155.

Sjodin, T. (1977). Circular dichroism studies on the inhibiting effect of oleic acid on binding of diazepam to human serum albumin. *Biochem. Pharmac.*, **26**, 2157–2161.

Sjolholm, C., Ekman, B., Kober, A., Ljungstedt-Dahlman, L., Sieving, B. and Sjodin, T. (1979). Binding of drugs to human serum albumin, XI. The specificity of three binding sites as studies with albumin immobilized in micro particles. *Molec. Pharmac.*, **16**, 767–777.

Smith, A. T., Bittencourt, P. R. M., Lloyd, D. S. L. and Richens, A. (1981). An efficient technique for determining characteristics of saccadic eye movements using a mini computer. *J. biomed. Engng*, **3**, 39–43.

Tedeschi, G., Smith, A. T., Dhillon, S. and Richens, A. (1983). Rate of entrance of benzodiazepines into the brain. *Brit. J. clin. Pharmac.* (in press).

Thiessen, S. S., Sellers, E. M., Denbeigh, P. and Dolman, L. (1976). Plasma protein binding of diazepam and tolbutamide in chronic alcoholics. *J. clin. Pharmac.* **16**, 345–351.

Tsutsumi, J. J., Sellers, E. M., Denbergh, P. and Dolman, P. R. (1975). The displacing effect of fatty acid on the binding of diazepam to human serum albumin. *Biochem. Pharmac.*, **24**, 1361–1362.

Viala, A., Caro, J. P., Dravet, L., Tassinani, C. A., Roger, J. and Angeletti-Phillipe, A. (1971). Bloodlevels of diazepam (Valium) and *N*-desmethyldiazepam in the epileptic child. A preliminary report. *Psychiatria Neurologica et Neurochirurgia*, **74**, 153–158.

Whelpton, R. (1979). Data compilation: benzodiazepine compounds. *Biopharmaceutics and Drug Disposition*, **1**, 37–45.

Wilkinson, G. R. (1980). Influence of liver disease on pharmacokinetics. In: *Applied Pharmacokinetics* (Eds Evans, W. E., Schentag, J. J. and Jusko, W. S.), Pub. Applied Therapeutics Inc. San Francisco, 57–76.

Wong, A. D. and Sellers, E. M. (1979). Intravascular factors affecting diazepam binding to human serum albumin. *Biochem. Pharmac.*, **28**, 3265–3270.

## DISCUSSION

## CHAIRMAN: DR M. TRIMBLE

DR. HERBERT: I want to ask you about the degree to which one can really correlate plasma levels with therapeutic effects. I ask this because we have recently been studying the distribution in the brain of another series of lipid-soluble compounds, the steroid hormones. They behave rather similarly to the benzodiazepines. The important thing is that you really cannot, without looking at the rate of clearance from the cerebrospinal fluid (rather than the plasma), say anything very sensible about the levels in the brain vis-à-vis those in the plasma. Although entry into the brain is predictable on the basis of their binding in the serum, or their lipid solubility, what is not predictable is their clearance, particularly in situations where there are fairly rapid changes in the serum levels.

I wondered if you have any information, therefore, on the clearance of benzodiazepines from the cerebrospinal fluid rather than from the plasma?

PROFESSOR RICHENS: No, not the clearance. Observations have been made on CSF concentrations of benzodiazepines but the purpose of those studies has been to look at binding. The concentration of the drug in the CSF mirrors that of the free concentration in the plasma.

I am not aware of any human studies in which the clearance of benzodiazepines has been studied. I am not sure how you are doing your steroid studies but it must be difficult making repeated sampling of CSF to look at clearance.

DR. HERBERT: I think that levels in the cerebrospinal fluid will relate to free levels in the serum only in situations of steady state. If you have a differential clearance rate, then there will rapidly be a very great discrepancy between the levels in the cerebrospinal fluid and the levels of the free drug in the serum if the drug is administered intermittently.

PROFESSOR RICHENS: Most studies that have been done of benzodiazepines and anticonvulsants, with which I am very familiar, show what you would predict in the way of the distribution between plasma and CSF namely that CSF concentrations correlate with the concentration of free drug in the plasma. So I think there may be a difference between steroids and these very lipid-soluble, freely diffusible drugs.

What has always bothered me about CSF studies though is that the brain itself is much closer to the blood than it is to the lumbar CSF, and very lipid-soluble drugs get in and out of the brain very quickly, whereas they do not get in and out of lumbar CSF very quickly.

DR. LASCELLES: Do we not have a special situation with the benzodiazepines in that they are very highly bound to protein and as the protein content of the CSF is low compared to brain and blood, the concentration of benzodiazepines must be very low too?

DR. HERBERT: The situation here is comparable to the steroid hormones which also bind in the blood to proteins; the ratio between blood and brain for a typical steroid is about 2% though it varies considerably between steroids.

DR. S. E. FILE: There is a very high correlation in both acutely and chronically treated rats between the brain concentrations and the plasma of all time periods, but zero correlation with behavioural effects. The plasma reflects perfectly what is going on in the brain; brain concentrations tell us nothing about the behavioural effects.

DR. M. SCHMUTZ: I want to stress the fact that in the literature there is some evidence that against pentylenetetrazole-induced seizures, the concentration of free diazepam in brain does not correlate at all with its time course of activity. What seems to correlate very well is the number of receptors occupied by diazepam.

DR. P. TYRER: I gather that about 95% of benzodiazepines are bound to plasma proteins. Is it only the free benzodiazepine that is actually available clinically, or is the bound also clinically active?

PROFESSOR RICHENS: Diazepam is something like 97–98% bound. Some of the other benzodiazepines are much less bound but in general the free drug is available for diffusion into tissues like the brain: it sets the concentration gradient driving the drug into the brain. From that point of view, the free drug concentration is what is pharmacologically active and not that bound to plasma proteins, although the latter comes off the plasma proteins extremely rapidly as the free drug goes into the tissues.

DR. TYRER: Do you think that in looking at the relationship between plasma levels and clinical effects one ought to be looking at the relationship of plasma levels of free drug only?

PROFESSOR RICHENS: To interpret a total plasma concentration you really need to know what the plasma albumin concentration is, what the free fatty acid concentration is, and possibly some other factors as well because these will influence the fraction that is bound. But, having said that, in practice the total concentration is quite a good measure because binding does not vary so much from one individual to another, or one time to another, such that the correlation between total level and effect is lost.

PROFESSOR M. LADER: There is a very high correlation between free (plasma water) benzodiazepine and CSF benzodiazepine concentrations. Another body fluid, saliva, is much more complicated. The correlation between clinical effects and plasma concentration is vitiated by the problems of tolerance. Several years ago we published data showing a correlation between plasma concentration and EEG effects, to which there is no tolerance, but no correlation between plasma concentration and clinical effect.

THE CHAIRMAN: Does the impairment or the slowing down of the saccadic velocity have any clinical relevance?

PROFESSOR RICHENS: The pathway we are studying is complex. Burst cells play down on to the motor neurons of the external occular muscles. They are situated in the reticular formation, and you could argue that we are just looking at an effect on the reticular formation which parallels the sedative action of benzodiazepines. We know that barbiturates also slow down saccadic movements in the same way, as does alcohol. On the other hand amphetamines will speed up saccadic velocity, particularly when it is slowed by a tiring effect. So as a pharmacological marker, which is what we are using it for, it seems to be extremely useful, but what it means in clinical terms I cannot say.

Benzodiazepines Divided
Edited by M. R. Trimble


# 15

# Clinical Laboratory Aspects of Therapeutic Monitoring for Benzodiazepines

PETER T. LASCELLES*

## INTRODUCTION

The use of benzodiazepines in therapeutic applications has increased exponentially over the last 20 years and they are now the most commonly prescribed of all groups of drugs (Klotz *et al.*, 1980; Lippa *et al.*, 1982; Lukas and Griffiths, 1982; Schütz, 1982a). Whilst many additional compounds have been synthesized and brought into use, the number of papers devoted to analysis and pharmacokinetics of the benzodiazepine group of compounds published per annum has risen from 10 in the year 1960 to 660 in 1979 (Schütz, 1982a). Recently, increased concern has been expressed about the possible overprescription of benzodiazepines in clinical practice and the ready availability of the drugs amongst the general public (Marks, 1978a; Williams, 1979, 1980; Rosser, 1982). Another recent development is the publication of reports describing the occurrence of a variety of symptoms in patients who have had the drugs withdrawn after taking benzodiazepines over a long period (Marks, 1978b; Balmer *et al.*, 1981; Hallstrom and Lader, 1981; Laughren *et al.*, 1982; Oswald *et al.*, 1982). Animal studies have confirmed that cessation of diazepam or chlordiazepoxide administration produces a typical barbiturate-like withdrawal syndrome (Cumin *et al.*, 1982; McNicholas and Martin, 1982; Rosenberg and Chiu, 1982). It is therefore recommended that changes in benzodiazepine therapy should be carried out slowly and with caution and with frequent monitoring of serum levels (Laughren *et al.*, 1982).

The clinical relevance of monitoring the serum concentration of benzodiazepines as a guide to therapy is not yet established (Tansella *et al.*, 1975;

*In conjunction with N. Ratnaraj and V. Goldberg.

Bittencourt and Dhillon, 1981; Bowden and Fisher, 1982); indeed, it has been claimed that such routine monitoring has no place in patient management (Bowden and Fisher, 1982). Some studies, however, have described a positive correlation between dose and serum concentration (Curry, 1974; Dasberg *et al.*, 1974), and recently a good objective correlation has been found between serum levels of temazepam and eye movements (Bittencourt and Dhillon, 1981; Bittencourt *et al.*, 1981). Therapeutic monitoring to date has been limited to establishing patient compliance or as a confirmation of suspected clinical intoxication.

No satisfactory therapeutic range for serum benzodiazepines has been established due to a variety of factors. These include:

1. the wide range of commercially available drugs possessing different pharmacokinetic characteristics;
2. altered pharmacokinetic characteristics in different age groups;
3. the existence of metabolites possessing variable biological activity;
4. the development of drug tolerance especially on long-term therapy;
5. difficulties in interpretation of serum levels as a result of drug interaction;
6. high and variable plasma protein binding of benzodiazepines;
7. some analytical problems associated with earlier laboratory techniques; and
8. difficulties in objective measurement of the clinical response in patients.

Moreover, the clinical response has been categorized as anxiolytic, muscle relaxant, anticonvulsant or sedative/hypnotic. The anticonvulsant properties, too, must be considered separately under headings of status epilepticus, and myoclonic movements in childhood, whilst the effects on seizures in adults should be viewed separately with respect to the 1,4- and 1,5-benzodiazepine compounds. In this context, the current emphasis on the development of radioreceptor assays (receptor binding assays) is of considerable importance (Dorow *et al.*, 1982; Mennini *et al.*, 1982). These assays are based on the occurrence in the central nervous system of receptors with a strong affinity for benzodiazepines (Braestrup *et al.*, 1977; Möhler and Okada, 1977a; Squires and Braestrup, 1977; Möhler *et al.*, 1978). They may allow the quantitative assessment of total benzodiazepine pharmacological activity in a sample and thus give a new insight into the mode of action of these drugs (Lader, 1978; Guidotti, 1981; Skolnick and Paul, 1982; Study and Barker, 1982).

## RECENT DEVELOPMENTS IN METHODOLOGY

The analysis of benzodiazepines in body fluids has proved to be difficult in practice because of the complexity of the benzodiazepine molecular structure and the low doses given to patients (Greenblatt and Shader, 1981; Ratnaraj *et al.*, 1981). Techniques such as gas liquid chromatography (GLC), high performance liquid chromatography (HPLC) and immunoassay are widely used in routine practice, and improvements in technique and instrumentation have allowed many new compounds to be accurately and reliable assayed. Nevertheless, these methods have their limitations, which may be overcome to some extent by the use of radioreceptor assays.

Several reviews of the methodology have already been published (Clifford and Smyth, 1974; Hailey, 1974; de Silva, 1978; Greenblatt and Shader, 1981; Dixon, 1982; Schütz, 1982b; Goldberg *et al.*, 1983) and the following account of methods together with data of our own summarizes the position at the present time.

## Chromatographic methods

Recent developments in gas chromatography include the introduction of pulsed [$^{63}$Ni] electron capture detectors which are linear over a wide range and more stable than earlier [$^{3}$H] models (Greenblatt and Shader, 1981; Toseland and Wicks, 1981). These detectors are now in general use and a number of new procedures have been described for 1,4-benzodiazepines and related compounds such as diazepam (Löscher, 1982), flunitrazepam (Greenblatt *et al.*, 1982; Jochemsen and Breimer, 1982), clonazepam (Badcock and Pollard, 1982), flurazepam (Cooper and Drolet, 1982), the water-soluble imidazole benzodiazepine, midazolam (Coassolo *et al.*, 1982), the 1,5-benzodiazepine, clobazam (Riva *et al.*, 1981), and SAS 643 (Mardente *et al.*, 1981). The design of nitrogen-specific detectors has also been greatly improved (Toseland and Wicks, 1981), and this type of detector has been used with success for the analysis of diazepam (Debruyne *et al.*, 1980) and midazolam (Vasiliades and Sahawneh, 1982).

The increasing use of specialized column-packing materials such as SP2250, SP2510-DA and Apolar 87 (Kovats 87), and support-coated open tubular columns have also improved the sensitivity and specificity of GLC procedures (Debruyne *et al.*, 1980; Toseland and Wicks, 1981; Riva *et al.*, 1981; Badcock and Pollard, 1982; Jochemsen and Breimer, 1982; Löscher, 1982; Vasiliades and Sahawneh, 1982). Detection limits for benzodiazepines and related compounds ranging from 500 pm ml$^{-1}$ to 50 ng ml$^{-1}$ can now regularly be achieved (Goldberg *et al.*, 1983).

The use of a mass spectrometer as a detector for a gas chromatograph (GC/MS) is a well established procedure (McCamish, 1980; Garland and Powell, 1981), and the technique has such sensitivity that it can be used to quantitate benzodiazepines in biological fluids in the low picogram range. For example, new methods have recently been reported for the determination of midazolam by GC/MS in the electron impact and chemical ionization modes (Coassolo *et al.*, 1982; Vasiliades and Sahawneh, 1982) and the recently introduced benzodiazepine derivative, tofisopam, can also be analysed by electron impact GC/MS (Tomori *et al.*, 1982). Use of a more specialized technique, gas chromatography negative ion mass spectrometry, is of particular relevance in the analysis of benzodiazepines which have a strong electron-capture capability (Garland and Min, 1979; McCamish, 1980; Miwa *et al.*, 1981).

GC/MS has very great specificity and sensitivity, although care must be taken to carry out adequate sample clean-up and devise correct search and scanning programmes in the analysis of multicomponent mixtures (Rosenthal, 1982). Unfortunately, however, the technique is limited by the fact that some benzodiazepines are difficult to chromatograph by GLC. By contrast, HPLC is being increasingly used in the particular circumstances when drugs and metabolites are thermally unstable or can only be chromatographed with difficulty, or when decomposition of metabolites makes it difficult to resolve them from the parent compound (Greenblatt and Shader, 1981; Puglisi and de Silva, 1981; Clark *et al.*, 1982; Lensmeyer *et al.*, 1982; Sumirtapura *et al.*, 1982; Goldberg *et al.*, 1983). Recently HPLC analyses have been devised for a number of benzodiazepines including diazepam (Ratnaraj *et al.*, 1981; Kinberger and Wahrgren, 1982; Lensmeyer *et al.*, 1982; Rao *et al.*, 1982), nitrazepam (Kelly *et al.*, 1982), clobazam (Brachet-Liermain *et al.*, 1982), midazolam (Vasiliades and Sahawneh, 1982) and lorazepam (Walmsley and Chasseaud, 1981), and their major metabolites, with sensitivity in the low nanogram range and sample sizes less than 500 $\mu$l. Generally, a reverse-phase mode is used with ultraviolet spectrophotometric detection, because the benzodiazepine group of compounds absorbs strongly in the ultraviolet (Goldberg *et al.*, 1983). An interesting development, however, is the analysis of 7-aminoflunitrazepam and 7-aminodesmethylflunitrazepam by an HPLC method with fluorimetric detection, which is potentially more sensitive than ultraviolet detection (Sumirtapura *et al.*, 1982). An HPLC method using a polarographic detector has been devised for the analysis of nitrazepam, and this type of detector may be brought into routine use with improvements in apparatus design (Brooks, 1980; Rooney, 1980; Harekamp *et al.*, 1981; Smyth, 1982).

Chromatographic methods have now developed so that suitable procedures can be rapidly devised to analyse many benzodiazepines and their metabolites with a high degree of sensitivity, but a number of the published procedures suffer from the limitation that interference from co-prescribed drugs has not been fully documented, and some internal standards employed are inappropriate since they consist of drugs commonly prescribed in neurological practice. Consequently, these methods are of limited use in therapeutic drug monitoring, though they can be used in pharmacokinetic studies (Coassolo *et al.*, 1982; Cooper and Drolet, 1982; Greenblatt *et al.*, 1982; Jochemsen and Breimer, 1982; Tomori *et al.*, 1982; Vasiliades and Sahawneh, 1982). In addition, since complicated techniques for sample preparation including back extraction and derivatization procedures may be necessary, some chromatographic methods are slow and labour intensive compared with other methods.

In this context, the use of short reverse-phase $C_{18}$ columns such as Bond ELUT[Tm] columns for sample preparation (Rao *et al.*, 1982) and the development of the Technicon FAST system of automatic sample extraction for HPLC (Bonnafe, 1980; Van der Wal and Snyder, 1981) are of considerable importance.

## Immunoassay techniques

Radioimmunoassay has the advantages of great sensitivity, simplicity, and minimal interferences from biological materials because of the nature of the radioactive label (Bolton, 1981). A major disadvantage, which this method shares to some extent with enzyme immunoassay, is the difficulty in producing antibodies entirely specific for the antigen, particularly in the case of compounds like the benzodiazepines and their metabolites which have a closely related structure (Dixon, 1982). Nevertheless, specific and sensitive assays have recently been described for diazepam (Rutterford and Smith, 1980), lormetazepam (Hümpel *et al.*, 1980), and nitrazepam (Dixon *et al.*, 1981). A radioimmunoassay technique suitable for the rapid screening for benzodiazepines such as diazepam, clonazepam, and nitrazepam and their metabolites in body fluids has also been reported (Robinson *et al.*, 1980).

The enzyme immunoassay kits EMIT dau and EMIT tox produced by the SYVA company give satisfactory results when used semi-quantitatively to screen for benzodiazepine activity in body fluids (Poklis, 1981; Pegon *et al.*, 1982; Slightom *et al.*, 1982). Results are obtained very quickly using these methods, and immunoassay techniques will undoubtedly become increasingly important in toxicology for the rapid screening of benzodiazepines in serum or urine in cases of suspected drug overdose (Slightom *et al.*, 1982).

## Polarography

Polarography is a technique with advantages of convenience and speed and it continues to be used for the analysis of benzodiazepines despite the fact that it requires comparatively large quantities of serum (Brooks, 1980; Zimak *et al.*, 1980). Recently, a full polarographic examination of flurazepam has been carried out (Groves and Smyth, 1981) and a method of analysis described (Smyth and Groves, 1981). The development of a polarographic detector for HPLC applications has overcome the problems of poor selectivity in polarographic methods (Harekamp *et al.*, 1981).

Since most endogenous materials present in body fluids are polarographically inactive, the method can be used for the direct determination of drugs in body fluids, and recent improvements in apparatus design have raised the possibility of examining the metabolism of drugs *in vivo* (Rooney, 1980; Pinkerton and

Lawson, 1982). This is a development of great potential importance in the field of benzodiazepine pharmacokinetics.

**Radioreceptor assays**

The introduction of radioreceptor assays (RR assays, receptor binding assays) constitutes a major advance in the field of benzodiazepine analysis. The procedures already described here assay the concentration in body fluids of parent drug alone or parent drug and major metabolites, without reference to pharmacological activity. Receptor binding assays, on the other hand, have the advantage that they measure total benzodiazepine activity in a sample because they estimate only those parent drugs and metabolites which have pharmacological activity.

The first RR assay was developed for phenothiazines by Snyder and co-workers (Creese and Snyder, 1977; Tune *et al.*, 1980) following the observation that neuroleptic drugs exert antischizophrenic therapeutic effects by blocking brain dopamine receptors (Creese *et al.*, 1976). Shortly afterwards, Squires and Braestrup (1977) and Möhler and Okada (1977a) observed highly specific receptors for benzodiazepines in rat brain, which were characterized by high affinity [$^3$H] diazepam binding. The receptors were shown to be located in the synaptic membranes and to be stereospecific (Möhler and Okada, 1977a; Squires and Braestrup, 1977), and the greatest density of receptors was found to occur in the cortical, cerebellar and hippocampal regions in rat and human brain (Braestrup *et al.*, 1977; Möhler and Okada, 1977a). While the distribution of the benzodiazepine receptors closely parallels the distribution of GABA receptors, GABA itself was found to have no activity in displacing [$^3$H] diazepam from the binding sites (Squires and Braestrup, 1977; Möhler *et al.*, 1978).

The specific binding of [$^3$H] diazepam to the benzodiazepine receptors was saturable while non-specific binding, measured by carrying out the assay with [$^3$H] diazepam in the presence of a large excess of unlabelled diazepam, was not saturable, and amounted to less than 10% of the total receptor binding (Braestrup and Squires, 1977; Möhler and Okada, 1977a,b; Squires and Braestrup, 1977). The benzodiazepines with the most pharmacological activity were found to have the highest affinity for the benzodiazepine receptors, which supported the views that these receptors constitute the site of action of benzodiazepines in the central nervous system (Braestrup and Squires, 1977; Braestrup *et al.*, 1977; Möhler and Okada, 1977a,b; Squires and Braestrup, 1977; Möhler *et al.*, 1978).

In 1979, several groups of workers separately reported RR assays which were based on the principle of competition between [$^3$H] diazepam and unlabelled benzodiazepines in serum for binding sites on isolated brain membrane preparations (Hunt, 1979; Hunt *et al.*, 1979; Owen *et al.*, 1979;

Skolnick *et al.*, 1979). Good correlation was found between the concentration of parent and drug and pharmacologically active metabolites as measured by RR assay and as calculated from results obtained for the same compounds using well established GLC methods (Owen *et al.*, 1979; Skolnick *et al.*, 1979). The original techniques used to obtain the receptor preparations were extremely time-consuming, involving as they did dissection of rat brains, homogenization of tissue in ice-cold 0.32 M sucrose, centrifugation and ultracentrifugation at 0 °C. This was followed by several washes with buffer and final resuspension of the pellet thus obtained in buffer at ph 7.4 (Möhler and Okada, 1977a,b; Squires and Braestrup, 1977). In addition, it was found to be necessary to extract benzodiazepines from serum using an organic solvent such as ether, chloroform, or ethyl acetate before carrying out the assay because a component of serum inhibited receptor binding, though there was considerable intersubject variation in this respect (Owen *et al.*, 1979). RR assays thus seemed to have only a limited scope for routine use, although the lack of cross-reactivity of other drugs had suggested that receptor binding techniques could form the basis of an assay for the routine monitoring of the serum levels of benzodiazepines and their pharmacologically active metabolites (Lader, 1978). The introduction of dry stable rat brain membrane receptor preparations, which were found to be fully equivalent in activity to fresh membranes, therefore constituted a major breakthrough in technique (Lund, 1981). Then the availability of [$^3$H] flunitrazepam, which has a much lower rate dissociation constant than [$^3$H] diazepam allowed the assays to be carried out at room temperature rather than 0 °C (Duka *et al.*, 1979; Lund, 1981). These factors, together with other improvements in technique and apparatus design (Freundlich and Taylor, 1980, 1981; Hung *et al.*, 1982) facilitated the development of assays for a number of benzodiazepines in serum including diazepam, nitrazepam, and clobazam, together with investigations into the mode of action of benzodiazepines at the cellular level (Dorow *et al.*, 1982; Jochemsen *et al.*, 1982; Mennini *et al.*, 1982; Schacht and Baecker, 1982).

In our own laboratory, we are preparing RR assays for several benzodiazepines including diazepam and clobazam for pharmacokinetic studies and the investigation of drug interactions between benzodiazepines and the most commonly prescribed anticonvulsant drugs.

## RESULTS AND DISCUSSION

The RR assay for diazepam and desmethyldiazepam was performed using a modification of the method developed by Lund (1981) (Ratnaraj *et al.*, 1983), and HPLC was carried out according to the method of Ratnaraj *et al.* (1981). It can be seen from Figures 1 and 2 that both methods give linear calibration curves. Since the curve for the RR assay (Figure 1) is linear when the specific binding value ($C_x$) is between 20 and 80% of the specific binding value of the

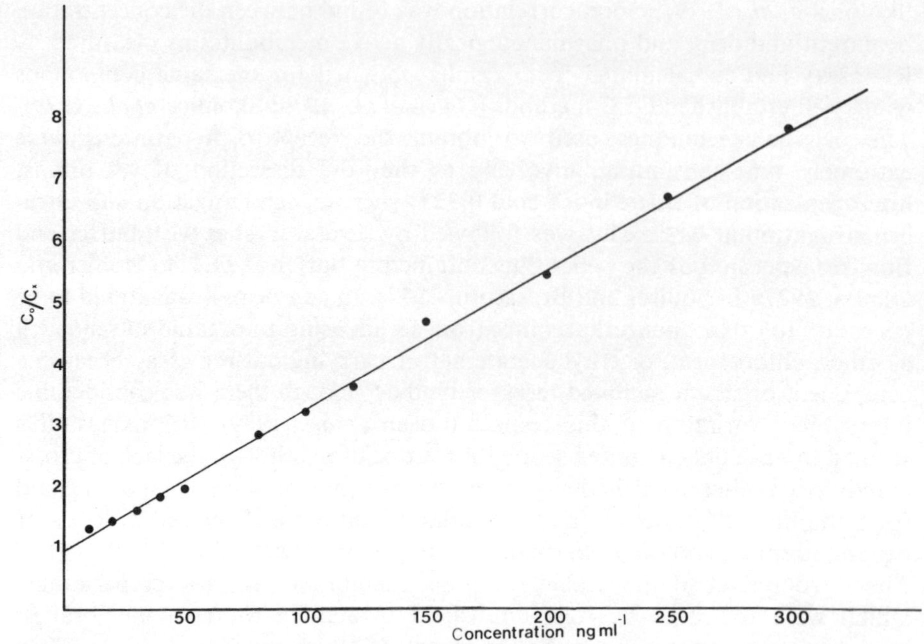


Figure 1 Calibration graph for diazepam by radioreceptor assay. $C_o$, specific binding in the zero standard; $C_x$, specific binding in the standard or sample. Reproduced by permission of the Royal Society of Chemistry

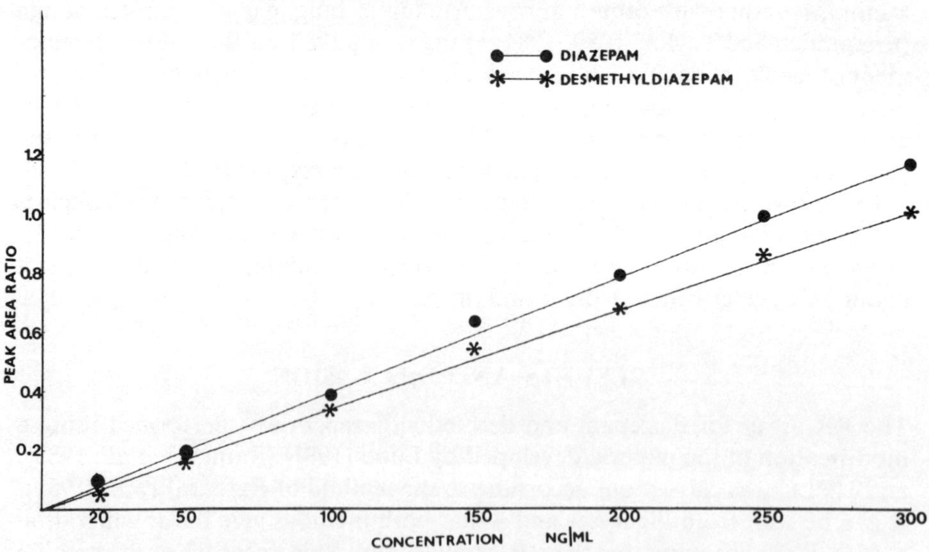


Figure 2 Calibration graph for diazepam and desmethyldiazepam by HPLC

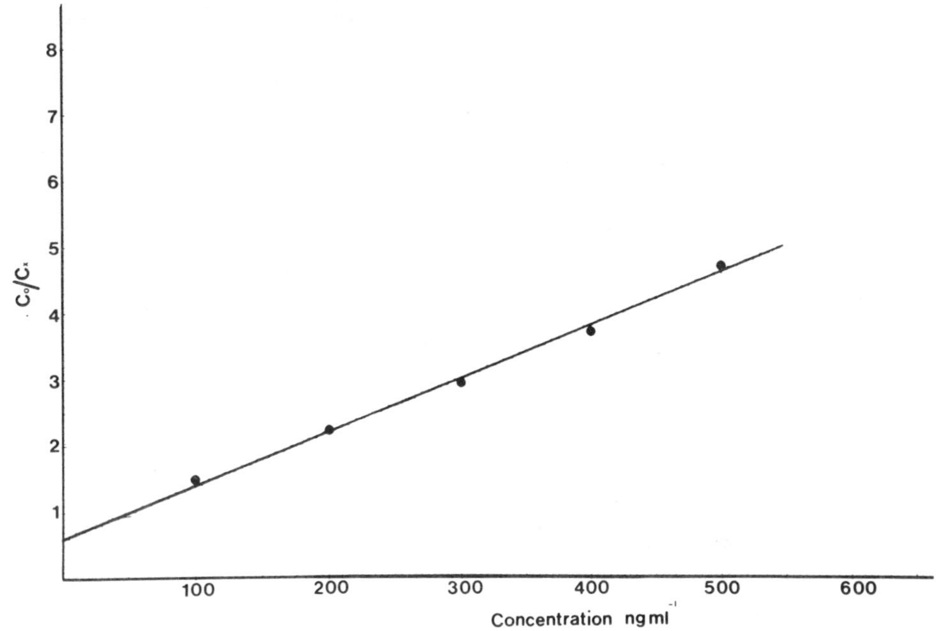


Figure 3 Calibration graph for clobazam by radioreceptor assay

zero standard ($C_0$), the amount of biological fluid used for each assay must be selected to give a value for $C_x$ within these limits.

Clobazam is the first 1,5-benzodiazepine to be used in clinical practice in Europe (Schacht and Baecker, 1982). Radioreceptor and HPLC analyses for clobazam and desmethylclobazam were also carried out using a modification of methods previously described (Lund, 1981; Ratnaraj *et al.*, 1981, 1983). It can be seen from Figures 3 and 4 that both methods give linear calibration curves between 10 and 800 ng $ml^1$ but Figure 5 shows that at very high concentrations (more than 100 ng $ml^1$) the standard curve for the RR assay for clobazam and desmethylclobazam tends to follow a saturation kinetic pattern.

The correlation beteen RR assay and HPLC for diazepam and desmethyldiazepam (Figure 6) and clobazam and desmethylclobazam (Figure 7) is quite acceptable, with a correlation coefficient of 0.97 for diazepam and 0.81 for clobazam. Nevertheless, some differences in what is being measured do exist in biological terms, and it is likely that these differences when closely investigated in the future will be of even greater usefulness than the similarities.

A useful application for RR assays would seem to be in the situation when new benzodiazepines are introduced into clinical practice. This would allow the relative contributions of the parent drug and its metabolites to the pharmacological activity of the whole system to be quantified. Used in

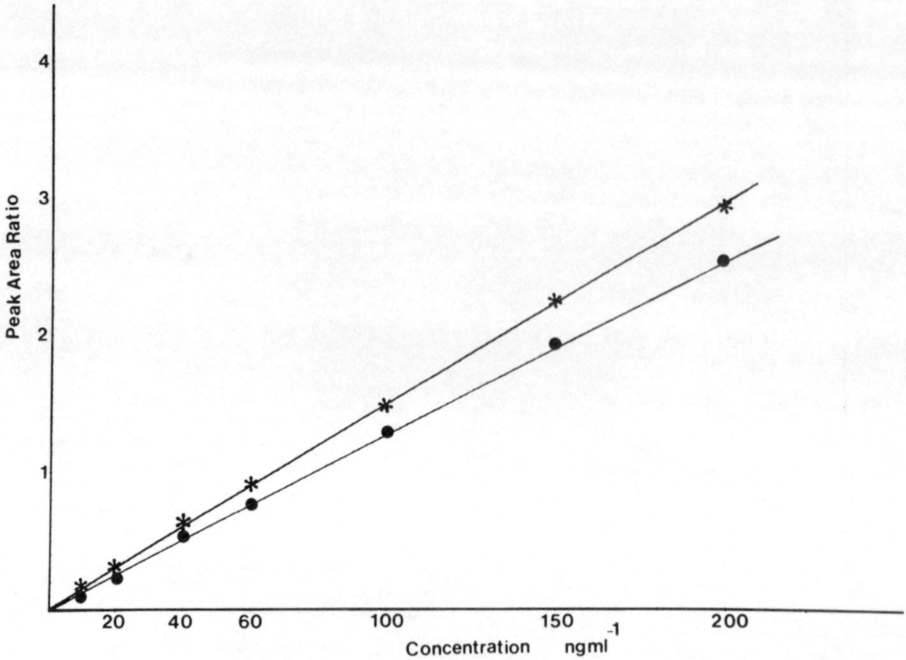


Figure 4 Calibration graph for clobazam and desmethylclobazam by HPLC. ●—● clobazam; *—* desmethylclobazam

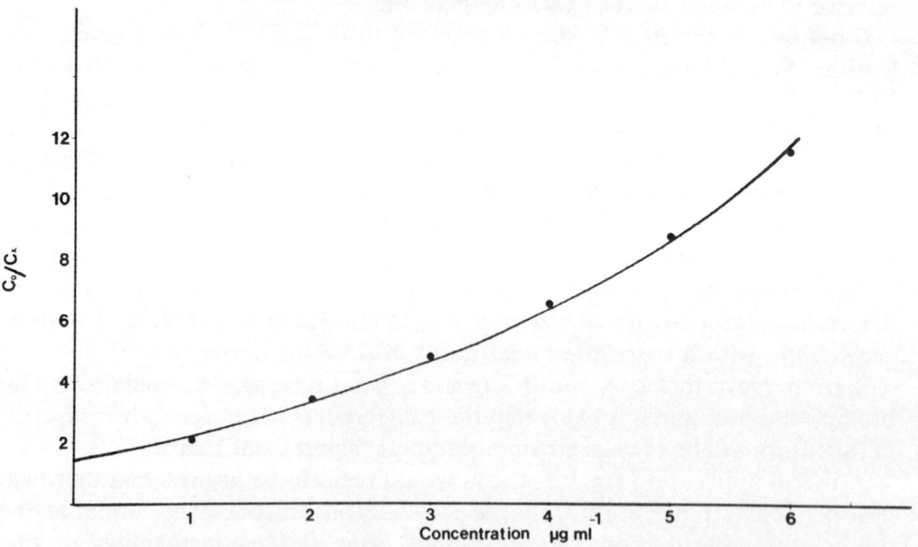


Figure 5 Calibration graph for clobazam at high concentration by radioreceptor assay

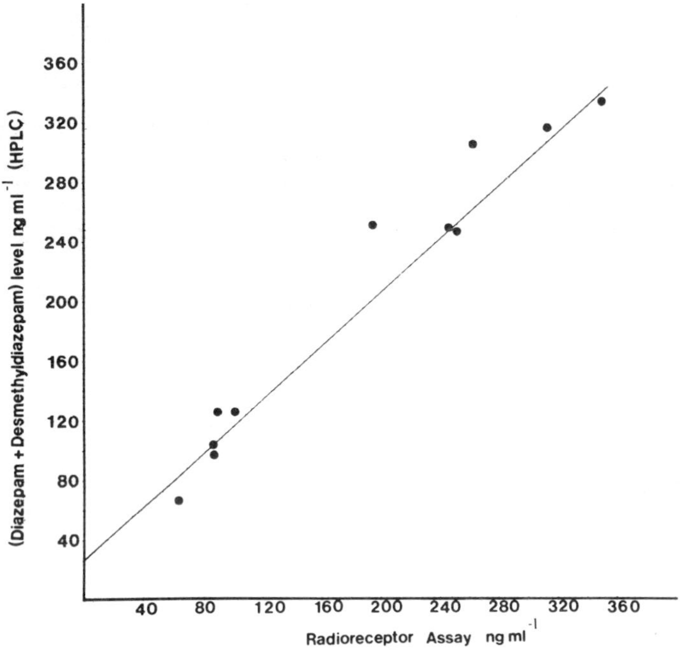


Figure 6 Correlation between plasma concentration of diazepam + desmethyldiazepam measured by HPLC and radioreceptor assay. Correlation coefficient 0.97. Reproduced by permission of the Royal Society of Chemistry

conjunction with HPLC at that stage, RR assays could provide valuable pharmacokinetic data, although application in routine therapeutic drug monitoring at a later stage would seem to be limited. Benzodiazepine agonists and antagonists such as barbiturates, caffeine, $\beta$-carbolines and biciculline are known to interact with benzodiazepine receptors (Tallman *et al.*, 1978; Braestrup *et al.*, 1979, 1980; Nielsen and Braestrup, 1980; Boulenger *et al.*, 1982; De Angelis *et al.*, 1982; File *et al.*, 1982; Skolnick *et al.*, 1982). This would necessarily lead to caution in the interpretation of results obtained by RR assays, except under controlled conditions. These two methods of analysis, RR and HPLC assay, are complementary and must be viewed in a different light dependent upon the particular problem under investigation.

When preparations of benzodiazepine receptors are used primarily as a tool in routine therapeutic monitoring, little or no information can be obtained as to the nature and structure of the receptors and the nature of the bond between receptors and drug. It is clear, however, from reviews of this topic published recently (Olsen, 1981; Costa, 1982; Gallager, 1982; Lippa *et al.*, 1982; Mennini and Garattini, 1982; Müller, 1982; Skolnick and Paul, 1982; Tallman, 1982) that the technique of receptor binding has an enormous potential use

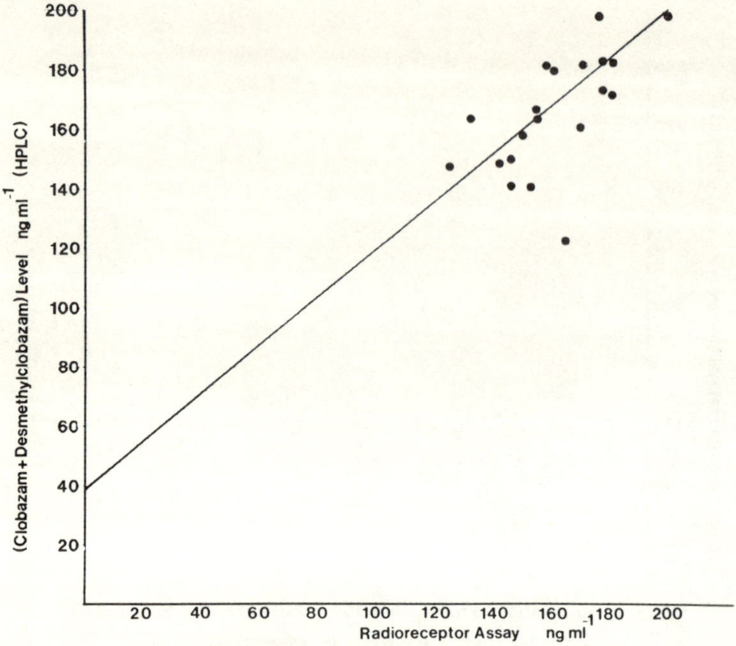


Figure 7 Correlation between plasma concentration of clobazam + desmethylclobazam measured by HPLC and radioreceptor assay. Correlation coefficient 0.81

in structural studies of this kind, and in the elucidation of relationships within the benzodiazepine–GABA receptor complexes in the central nervous system.

## REFERENCES

Badcock, N. R. and Pollard, A. C. (1982). Microdetermination of clonazepam in plasma or serum by electron-capture gas–liquid chromatography. *J. Chrom.*, **230**, 353–361.

Balmer, R., Battegay, R. and von Marschall, R. (1981). Long-term treatment with diazepam. Investigation of consumption habits and the interaction between psychotherapy and psychopharmacotherapy; a prospective study. *Int. Pharmacopsychiat.*, **16**, 221–234.

Bittencourt, P. R. M. and Dhillon, S. (1981). Benzodiazepines: clinical aspects. In: *Therapeutic Drug Monitoring*, pp.255–271 (Eds. Richens, A. and Marks, V.), Churchill Livingstone, London.

Bittencourt, P. R. M., Wade, P., Smith, A. T. and Richens, A. (1981). The relationship between peak velocity of saccadic eye movements and serum benzodiazepine concentration. *Brit. J. clin. Pharmac.*, **12**, 523–533.

Bolton, A. E. (1981). Immunoassay. In: *Immunoassays for the '80s*, pp.69–83 (Eds. Voller, A., Bartlett, A. and Bidwell, D.), M.T.P. Press Ltd., Lancaster.

Bonnafe, M. (1980). *Benzodiazepines in Serum*. Technicon International Divn. Report, FAST-LC Research System.

Boulenger, J.-P., Patel, J. and Marangos, P. J. (1982). Effects of caffeine and theophylline on adenosine and benzodiazepine receptors in human brain. *Neurosci. Lett.*, **30**, 161–166.

Bowden, C. L. and Fisher, J. G. (1982). Relationship of diazepam serum level to antianxiety effects. *J. clin. Psychopharmac.*, **2**, 110–114.

Brachet-Liermain, A., Jarry, Ch., Faure, O., Guyot, M. and Loiseau, P. (1982). Liquid chromatographic determination of clobazam and its major metabolite *N*-desmethylclobazam in human plasma. *Ther. Drug Mon.*, **4**, 301–305.

Braestrup, C., Albrechtsen, R. and Squires, R. F. (1977). High densities of benzodiazepine receptors in human cortical areas. *Nature*, **269**, 702–704.

Braestrup, C., Nielson, M., Krogsgaard-Larsen, P. and Falch, C. (1979). Partial agonists for brain GABA/benzodiazepine receptor complex. *Nature*, **280**, 331–332.

Braestrup, C., Nielson, M. and Olsen, C. E. (1980). Urinary and brain β-carboline-3-carboxylates as potent inhibitors of brain benzodiazepine receptors. *Proc. Natl Acad. Sci. USA*, **7**, 2288–2292.

Braestrup, C. and Squires, R. F. (1977). Specific benzodiazepine receptors in rat brain characterized by high-affinity [$^3$H] diazepam binding. *Proc. Natl Acad. Sci. USA*, **74**, 3805–3809.

Brooks, M. A. (1980). Trace level polarographic analysis of drugs in body fluids. In: *Electroanalysis in Hygiene, Environmental, Clinical and Pharmaceutical Chemistry*, pp.287–298 (Ed. Smyth, W. F.), Elsevier, Amsterdam.

Clark, C. R., Ravis, W. R., Dockens, R., Barksdale, J. M., Arrington, H. S. and D'Andrea, G. H. (1982). Liquid chromatographic determination of chlorazepate decomposition rates. *J. Chrom.*, **240**, 196–201.

Clifford, J. M. and Smyth, W. F. (1974). The determination of some 1,4-benzodiazepines and their metabolites in body fluids: a review. *The Analyst*, **99**, 241–272.

Coassolo, P., Aubert, C., Sumirtapura, Y. and Cano, J. P. (1982). Determination of midazolam and its major hydroxy metabolite in plasma by gas liquid chromatography. Application to a pharmacokinetic study. *J. High Res. Chrom. and Chrom. Comm.*, **5**, 31–37.

Cooper, S. F. and Drolet, D. (1982). Gas liquid chromatographic determination of flurazepam and its major metabolites in plasma with electron-capture detection. *J. Chrom.*, **231**, 321–331.

Costa, E. (1982). Do benzodiazepines act through a GABA-ergic mechanism? In: *The Chemical Regulation of Biological Mechanisms*, pp.77–91 (Eds. Creighton, A. M. and Turner, S.), The Royal Society of Chemistry, London.

Creese, I., Burt, D. R. and Snyder, S. H. (1976). Dopamine receptor binding predicts clinical and pharmacological potencies of antischizophrenic drugs. *Science*, **192**, 481–483.

Creese, I. and Snyder, S. H. (1977). A simple and sensitive radioreceptor assay for antischizophrenic drugs in blood. *Nature*, **270**, 180–182.

Cumin, R., Bonetti, E. P., Scherschlicht, R. and Haefely, W. E. (1982). Use of the specific benzodiazepine antagonist Ro15-1788, in studies of physiological dependence on benzodiazepines. *Experientia*, **38**, 833–834.

Curry, S. H. (1974). Concentration–effect relationships with major and minor tranquilisers. *Clin. Pharmac. Ther.*, **16**, 192–197.

Dasberg, H. H., van der Kleijn, E., Guelen, P. J. R. and van Praag, H. M. (1974). Plasma concentrations of diazepam and of its metabolite *N*-desmethyldiazepam in relation to anxiolytic effect. *Clin. Pharmac. Ther.*, **15**, 473–483.

De Angelis, L., Bertolissi, M., Nardini, G., Traversa, U. and Vertua, R. (1982). Interaction of caffeine with benzodiazepines: behavioral effects in mice. *Arch. int. Pharmacodyn.*, **255**, 89–102.

Debruyne, D., Moulin, M. A., Camsonne, R. and Bigot, M.-C., (1980). Wall-coated open tubular column coupled with nitrogen-selective detector for routine GLC determination of diazepam, meprobamate, phenylbutazone, and thioridazine in serum. *J. Pharm. Sci.*, **69**, 835–838.

De Silva, J. A. F. (1978). Electron capture-GLC in the quantitation of 1,4-benzodiazepines. In: *Antiepileptic drugs: Quantitation and Interpretation*, pp.111–138 (Eds. Pippenger, C. E., Penry, J. K. and Kutt, H.), Raven Press, New York.

Dixon, R. (1982). Radioimmunoassay of benzodiazepines. In: *Methods in Enzymology*, Vol. 84, *Immunochemical Techniques*, Part D. *Selected Immunoassays*, pp.490–515 (Eds. Langone, J. J. and van Vunakis, H.), Academic Press, New York.

Dixon, R., Glover, W. and Earley, J. (1981). Specific radioimmunoassay for flunitrazepam. *J. Pharm. Sci.*, **70**, 230–231.

Dorow, R. G., Seidler, J. and Schneider, H. H. (1982). A radioreceptor assay to study the affinity of benzodiazepines and their receptor binding activity in human plasma including their active metabolites. *Brit. J. clin. Pharmac.*, **13**, 561–565.

Duka, T., Höllt, V. and Herz, A. (1979). In vivo receptor occupation by benzodiazepines and correlation with pharmacological effect. *Brain Res.*, **179**, 147–156.

File, S. E., Bond, A. J. and Lister, R. G. (1982). Interaction between effects of caffeine and lorazepam in performance tests and self-ratings. *J. clin. Psychopharmac.*, **2**, 102–106.

Freundlich, R. and Taylor, D. B. (1980). Two swinging-bucket ultracentrifugal filters for receptor binding assays. *Anal. Biochem.*, **105**, 268–273.

Freundlich, R. and Taylor, D. B. (1981). An improved swinging-bucket ultracentrifugal filter for receptor-binding assays. *Anal. Biochem.* **114**, 103–104.

Gallagher, D. W. (1982). Benzodiazepines and $\gamma$-aminobutyric acid. *Sleep*, **5** (suppl. 1), S3–S11.

Garland, W. A. and Min, B. H. (1979). Determination of clonazepam in human plasma by gas chromatography—negative ion chemical ionization mass spectrometry. *J. Chrom.*, **172**, 279–286.

Garland, W. A. and Powell, M. L. (1981). Quantitative selected ion monitoring (QSIM) of drugs and/or drug metabolites in biological matrices. *J. Chrom. Sci.*, **19**, 392–434.

Goldberg, V. D., Ratnaraj, N., Elyas, A. and Lascelles, P. T. (1983). Recent developments in therapeutic drug monitoring. In: *Research Progress in Epilepsy*, pp.462–483 (Ed. Rose, C.), Pitman Books Ltd., London.

Greenblatt, D. J., Ochs, H. R., Locniskar, A. and Lauven, P. M. (1982). Automated electron-capture gas chromatographic analysis of flunitrazepam in plasma. *Pharmacology*, **24**, 82–87.

Greenblatt, D. J. and Shader, R. I. (1981). Benzodiazepines: analytic techniques. In: *Therapeutic Drug Monitoring*, pp.272–280 (Eds. Richens, A. and Marks, V.), Churchill Livingstone, London.

Groves, J. A. and Smyth, W. F. (1981). Polarographic study of flurazepam and its major metabolites. *Analyst*, **106**, 890–897.

Guidotti, A. (1981). Interaction between benzodiazepine and GABA receptors: a base for the therapeutic action of benzodiazepines. *Neuro-Receptors. Basic and Clinical Aspects*, pp.189–197 (Eds. Usdin, E., Bunney, W. E. (Jr.) and Davis, J. M.), Wiley Interscience, New York.

Hailey, D. M. (1974). Chromatography of the 1,4-benzodiazepines. *J. Chrom.*, **98**, 527–568.

Hallstrom, C. and Lader, M. (1981). Benzodiazepine withdrawal phenomena. *Int. Pharmacopsychiat.*, **16**, 235–244.

Harekamp, H. B., Voogt, W. H., Frei, R. W. and Bos, P. (1981). Continuous flow alternating current polarographic detection of nitrazepam in liquid chromatography. *Anal. Chem.*, **53**, 1362–1365.

Hümpel, M., Nieuweboer, B., Milius, W., Hanke, H. and Wendt, H. (1980). Kinetics and biotransformation of lormetazepam II. Radioimmunologic determinations in plasma and urine of young and elderly subjects: first-pass effect. *Clin. Pharmac. Ther.*, **28**, 673–679.

Hung, C.-R., Hong, J.-S. and Bondy, S. C. (1982). The prevention of an artifact in receptor binding assay by an improved technique. *Life. Sci.*, **30**, 1713–1720.

Hunt, P. (1979). Assay of clobazam in human serum by a radioreceptor technique. *Brit. J. clin. Pharmac.*, 7(suppl. 1), 375–405.

Hunt, P., Husson, J.-M. and Raynaud, J-P. (1979). A radioreceptor assay for benzodiazepines. *J. Pharm. Pharmac.*, **31**, 448–451.

Jochemsen, R. and Breimer, D. D. (1982). Assay of flunitrazepam, temazepam and desalkylflurazepam by capillary gas chromatography with electron capture detection. *J. Chrom.*, **227**, 199–206.

Jochemsen, R., Horbach, G. J. M. J. and Breimer, D. D. (1982). Assay of nitrazepam and triazolam in plasma by a radioreceptor technique and comparison with a gas chromatographic method. *Res. Comm. Chem. Path. Pharmac.*, **35**, 259–273.

Kelly, H., Huggett, A. and Dawling, S. (1982). Liquid-chromatographic measurement of nitrazepam in plasma. *Clin. Chem.*, **28**, 1478–1481.

Kinberger, B. and Wahrgren, P. (1982). Determination of benzodiazepines in serum by high performance liquid chromatography using radially compressed columns and an aqueous methanolic mobile phase. *Analyt. Lett.*, **15(B6)**, 549–557.

Klotz, U., Kangas, L. and Kanto, J. (1980). Clinical pharmacokinetics of benzodiazepines. *Prog. Pharmac.*, **3(no.3)**, 1–71.

Lader, M. (1978). Correlation of plasma concentrations of benzodiazepines with clinical effects. In: *Sleep Research*, pp.99–108 (Eds. Priest, R. G., Pletscher, A. and Ward, J.), M.T.P. Press Limited, Lancaster.

Laughren, T. P., Battey, Y., Greenblatt, D. J. and Harrop, D. S., III (1982). A controlled trial of diazepam withdrawal in chronically anxious outpatients. *Acta psychiat. scand.*, **65**, 171–191.

Lensmeyer, G. L., Rajani, C. and Evenson, M. A. (1982). Liquid-chromatographic procedure for simultaneous analysis for eight benzodiazepines in serum. *Clin. Chem.* **28(11)**, 2274–2278.

Lippa, A. S., Meyerson, L. R. and Beer, B. (1982). Minireview. Molecular substrates of anxiety: clues from the heterogeneity of benzodiazepine receptors. *Life Sci.*, **31**, 1409–1417.

Löscher, W. (1982). Rapid gas chromatographic measurement of diazepam and its metabolites desmethyldiazepam, oxazepam and 3-hydroxydiazepam (temazepam) in small samples of plasma. *Ther. Drug. Mon.*, **4**, 313–318.

Lukas, S. E. and Griffiths, R. R. (1982). Precipitated withdrawal by a benzodiazepine receptor antagonist (Ro15-1788) after seven days of diazepam. *Science*, **217**, 1161–1163.

Lund, J. (1981). Radioreceptor assay for benzodiazepines in biological fluids, using a new dry and stable receptor preparation. *Scand. J. clin. lab. Invest.*, **41**, 275–280.

Mardente, S., Bicchi, C. and Mano, G. M. (1981). GLC-ECD determination of 1-(2-hydroxyethyl)-3-hydroxy-7-chloro-1,3-dihydro-5-(O-fluorophenyl)-2H-1,4-benzodiazepin-2-one (SAS 643) in plasma and urine identification of its main biotransformation products. *Ther. Drug Mon.*, **3**, 351–356.

Marks, J. (1978a). The level of use. In: *The Benzodiazepines: Use, Overuse, Misuse, Abuse,* pp.51–57 (Ed. Marks, J.), M.T.P. Press Limited, Lancaster.

Marks, J. (1978b). Clinical description of benzodiazepine dependence. In: *The*

*Benzodiazepines: Use, Overuse, Misuse, Abuse*, pp.35–37 (Ed. Marks, J.), M.T.P. Press Limited, Lancaster.

McCamish, M. (1980). Quantitative mass spectrometry in pharmacological science. *Eur. J. Mass Spectr.*, **1**, 7–31.

McNicholas, L. F. and Martin, W. R. (1982). The effect of a benzodiazepine antagonist Ro15-1788 in diazepam dependent rats. *Life Sci.*, **31**, 731–737.

Mennini, T., Cotecchia, S., Caccia, S. and Garattini, S. (1982). Benzodiazepines: relationship between pharmacological activity in the rat and in vivo receptor binding. *Pharmac. Biochem. Behav.*, **16**, 529–532.

Mennini, T. and Garattini, S. (1982). Minireview. Benzodiazepine receptors: correlation with pharmacological responses in living animals. *Life Sci.*, **31**, 2025–2036.

Miwa, B. J., Garland, W. A. and Blumenthal, P. (1981). Determination of flurazepam in human plasma by gas chromatography-electron capture negative chemical ionization mass spectrometry. *Anal. Chem.*, **53**, 793–797.

Möhler, H. and Okada, T. (1977a). Benzodiazepine receptor: demonstration in the central nervous system. *Science*, 198, 849–851.

Möhler, H. and Okada, T. (1977b). Properties of $^3$H-diazepam binding to benzodiazepine receptors in rat cerebral cortex. *Science*, **20**, 2101–2110.

Möhler, H., Okada, T., Heitz, P. and Ulrich, J. (1978). Biochemical identification of the site of action of benzodiazepines in human brain by $^3$H-diazepam binding. *Life Sci.*, **22**, 985–995.

Müller, W. E. (1982). The benzodiazepine receptor: a summary. In: *Neuroreceptors. Proceedings of the Symposium, Berlin (West), September 28–29, 1981*, pp.3–41 (Ed. Hucho, F.), Walter de Gruyter & Co., Berlin.

Nielsen, M. and Braestrup, C. (1980). Ethyl β-carboline-3-carboxylate shows differential benzodiazepine receptor interactions. *Nature*, **286**, 606–607.

Olsen, R. W. (1981). Short review. GABA–benzodiazepine–barbiturate receptor interactions. *J. Neurochem.*, **37**, 1–13.

Oswald, I., French, C., Adam, K. and Gilham, J. (1982). Benzodiazepine hypnotics remain effective for 24 weeks. *Brit. med. J.*, **284**, 860–863.

Owen, F., Lofthouse, R. and Bourne, R. C. (1979). A radioreceptor assay for diazepam and its metabolites in serum. *Clin. Chem. Acta*, **93**, 305–310.

Pegon, Y., Pourcher, E. and Vallon, J. J. (1982). Evaluation of the EMIT Tox enzyme immunoassay for toxicological analysis of benzodiazepines. *J. Anal. Tox.*, **6**, 1–3.

Pinkerton, T. C. and Lawson, B. C. (1982). Analytical problems facing the development of electrochemical transducers for in vivo drug monitoring: an overview. *Clin. Chem.*, **28**, 1946–1955.

Poklis, A. (1981). An evaluation of EMIT-dau benzodiazepine metabolite assay for urine drug screening. *J. Anal. Tox.*, **5**, 174–176.

Puglisi, C. V. and de Silva, J. A. F. (1981). Determination of the anxiolytic agent 8-chloro-6-(2-chlorophenyl)-4H-imidazo-[1,5-α] [1,4]-benzodiazepine-3-carboxamide in whole blood, plasma or urine by high-performance liquid chromatography. *J. Chrom.*, **226**, 135–146.

Rao, S. N., Dhar, A. K., Kutt, H. and Okamoto, M. (1982). Determination of diazepam and its pharmacologically active metabolites in blood by Bond ELUT$^{Tm}$ column extraction and reversed phase high-performance liquid chromatography. *J. Chrom.*, **231**, 341–348.

Ratnaraj, N., Goldberg, V. and Lascelles, P. T. (1981). Determination of diazepam and its major metabolites using high performance liquid chromatography. *Analyst*, **106**, 1001–1006.

Ratnaraj, N., Goldberg, V. and Lascelles, P. T. (1983). Receptor binding assay—a new biological method for the determination of drugs in body fluids. *Anal. Proc.* (in press).

Riva, R., Tedeschi, G., Albani, F. and Baruzzi, A. (1981). Quantitative determination of clobazam in the plasma of epileptic patients by gas–liquid chromatography with electron-capture detection. *J. Chrom.*, **225**, 219–224.

Robinson, K., Rutterford, M. G. and Smith, R. N. (1980). A sensitive benzodiazepine radioimmunoassay of broad specificity. *J. Pharm. Pharmac.*, **32**, 773–777.

Rooney, R. (1980). Polarography: don't wait for the renaissance. *Lab. Equip. Digest.*, **18**, 75–79.

Rosenberg, H. C. and Chiu, T. H. (1982). An antagonist-induced benzodiazepine abstinence syndrome. *Eur. J. Pharmac.*, **81**, 153–157.

Rosenthal, D. (1982). Theoretical limitations of gas chromatographic/mass spectrophotometric identification of multicomponent mixtures. *Anal. Chem.*, **54**, 63–66.

Rosser, W. W. (1982). Benzodiazepine prescription to middle-aged women. *Postgrad. Med.*, **71**, 115–120.

Rutterford, M. G. and Smith, R. N. (1980). Radioimmunoassay of diazepam in samples of forensic interest. *J. Pharm. Pharmac.*, **32**, 449–452.

Schacht, U. and Baecker, G. (1982). Effects of clobazam in receptor binding assays. *Drug Devel. Res.*, Suppl. 1, 83–93.

Schütz, H. (1982a). Preface. In: *Benzodiazepines: A Handbook*, p.5 (Ed. Schütz, H.), Springer-Verlag, Berlin.

Schütz, H. (1982b). Presentation of analytical methods. In: *Benzodiazepines. A Handbook*, pp.123–204 (Ed. Schütz, H.), Springer-Verlag, Berlin.

Skolnick, P., Goodwin, F. K. and Paul, S. M. (1979). A rapid and sensitive radioreceptor assay for benzodiazepines in plasma. *Arch. gen. Psychiat.*, **36**, 78–80.

Skolnick, P. and Paul, S. M. (1982). Benzodiazepine receptors in the central nervous system. *Int. Rev. Neurobiol.*, **23**, 103–140.

Skolnick, P., Rice, K. C., Barker, J. C. and Paul, S. M. (1982). Interactions of barbiturates with benzodiazepine receptors in central nervous system. *Brain. Res.*, **233**, 143–156.

Slightom, E. L., Cagle, J. C., McCurdy, H. H. and Castagna, F. (1982). Direct and indirect homogeneous enzyme immunoassay of benzodiazepines in biological fluids and tissues. *J. Anal. Tox.*, **6**, 22–25.

Smyth, W. F. (1982). Electroanalysis of selected organic and organometallic molecules and their metabolites in clinical and environmental chemistry. *Anal. Proc.*, **19**, 82–86.

Smyth, W. F. and Groves, J. A. (1981). The solvent extraction of flurazepam and its major metabolites and their determination by polarography. *Anal. Chim. Acta*, **123**, 175–186.

Squires, R. F. and Braestrup, C. (1977). Benzodiazepine receptors in rat brain. *Nature*, **266**, 732–734.

Study, R. E. and Barker, J. L. (1982). Cellular mechanisms of benzodiazepine action. *J. Am. med. Ass.*, **247**, 2147–2151.

Sumirtapura, Y. C., Aubert, C., Coassolo, Ph. and Cano, J. P. (1982). Determination of 7-amino-flunitrazepam (R020-1815) and 7-amino-desmethylflunitrazepam (R05-4650) in plasma by high performance liquid chromatography and fluorescence detection. *J. Chrom.*, **232**, 111–118.

Tallman, J. F. (1982). From receptor to function in sleep. *Sleep*, **5** (Suppl. 1), S12–S17.

Tallman, J. F., Thomas, J. W. and Gallagher, D. W. (1978). GABAergic modulations of benzodiazepine binding site sensitivity. *Nature*, **274**, 383–385.

Tansella, M., Siciliani, O., Burti, L. *et al.* (1975). *N*-Desmethyldiazepam and amylobarbitone sodium as hypnotics in anxious patients. Plasma levels, clinical efficacy and residual effects. *Psychopharmacologia*, **41**, 81–85.

Tomori, É., Horváth, Gy., Elekes, I., Láng, T. and Körösi, J. (1982). Investigation of the metabolites of tofizopam in man and animals by gas–liquid chromatography-mass spectrometry. *J. Chrom.*, **241**, 89–99.

Toseland, P. A. and Wicks, J. F. C. (1981). Gas chromatography. In: *Therapeutic Drug Monitoring*, pp.85–109 (Eds. Richens, A. and Marks, V.), Churchill Livingstone, London.

Tune, L. E., Creese, I., DePaulo, P. R. *et al.* (1980). Clinical state and serum neuroleptic levels measured by radioreceptor assay in schizophrenia. *Am. J. Psych.*, **137**, 187–190.

Van der Wal, S. J. and Snyder, L. R. (1981). Precision of 'high performance' liquid chromatographic assays with sample pre-treatment. Error analysis for the Technicon 'FAST-LC' system. *Clin. Chem.*, **27**, 1233–1240.

Vasiliades, J. and Sahawneh, T. (1982). Midazolam determination by gas chromatography, liquid chromatography and gas chromatography–mass spectometry. *J. Chrom.*, **228**, 195–203.

Walmsley, L. M. and Chasseaud, L. F. (1981). High-performance liquid chromatographic determination of lorazepam in monkey plasma. *J. Chrom.*, **226**, 155–163.

Williams, P. (1979). Psychotropic drug prescription. In: *Psychosocial Disorders in General Practice*, pp.151–160 (Eds. Williams, P. and Clare, A. W.), Academic Press, London.

Williams, P. (1980). Recent trends in the prescribing of psychotropic drugs. *Health Trends*, **12**, 6–7.

Zimak, J., Gasparic, J. and Volke, J. (1980). Polarographie 1,4-benzodiazepinu. *Cesk Farm Praha*, **29**, 353–362.

## DISCUSSION

## CHAIRMAN: DR M. TRIMBLE

PROFESSOR A. RICHENS: In the studies in which the radioreceptor assay has been compared with the HPLC assay, have you looked at clinical effects? Does your radioreceptor assay relate better to clinical effects than other types of assay?

DR. P. LASCELLES: No, this has not been done but it should now be done.

PROFESSOR M. LADER: You asked the clinicians to give you some feedback about the usefulness of therapeutic monitoring.

The greatest use for therapeutic monitoring is with a drug with a low therapeutic index. The best example is lithium. In psychiatry if you cannot monitor lithium you do not give it. The benzodiazepines are not in that category.

Second is compliance, but with the benzodiazepines one is not so concerned about it.

Third is with a delayed therapeutic effect where you are having to manipulate the dosage of the drug to what you think is going to be the correct therapeutic level; but you cannot predict that quickly because the effects are delayed. The anticonvulsants are an example, where it may take a year before you know whether your manipulation of dose in somebody with infrequent fits has been beneficial or deleterious. Again, however, with the benzodiazepines that is not an important aspect.

The final main use is where people postulate an inverted U-shaped curve of therapeutic response, where failure to respond can be due either to too low a bodily concentration, or more controversially where the plasma concentrations are too high, perhaps with the antidepressants. This again has not been established for the benzodiazepines.

DR. P. TYRER: Could I interject with one more possible use of monitoring, particularly in view of the fact that low grade dependence exists with benzodiazepines? I have found it useful in clinical practice, particularly when I suspect patients to be taking medication from more than one source, to take blood levels. As you have already shown, dosage is one of the few things that does correlate with the blood levels. If the plasma levels are beyond a certain point, and this is wholly inconsistent with the dosage that the patient is allegedly taking, then I can challenge him and say, 'You have been taking more tablets than you have been prescribed'. So detection of abuse is a possibility that may be useful clinically.

Benzodiazepines Divided
Edited by M. R. Trimble


# 16

# Long- and Short-acting Benzodiazepines—A Review of the Role of Benzodiazepines

JAY B. COHN

My objective is to address some clinical aspects of long-acting *v.* short-acting benzodiazepines. First, however, I would like to amend the classifications to include not only short-acting and long-acting, but intermediate-acting benzodiazepines, as well (see Table 1). I want to use some well-known agents as prototypes. Triazolam, with a half-life of 1.2–3.3 hours, is a prototype for the short-acting benzodiazepine group. Ketazolam, with metabolites which increase the half-life from 6 to 25 hours, is a prototype for the intermediate-acting group. This compound is similar to oxazepam, which also has a 6–25 hour half-life. In the long-acting group, diazepam is the representative; diazepam's half-life ranges between 24 and 48 hours (Breimer *et al.*, 1980). An important variable is the presence or absence of long-acting metabolites like desmethyldiazepam, which lengthens the half-life from 36 to 200 hours. Thus the duration of action is dependent on the parent compound, the metabolites, and the pharmacokinetics of both.

With this preface, I would like to discuss briefly the results of a clinical research investigation. Our research team conducted a 200 patient double-blind study comparing alprazolam, lorazepam and placebo. This was a 32 week study, with a single-blind placebo period during weeks 25 through 28. The study inclusionary criteria conformed to the DSM-III guidelines for chronic anxiety states including both somatic and psychological symptoms. The patients were required to have a score on the Hamilton Anxiety Rating Scale of greater than 26 and a score on the 35-item Self-Rating Symptom Scale of greater than 80. The one month of withdrawal, beginning at week 25 and ending at the completion of week 28, provided the opportunity to examine the withdrawal effects in these third and fourth generation drugs of the intermediate-acting class. As part of the prestudy informed consent, patients

Table 1 Pharmacokinetic classification of benzodiazepine derivatives*

| Parent compound | Clinically important active metabolites |
|---|---|
| *Long (effective half-life usually > 24 h)* | |
| Chlordiazepoxide (5–30) | Desmethylchlordiazepoxide |
| | Demoxepam |
| | Desmethyldiazepam (36–200) |
| Diazepam (20–100) | Desmethyldiazepam (36–200) |
| [Clorazepate]† | Desmethyldiazepam (36–200) |
| [Prazepam]† | Desmethyldiazepam (36–200) |
| Medazepam | Desmethylmedazepam |
| | Diazepam |
| | Desmethyldiazepam (36–200) |
| Clobazam (12–60) | Desmethylclobazam |
| [Flurazepam]† | Desalkylflurazepam (40–250) |
| *Intermediate—short (half-life 5–24 h)* | |
| Nitrazepam (15–38) | |
| Flunitrazepam (20–30) | Desmethylflunitrazepam |
| Estazolam (10–30) | ? of hydroxylated metabolite |
| Bromazepam (10–20) | ? 3-hydroxybromazepam |
| Alprazolam (6–20) | |
| Lorazepam (10–20) | |
| Temazepam (8–22) | |
| Oxazepam (4–15) | |
| *Ultrashort (half-life < 5 h)* | |
| Triazolam | |
| Midazolam | |

*Approximate range of elimination half-life values is shown in parentheses when the data are available.

†Brackets indicate prodrugs or drug precursors that do not reach the systemic circulation as such in clinically important amounts.

were informed that there would be a blind placebo period at some time during the protocol. In general, the reported complaints and withdrawal symptoms during that 4 week placebo period conformed to those listed by Rickels *et al.* (1982) and Petursson and Lader (1981) (see Table 2). Rickels found only 20 out of 158 patients (13%) had symptoms; these results are indeed similar to ours.

Seventy-two patients entered the seventh month, the placebo period, of our study. More than half (53%) made no comments regarding any significant change in their mental or physical status. Of the remaining half (47%), 24 patients dropped from the study. Of those 24 patients, only six required immediate examination and/or telephone intervention. Of those six, four patients had symptoms which required more than encouragement, reassurance

Table 2 Withdrawal symptoms and numbers of patients experiencing them

| | No. of cases | | No. of cases |
|---|---|---|---|
| Anxiety, tension | 16 | Loss of appetite | 9 |
| Agitation, restlessness | 16 | Nausea, dry retching | 9 |
| Bodily symptoms of anxiety | 16 | Depression | 8 |
| Irritability | 9 | Perspiration | 7 |
| Lack of energy | 6 | Metallic taste, hyperosmia | 12 |
| Impaired memory and concentration | 4 | Blurred vision, sore eyes, photophobia | 9 |
| Depersonalization, derealization | 4 | Incoordination, vertigo | 9 |
| Sleep disturbance | 16 | Hyperacusis | 6 |
| Tremor, shakiness | 13 | Paraesthesia | 5 |
| Headache | 12 | Hypersensitivity to touch, pain | 4 |
| Muscle pains, aches, twitchings | 10 | Paranoid reaction | 2 |

Table 3 Symptoms or side-effects emerging or worsening during withdrawal from alprazolam

| | No. of reports | | No. of reports |
|---|---|---|---|
| Fatigue | 6 | Sedation | 1 |
| Weakness | 8 | Confusion | 1 |
| Dizziness | 9 | Nausea | 7 |
| Faintness | 4 | Abdominal pain | 1 |
| Unsteadiness | 4 | Constipation | 1 |
| Palpitations | 7 | Headache | 4 |
| Hand tremor | 1 | Blurred vision | 4 |
| Lightheadedness | 7 | Bad taste in mouth | 1 |
| Change in appetite | 4 | Nasal congestion | 1 |
| Depression | 1 | Eye burning | 1 |
| Sleep disturbance | 3 | | |

Table 4 Symptoms or side-effects emerging or worsening during withdrawal from lorazepam

| | No. of reports | | No. of reports |
|---|---|---|---|
| Fatigue | 1 | Nausea | 3 |
| Weakness | 3 | Stomach discomfort | 1 |
| Dizziness | 1 | Diarrhoea | 3 |
| Unsteadiness | 1 | Headache | 1 |
| Lightheadedness | 1 | Tinnitus | 1 |
| Ataxia | 5 | Blurred vision | 3 |
| Palpitations | 2 | Numbness | 1 |
| Change in appetite | 6 | Concentration difficulty | 1 |
| Excessive weight loss | 1 | Sleep disturbance | 2 |

and/or explanation. These four patients were given small doses of lorazepam for several days to help them with their symptoms. The doses did not exceed 1.0 m of lorazepam twice daily, for 4 days.

Shown in Tables 3 and 4 are the symptoms of patients in both the alprazolam and lorazepam treatment groups. The symptoms were approximately equal in frequency and severity for both. Some symptoms were due to a resurgence of the anxiety process and, therefore, were independent of drug discontinuance. It is significant that there were no serious side-effects which required intervention. Especially, there were no convulsions, no psychoses, and no neurological sequelae. As a result of this study, we believe we have developed additional evidence that therapeutic doses (not abuse or toxic doses) of the intermediate-acting benzodiazepines, when used for a period of 6 months, produce relatively few serious withdrawal effects.

There are several clinical indications for shorter-acting drugs. Obviously, use as an hypnotic is a prime consideration. Additional indications include anxiety, detoxification in alcohol related problems, and as a preoperative medication, prior to surgery. As Nicholson (1981) has indicated:

> 'Some benzodiazepines may not lead to obvious effects on performance, such as nordiazepam and clobazam, and the persistence of residual sequelae may not relate obviously to eliminate half-lives (as with diazepam and possibly flunitrazepam). However, benzodiazepines with mean half-lives of less than 8 hours may have residual sequelae, whereas hypnotics with mean half-lives that are greater than 16 hours are likely to lead to impaired performance and/or anxiolytic effects the next day.'

The intermediate class, therefore, has a place in sleep disorders in which patients have both difficulty in falling asleep (latency) and difficulty in staying asleep (maintenance). Additional indications for the 'intermediate' group include muscle relaxation and, of course, anxiety, particularly where frequent dosing may present a problem of compliance.

Long-acting first generation drugs, or drugs that break down to their metabolites (such as diazepam), are widely used for sedation. Where the lipid solubility is connected with the patient's awareness of being on a drug we see the 'drug effect' noted by patients. Hollister (1981a) discussed a preference for diazepam and its long-acting characteristics. He stated,

> 'I suspect that physical, chemical and pharmacokinetic factors are involved. Diazepam is the most highly lipid-soluble drug in the (benzodiazepine) group; and, lipid solubility facilitates passage across membranes of the gut and the brain. Thus, the drug is rapidly absorbed and rapidly reaches the target organ. Patients

quickly know they have a drug effect. However, the presence of a moderately long parent drug and an even longer acting metabolite permits accumulation of the drug during chronic dosing. Thus one attains a sustained drug effect that requires infrequent dosing. The rapid onset of action may be predisposed to some abuse of the drug but accumulation with repeated doses would tend to mitigate that possibility.'

Hollister (1981b) also stated:

> 'The problem is that the withdrawal reactions following abuse are much more severe and abrupt with the short-acting drugs, because the rapidity of onset and the severity of withdrawal reactions are functions of the rate of decline from high plasma concentrations. The longer-acting drugs have a built-in tapering off action that allows some restitution to be made before it gets out of control, which the short-acting drugs lack.'

We agree with Breimer (Breimer *et al.*, 1980) who stated that metabolic rate differences:

> 'may be very important clinically because pharmacokinetic factors will determine the duration of drug effect and pharmacokinetic parameters constitute the basis for a rational dosage regimen. For the various clinical indications of benzodiazepines that required duration of drug action differs quite fundamentally. In anticonvulsant and antianxiety treatment, continuous treatment is pursued, so that compounds with long elimination half-lives of parent drug or active metabolites are of advantage. If, on the other hand, a benzodiazepine is taken as a hypnotic, the duration of action should be restricted to the night, hence a compound with a short elimination half-life is to be preferred.'

Having reviewed some of the relevant literature, and having our experience with withdrawal reactions and a long list of clinical studies with various benzodiazepines, I have a preference for the shorter acting, shorter half-life, fourth generation, newer, cleaner benzodiazepines. These include alprazolam (Cohn, 1982), ketazolam and triazolam rather than the first generation diazepam. In utilizing shorter acting benzodiazepines, I am able to mitigate the metabolite accumulation which is associated with the first generation drugs; thus, the shorter acting benzodiazepines are, in my opinion, significantly safer. As usual, there is an exception to this generalization. Patients who are using high level benzodiazepines for periods in excess of 4 months are a special group.

Their withdrawal and drug interaction complications will be diminished on the first generation, longer acting drugs. Thus, in drug abuse, non-therapeutic, high level, long-duration use, the withdrawal reactions and the drug interactions will be less troublesome with the first generation, longer acting diazepam. The metabolites remain in the blood up to 200 hours, and therefore smooth out the withdrawal. It is thus a pharmacokinetic withdrawal rather than a dosage withdrawal effect which allows for a smoother withdrawal from that particular drug.

## ACKNOWLEDGEMENT

Special thanks to Ms Betty Porter for her work in the writing of this chapter.

## REFERENCES

Breimer, D. D., Jochemsen, R. and Von Albert, H. H. (1980). Pharmacokinetics of benzodiazepines short-acting vs. long-acting. *Arzneim-Forsch./Drug Res.*, **30 (1)**, Nr. 5a.

Cohn, J. B. (1982). Multicenter double-blind efficacy and safety study comparing alprazolam, diazepam and placebo in clinically anxious patients. *J. clin. Psychiat.*, **42**, 347–351.

Hollister, L. E. (1981a). Benzodiazepines—an overview. *Brit. J. Clin. Pharmac.*, **11** (Suppl.), 117s–119s.

Hollister, L. E. (1981b). Management of the anxious patient prone to drug abuse. *J. clin. Psychiat.*, **42**, 35–39.

Nicholson, A. N. (1981). The use of short- and long-acting hypnotics in clinical medicine. *Brit. J. clin. Pharmac.*, **11**, 615–695.

Petursson, H. and Lader, M. H. (1981). Withdrawal from long-term benzodiazepines treatment. *Brit. med. J.*, **285**, 643–645.

Rickels, K., Case, W. and Downing, R. (1982). Issues in long-term treatment with diazepam. *Psychopharmac. Bull.*, **18**, 38–41.

## DISCUSSION

## CHAIRMAN: PROFESSOR A. RICHENS

THE CHAIRMAN: Could I bring us back to this question of the short-acting drugs and rebound phenomenon which one might get with use in anxiety.

DR. COHN: I see the anxiety they have from the rebound of a very short-acting drug as useful for people to get started in the morning. If it is disabling during the day-time then I think the patient is on the wrong drug.

PROFESSOR I. OSWALD: I should perhaps explain that in our studies we were doing a whole lot of laboratory tests of skills, in the morning, at lunch time, and in the late afternoon. There was still some residual impairment in the morning, very slight from triazolam and from loprazolam, not in the afternoon. The anxiety ratings were made on the basis of the whole day. I am sure the anxiety feelings were arising in the late afternoon and evening, not in the morning.

DR. P. TYRER: Both the patients that Malcolm Lader and I have studied independently have been patients who have not abused their benzodiazepines at all. They have been given therapeutic doses and they have still had significant withdrawal symptoms when the drugs have been stopped. I found your results very interesting, although in some ways still a little bit disturbing as the patients were taking drugs regularly for 6 months and a significant proportion of them have symptoms on withdrawal. In clinical practice these patients who get minor withdrawal symptoms, unless they are warned about it in advance, would think that their anxiety was coming back and therefore continue their tablets. It could therefore set off a cycle of dependence.

I wondered if you had any experience at all about the differences between the intermediate and the long-acting drugs because we found in our study that lorazepam produced a significantly higher number of withdrawal symptoms than diazepam and this may be related to its elimination half-life.

DR. COHN: Unfortunately, both of the drugs here were really intermediate- to short-acting, and if we could have done it against diazepam with the same group we would have had much more information.

PROFESSOR OSWALD: Can I address a question to our receptor experts here? We have been talking about withdrawal effects this morning. As I see it, if the brain is exposed to a drug—let us say one that will enhance sleep—then over a period of time the brain changes its machinery to counteract that drug, to produce the something created that will reduce sleep. You take the drug away and you are left with that which has been created, that is to say something that will reduce sleep and so you have less sleep for a period until, through turnover, recovery naturally occurs. Is it possible to put this into a coherent form for what happens in the brain?

DR. L. L. IVERSEN: It is basically a phenomenon that we do not understand. At the moment I do not think the pharmacologists can offer any good advice, except tapering off; it seems to be better than abrupt withdrawal.

PROFESSOR OSWALD: Are we obliged to think in terms of receptors on the surface of the cell, or can we think of something going on inside?

DR. L. L. IVERSEN: The benzodiazepine receptors on the surface of target cells do not seem to adapt; there are no obvious changes in either their number or properties after chronic drug treatment in animal studies. The dependence syndrome, therefore, depends on changes at some stage removed from the primary drug–receptor interaction.

PROFESSOR OSWALD: It is really a kind of learning, and we do not know what is the change in the brain cells that underlies a memory.

DR. STRAW: We have some data comparing alprazolam to diazepam, and, as you know, the half-life of alprazolam is similar to that of lorazepam. Again, these patients were dosed for 6 month periods, and then followed up with a 2 week placebo withdrawal period. The design of the study could perhaps be criticized in that we did not look at the patients except for once at the end of that 2 week withdrawal, but at least, based on that information, the symptom emergence that occurred during that period of time was similar for both alprazolam and diazepam.

DR. TYRER: When we compared blood levels in patients being withdrawn from diazepam those who had a gradual reduction in blood levels of desmethyldiazepam had fewer withdrawal symptoms than those who had a rapid reduction. My very primitive concept of what is going on is the old one of homoeostasis at a physiological level: if, in fact, you can have gradual change in a physiological system when there is a withdrawal of an exogenous agent, then there is much less likelihood of major reaction. Whether or not that occurs at a receptor level or a cellular level is obviously unclear.

THE CHAIRMAN: What do we know about the time course of the development of tolerance? Is 6 weeks' any different from 6 years' treatment? Are the withdrawal effects any different in the two cases?

DR. TYRER: The evidence is that the longer patients are taking the drug the higher the risk of withdrawal, but once you get beyond a year it does not seem to make much difference. The risk is conventionally regarded as between 6 months and a year.

PROFESSOR OSWALD: We have done many studies of people's sleep with many different drugs. I am sorry to refer to triazolam again, but we did use a very large dose by British standards, and with 3 weeks' taking of triazolam 0.5 mg we encountered the worst withdrawal insomnia that I have ever encountered, with people getting as little as 40 minutes of sleep in a night and an average of 270 minutes on the first withdrawal night when they went on to a placebo.

DR. STRAW: There are studies in the literature to the contrary.

THE CHAIRMAN: Does that reflect the high dose that was used?

PROFESSOR OSWALD: I am sure it reflects the high dose. You saw the cortisol leap up immediately too.

THE CHAIRMAN: Yes, I know.

Benzodiazepines Divided
Edited by M. R. Trimble


# 17

# Benzodiazepines in the Treatment of Anxiety and Tension States

PETER TYRER

Anxiety and tension states are very common in all forms of clinical practice but their classification is not uniformly agreed. It is important to understand the main areas of controversy to determine the place of benzodiazepines in the treatment of these disorders. Both of the latest classificatory systems, ICD-9 (World Health Organization, 1978) and DSM-111 (American Psychiatric Association, 1980) separate stress and adjustment reactions with predominant anxiety from anxiety neurosis. DSM-111 also subdivides anxiety disorders into panic disorder and generalized anxiety disorder, and agoraphobia is also subdivided into two groups depending on the presence or absence of panic attacks. It is preferable to deal with the use of benzodiazepines in each of these conditions separately.

## ACUTE STRESS REACTIONS

Stress reactions (or post-traumatic stress disorder in the American literature) are transient disorders of mood occurring in apparently normal individuals in response to exceptional physical and mental stress. The clinician who is called upon to treat such anxiety usually has to act without full knowledge of the subject and the specific personal impact of the stress. He has to guess whether the disorder is short-lived or not and whether the sufferer was 'normal' prior to the stress. The significance of these decisions is that they determine both whether drug therapy is indicated and, if so, for how long.

Drug therapy may be considered ill-advised if the stress has important personal implications that need to be 'worked through'. There is an abundant literature on the necessity for grief and other emotions to be experienced openly after major loss if subsequent depressive illness is to be avoided (Freud,

1917; Lindemann, 1944; Bowlby, 1973). If a benzodiazepine is prescribed to alleviate the distress that immediately follows an unexpected bereavement it would probably help in the short-term but if it also aids the process of denial it may create long-term pathology. Benzodiazepines are popular in anaesthesia because they create anterograde amnesia for the events immediately following drug administration (Dundee and Pandit, 1972). This may be ideal to reduce the emotional impact of tooth extraction but a major handicap if it suppresses the memory of events after bereavement.

The treatments of stress reactions are rarely subjected to controlled trials of efficacy because of their unpredictability and emergency nature. If drug therapy is chosen, benzodiazepines are probably the drugs of choice although some still recommend barbiturates or paraldehyde for this purpose. As treatment rarely continues for more than a few days it is argued that such drugs are justified whereas they would not be considered for less acute disorders. This practice cannot be defended; barbiturates and other general depressant drugs offer no advantages over the benzodiazepines and their poor safety record and high predilection to dependence even in this population should prohibit their use.

The dosage of benzodiazepines in stress disorder should be flexible in both quantity and frequency. It is preferable to decide on an agreed maximum daily dosage before starting treatment and to take the drug in intermittent flexible dosage within the daily range. Because most stress reactions occur in individuals who have not been exposed to these drugs before, it is appropriate to set the maximum daily dosage at about 15 mg of diazepam or its equivalent per day. Severe insomnia occurring in response to stress may also be treated in the same way. It is unusual to continue therapy for longer than a few days and certainly no longer than one week. The danger of continuing beyond this point is that the pleasurable antianxiety qualities of benzodiazepines may so impress the patient that further prescriptions are requested long after the initial stress has been overcome.

## ANXIETY STATES

Anxiety states differ from stress and adjustment reaction in that they tend to be precipitated by less serious events than in acute stress reactions and occur in individuals who are more anxiety prone. The old concept of the 'neurotic constitution' (Slater, 1943) is now regarded as too simple, but is still an excellent way of demonstrating the relationship between personality, predisposition, and external stress (Figure 1).

The symptoms of anxiety include the psychological ones of irritability, apprehension, restlessness, and awareness of threat, and bodily ones, including muscular tension, trembling, palpitations, sweating, nausea, and

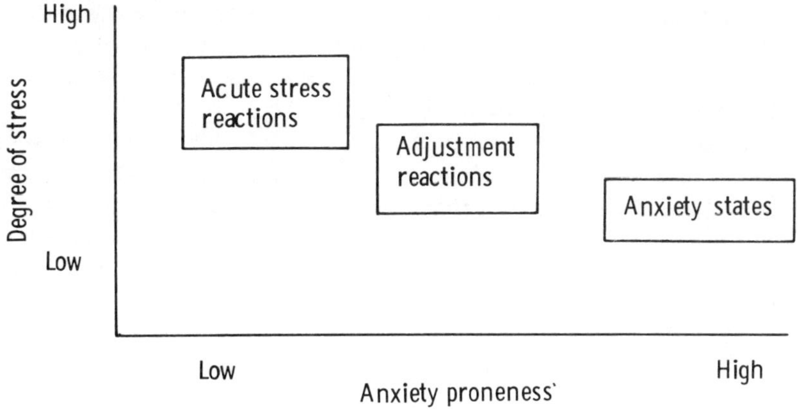


Figure 1 Relationship between stress, anxiety proneness, and pathological anxiety

giddiness. Anxiety therefore best illustrates one of the features of all psychiatric illness, the presence of both psychic and somatic components. There is great variation in the relative intensity of psychic and somatic symptoms and in the way they are interpreted by the sufferer. At one extreme is the old term 'anxiety hysteria', considered to be dissociation of anxiety in the form of phobias, and at the other are the anxious disorders expressed solely as bodily complaints, considered to be conversion phenomena or 'anxiety equivalents' (Freud, 1894) or somatosthenic anxiety (Tyrer, 1982). Nobody has satisfactorily explained this variation in symptomatology but it is important in management.

Benzodiazepines are probably the drug treatment of choice in most anxiety states but the evidence for this is rather less clear than many believe. There are some data from clinical trials that they are more effective than the barbiturates (Lader *et al.*, 1974), the propanediols (Rickels *et al.*, 1971), and low dosage antipsychotic drugs (Smith and Chassan, 1964), but in a review of 52 clinical trials of benzodiazepines versus other antianxiety agents in the treatment of anxiety neurosis only three showed the benzodiazepines to be superior (Greenblatt and Shader, 1974). In recent years antidepressants have also been shown to have antianxiety properties. Some studies of drug treatment of minor affective disorders have shown no difference between the antianxiety effects of tricyclic antidepressants and benzodiazepines (Johnstone *et al.*, 1980), and many of the newer antidepressants such as doxepin, dothiepin, trazodone and zimelidine have demonstrable antianxiety activity (Snyder and Yamamura, 1977; Montgomery *et al.*, 1981; Barnes and Bridges, 1983). These drugs may be preferred to benzodiazepines in the treatment of anxiety states if secondary depressive symptoms are prominent.

Anxiety symptoms presenting for the first time in middle or late life with no obvious relationship to severe stress are sometimes regarded as 'depressive equivalents' (West and Dally, 1959) or masked depression. On these grounds they should be regarded as suitable for antidepressant therapy. Pollit and Young (1971) support this notion from a review of the effectiveness of monoamine oxidase inhibitor antidepressants in different age groups. The evidence from these studies suggests that there is a type of anxiety state that is responsive to antidepressant drug therapy and therefore less appropriate to treat with benzodiazepines. The main differences between true and false anxiety states are illustrated (Table 1).

Table 1 Differences between true and false anxiety states

| True anxiety states | False anxiety states (primary diagnosis not that of anxiety) |
|---|---|
| Anxiety proneness common | Stable premorbid personality common |
| Diffuse phobic symptoms | Clear-cut phobic symptoms |
| True panic not very common (anxiety is predictable) | True panic common |
| No personality change | Personality change common |
| Depressive symptoms uncommon | Depressive symptoms may be prominent |

## PANIC DISORDER

Panic disorder is not recognized in the *International Classification of Disease* because it is subsumed under anxiety states. In the DSM-111 it is described as a disorder 'manifested by the sudden onset of intense apprehension, fear, or terror, often associated with feelings of impending doom'. If such attacks occur in patients with generalized anxiety the diagnosis is still that of panic disorder. The main reason for this diagnostic separation is the apparent differential response to behaviour therapy and drug treatment. The work of Klein has been largely responsible for the elevation of panic to a diagnostic category in its own right, and nearly 20 years ago he was one of the first to show that antidepressant drugs were of benefit in anxiety disorders characterized by panic as a major symptom (Klein, 1964). Soon afterwards, the apparent demonstration of experimentally induced panic by Pitts and McClure (1967) in some anxious patients also supported the validity of panic disorder as a separate diagnosis. Klein and his colleagues argue that panic disorder should not be treated with benzodiazepines as it is more responsive to antidepressant drug therapy. However, as he himself admits (Klein *et al.*, 1980), no controlled studies have been carried out on the effectiveness of drug treatment in panic disorder alone. On this side of the Atlantic, the presence of panic is not normally considered to be a contraindication to benzodiazepine therapy.

## PHOBIC DISORDERS

Agoraphobia and social phobias are appropriate for treatment with benzodiazepines but monosymptomatic phobias, such as those of spiders, dogs, and heights, are best treated by exposure techniques. In agoraphobia and social phobia benzodiazepines should never be thought of as sole therapy. Treatment should never be by a fixed dosage regimen as phobic disorders are characterized by situational anxiety. There is some doubt whether it is best to give the benzodiazepine some hours before exposure to the phobic stimulus in the hope that it will alleviate anticipatory anxiety, or to give the drug just before exposure so that anxiety at the time of phobic confrontation is reduced pharmacologically. In an early study it was found that reduction of anticipatory anxiety was more important, as better results were found with behaviour therapy when the benzodiazepine was taken 4 hours before phobic exposure (Marks *et al.*, 1972). However, in a later study, this positive 'waning diazepam effect' was not found (Hafner and Marks, 1976). As the evidence is unclear, it is better for each patient to experiment with the timing of benzodiazepine therapy to find the most appropriate pharmacological response.

The category of agoraphobic disorder with panic attacks described in DSM-111 has again been studied most closely by Klein and his co-workers. There have been more controlled trials of drug therapy with this disorder, and there is some evidence that imipramine is superior to at least one benzodiazepine, chlordiazepoxide, in treatment (McNair and Kahn, 1981). There is also good evidence that monoamine oxidase inhibitors are effective in the treatment of phobic disorders (Lipsedge *et al.*, 1973; Tyrer *et al.*, 1973; Ravaris *et al.*, 1976), although this evidence is based on placebo studies and no control comparisons with benzodiazepines have been published. However, it is fair to add that most phobic patients have received prolonged courses of benzodiazepines without significant effect before receiving antidepressants or monoamine oxidase inhibitors. This suggests that in chronic phobic disorders benzodiazepines are generally ineffective.

## COMPARISON OF BENZODIAZEPINES WITH NEWER ANTIANXIETY DRUGS

Until recently, benzodiazepines have been considered as the unequivocal first-choice drug treatment for anxiety states because of their specificity, safety, and low risk of dependence. The increasing evidence for low grade physical dependence with these drugs has altered the picture somewhat. Drugs which are not quite as effective as benzodiazepines may be preferable in patients if they have little or no risk of dependence. It has to be said that no drug satisfying these requirements has been shown to exist. Chlormethiazole is a non-benzodiazepine drug that has a simple structure developed from part of the vitamin B molecule. It is an effective antianxiety drug and as an hypnotic it has similar efficacy to temazepam (Briggs *et al.*, 1980). However, like the barbiturates and benzodiazepines, it facilitates GABA transmission, and may produce physical dependence (Hession *et al.*, 1979). Chlormezanone has been in clinical practice for many years and no reports of serious dependence have been published. In adequate dosage (e.g. 800 mg daily) it is equivalent to the benzodiazepines in efficacy but also produces more sedation (Rickels *et al.*, 1974). It is a reasonable alternative to the benzodiazepines if there is reason to suspect that the anxious patient is liable to become dependent on drug therapy. Benzoctamine has also been available for some years but it has never enjoyed much popularity. It has been too little used to give firm recommendations about its indications.

## DIFFERENCES BETWEEN BENZODIAZEPINES

Generally there are far too many benzodiazepines commercially available, and as a group their similarities vastly outweigh their differences. The major variants are pharmacokinetic ones and the division of benzodiazepines into short- and long-acting compounds (Committee on Review of Medicines, 1980) has been widely accepted. This division is more important in the treatment of insomnia than of anxiety. In healthy adults there is little evidence that a short-acting benzodiazepine is any way superior to a long-acting one, or vice versa. Differences that have been found between benzodiazepines can usually be accounted for, the drugs not being given in equivalent dosage. In the elderly, however, there may be some merits in giving a shorter acting compound because of the dangers of accumulation with long-acting ones. If, however, the benzodiazepine is given in intermittent flexible dosage these problems will not arise and any type of benzodiazepine can be used.

## OTHER ANTIANXIETY DRUG TREATMENTS

Beta-adrenoceptor blocking drugs probably act peripherally in relieving anxious symptoms. In low dosage they reduce tachycardia and tremor and may be particularly effective in somatosthenic anxiety, in which anxiety is perceived primarily as an abnormality in bodily symptomatology. In such patients beta-adrenoceptor blockade is at least as effective as treatment with benzodiazepines (Tyrer and Lader, 1974). Such forms of anxiety are not particularly common in psychiatric practice. Patients with mixed features of hypochondriacal concern over certain somatic symptoms, together with psychological symptoms of anxiety, are much more common. The combination of the benzodiazepine and a beta-adrenoceptor blocking drug is therapeutically useful in such patients, and shows some superiority over a benzodiazepine given alone (Hallstrom *et al.*, 1981). Beta-adrenoceptor blocking drugs also have the advantage of no potential for dependence.

Table 2 Effectiveness of benzodiazepines in different types of anxiety disorder

| Order of efficacy | Acute stress reactions | Generalized anxiety | Panic disorder | Agoraphobia | Agoraphobia with panic | Somatosthenic anxiety |
|---|---|---|---|---|---|---|
| 1 | Benzodiazepines | Benzodiazepines | No | MAOIs | MAOIs* | Benzodiazepines† |
| 2 | Neuroleptics | Neuroleptics | satisfactory | Tricyclic anti-depressants | Tricyclic anti-depressants* | Beta-blockers† |
| 3 | New anxiolytics | New anti-depressants | evidence | Benzodiazepines | Benzodiazepines | Tricyclic anti-depressants |
| 4 | Beta-blockers | Tricyclic anti-depressants | available | Neuroleptics | Neuroleptics | New anti-depressants |

* Equal efficacy
†Equal efficacy

Other non-benzodiazepine antianxiety drugs are likely to be available in the near future. They include buspirone, suriclone, and their analogues. There is little to suggest that they are more effective than benzodiazepines but they may be of value if they are less prone to dependence.

## CONCLUSION

Benzodiazepines are still the drug therapy of choice for most anxiety states but in cases of panic and agoraphobic disorder they are less effective than monoamine oxidase inhibitors and antidepressants (Table 2). The recent evidence that they predispose to low grade dependence in chronic dose means that they are no longer the automatic drug therapy for anxiety states. Nevertheless, an equally effective drug therapy has yet to be found.

## REFERENCES

American Psychiatric Association (1980). DSM-111. In: *Diagnostic and Statistical Manual of Psychiatric Disorders*, 3rd edition, American Psychiatric Association, Washington.

Barnes, T. R. E. and Bridges, P. (1983). New generation of antidepressant. In: *Drugs in Psychiatric Practice*, pp.219–248 (Ed. Tyrer, P.), Butterworths, London.

Bowlby, J. (1973). *Attachment and Loss, 2: Separation, Anxiety and Anger*. Hogarth Press, London.

Briggs, R. S., Castleden, C. M. and Kraft, C. A. (1980). Improved hypnotic treatment using chlormethiazole and temazepam. *Brit. med. J.*, **280**, 601–604.

Committee on the Review of Medicines (1980). Systematic review of the benzodiazepines. *Brit. med. J.*, **280**, 910–912.

Dundee, J. W. and Pandit, S. K. (1972). Anterograde amnesic effects of pethidine, hyoscine and diazepam in adults. *Brit. J. Pharmac.*, **44**, 140–144.

Freud, S. (1894). The justification for detaching from neurasthenia a particular syndrome: the anxiety neurosis. In: *Collected Papers*, **1**, 76–106, Hogarth Press, London.

Freud, S. (1917). Mourning and melancholia. In: *Collected Papers*, **IV**, Hogarth Press, London.

Greenblatt, D. J. and Shader, R. I. (1974). *Benzodiazepines in Clinical Practice*, Raven Press, New York.

Hafner, J. and Marks, I. (1976). Exposure in vivo of agoraphobics: contributions of diazepam, group exposure and anxiety evocation. *Psychol. Med.*, **6**, 71–88.

Hallstrom, C., Treasaden, I., Edwards, J. G. and Lader, M. (1981). Diazepam, propanolol and their combination in the management of chronic anxiety. *Brit. J. Psych.*, **139**, 417–421.

Hession, M. A., Verma, S. and Mohan Bhakta, K. G. (1979). Dependence on chlormethiazole and effects of its withdrawal. *Lancet*, **i**, 953–954.

Johnstone, E. C., Owens, D. G., Frith, C. D., McPherson, K., Dowie, C., Riley, G. and Gold, A. (1980). Neurotic illness and its response to axiolyic and antidepressant treatment. *Psychol. Med.*, **10**, 321–328.

Klein, D. F. (1964). Delineation of two drug-responsive anxiety syndromes. *Psychopharmacologia*, **5**, 397–408.

Klein, D. F., Gittelman, R., Quitkin, F. and Rifkin, A. (1980). *Diagnosis and Drug*

*Treatment of Psychiatric Disorders: Adults and Children*, 2nd edition, Williams and Wilkins, Baltimore.

Lader, M. H., Bond, A. J. and James, D. C. (1974). Clinical comparison of anxiolytic drug therapy. *Psychol. Med.*, **4**, 381–387.

Lindemann, E. (1944). Symptomatology and management of acute grief. *Am. J. Psychiat.*, **101**, 141–150.

Lipsedge, M. S., Hajioff, J., Huggins, P., Napier, L., Pearce, J., Pike, D. J. and Rich, M. (1973). The management of severe agoraphobia: a comparison of iproniazid and systematic desensitisation. *Psychopharmacologia*, **32**, 67–80.

Marks, I. M., Viswanathan, R., Lipsedge, M. S. and Gardner, R. (1972). Enhanced relief of phobias by flooding during waning diazepam effect. *Brit. J. Psychiat.*, **121**, 493–505.

McNair, D. M. and Kahn, R. J. (1981). Imipramine compared with a benzodiazepine for agoraphobia. In *Anxiety: New Research and Changing Concepts*, pp.69–80 (Eds. Klein, D. F. and Rabkin, J. G.), Raven Press, New York.

Montgomery, S. A., McAuley, R., Rani, S. J., Roy, D. and Montgomery, D. B. (1981). A double blind comparison of zimelidine and amitriptyline in endogenous depression. *Acta psychiat. scand.*, **63**, Suppl. 290, 314–327.

Pitts, F. and McClure, J. (1967). Lactate metabolism in anxiety neurosis. *New Engl. J. Med.*, **277**, 1329–1336.

Pollitt, J. and Young, J. (1971). Anxiety state or masked depression? A study based on the action of monoamine oxidase inhibitors. *Brit. J. Psychiat.*, **119**, 143–149.

Ravaris, C. L., Nies, A., Robinson, D. S., Ives, J. O., Lamborn, K. R. and Korson, L. (1976). A multiple dose, controlled study of phenelzine in depression-anxiety states. *Arch. gen. Psychiat.*, **37**, 347–350.

Rickels, K., Lipman, R. S., Park, L. C., Covi, L., Uhlenhuth, E. H. and Mock, J. E. (1971). Drug, doctor warmth, and clinic setting in the symptomatic response to minor tranquilizers. *Psychopharmacologia*, **20**, 128–152.

Rickels, K., Pereira-ogan, J. A., Case, W. G., Csanalosi, I., Mirman, M. J., Nathanson, J. E. and Parish, L. C. (1974). Chlormezanone in anxiety: a drug rediscovered. *Am. J. Psychiat.*, **131**, 592–595.

Slater, E. (1943). The neurotic constitution: a statistical study of two thousand neurotic soldiers. *J. Neurol. Psychiat.*, **6**, 1–16.

Smith, M. E. and Chassan, J. B. (1964). Comparison of diazepam, chlorpromazine and trifluoperazine in a double-blind clinical investigation. *J. Neuropsychiat.*, **5**, 593–600.

Snyder, S. H. and Yamamura, H. I. (1977). Antidepressants and the muscarinic receptor. *Arch. gen. Psychiat.*, **34**, 236–239.

Tyrer, P. (1982). The concept of somatic anxiety. *Brit. J. Psychiat.* **140**, 325.

Tyrer, P., Candy, J. and Kelly, D. (1973). A study of the clinical effects of phenelzine and placebo in the treatment of phobic anxiety. *Psychopharmacologia*, **32**, 237–254.

Tyrer, P. J. and Lader, M. H. (1974). Response to propranolol and diazepam in somatic and psychic anxiety. *Brit. med. J.*, **2**, 14–16.

West, E. D. and Dally, P. J. (1959). The effects of iproniazid in depressive syndromes. *Brit. med. J.*, **1**, 1491–1494.

World Health Organization (1978). *International Classification of Disease*, ninth revision, Geneva, WHO.

## DISCUSSION

## CHAIRMAN: PROFESSOR A. RICHENS

PROFESSOR HAMILTON: What about 'autonomic dystonia'?

DR. TYRER: I think there is an amazing plethora of names for these different conditions with disorders that are variously labelled 'hyperdynamic beta-adrenergic circulatory state', hyperdynamic heart syndrome', 'hyperventilation syndrome', 'neurocirculatory asthenia', 'nervous heart complaints', 'da Costa syndrome'. Many of these I would regard primarily as somatasthenic anxiety, anxiety in which one or more symptoms are given special prominence both by the doctor and by the patient.

DR. COBB: I think one of the things wrong with the term 'anxiety state' or 'free floating anxiety' which I think is not wrong about the term 'dystonia' is that if you get patients to keep a diary and measure their anxiety levels during the day using a visual analogue scale, you find it fluctuates. This is true of people who work at high and at low levels of anxiety, so that the idea of the anxiety state which is something which goes continuously through the day is, I think, usually clinically erroneous.

You mentioned that anxiety is intermittent but I think you probably meant it is intermittent on a week by week basis. But it is also intermittent on an hour by hour basis. If you take it a step further and say to the patients, 'Now what level of anxiety can you tolerate?', they can then mark a level which usually shows that for most of the day they can put up with the anxiety which they are experiencing, but there are certain times during the day when it becomes uncomfortable. Then, rather than altering their level of arousal continuously, the problem becomes how they are going to deal with those times during the day when their anxiety actually causes them distress and makes them feel that they are not functioning properly.

THE CHAIRMAN: So you are supporting the concept of a quick acting antianxiety drug when symptoms get too much?

DR. COBB: That would be one possibility though in my view there are psychological methods which are also effective. You can then say to the patient, 'O.K., you are getting your intermittent episodes of panic or high anxiety during the day. How do you want to deal with it? Do you want to deal with it with a pill or do you want to find some other way of coping with it?'

PROFESSOR HAMILTON: If I may comment on this, that in fact is the way the experience of humanity has devised for coping with this problem. It is well known that those who are about to stand up before an audience, say actors or performers of some kind, will take a quick drink beforehand to allay their anxiety and enable them to keep it under control during that period of stress. We know it is also medical tradition that for patients who are liable to a sudden increase in anxiety under certain situations, you gave them a capsule of sodium amytal and said, 'Keep that and take it just beforehand', and very often the fact that they had it was itself sufficient help to avoid using it.

DR. TYRER: It seems to me that the ideal antianxiety drug would be one that only had a duration of action of an hour. But, of course, if we are going to give a drug of that nature and it is similar to or is a benzodiazepine, which produces a rebound effect immediately afterwards, that will be counterproductive. However, I would think that if one had a short duration of action like that and no after-effects, one would have the ideal drug.

DR. COBB: If you ask the patient to measure how long the intolerable anxiety lasts it is usually about 20 minutes. If they can get through that 20 minutes, then the level comes down.

THE CHAIRMAN: But has this rebound anxiety been demonstrated with daytime use of a short-acting benzodiazepine drug?

PROFESSOR OSWALD: No.

PROFESSOR M. LADER: What are your views on mitral valve prolapse?

DR. TYRER: Mitral valve prolapse is something which has caused great interest in the United States, because it seems to simulate the symptoms of anxiety neurosis. When it was first detected there was a wild suggestion that perhaps all our patients with anxiety neurosis had mitral valve prolapse. If that were true, mitral valve prolapse would be a significant clinical syndrome because anxiety is so common. I really am quite bemused by the literature from the other side of the Atlantic on that subject.

Benzodiazepines Divided
Edited by M. R. Trimble


# 18

# Benzodiazepines in Depression

DON A. W. JOHNSON

The presence of an association between depression and the benzodiazepines is a matter for frequent comment. An inspection of the literature will reveal that the nature of this association, and the clinical effects claimed, is anything but constant. Some authorities state that the benzodiazepines are effective as an antidepressant, others only that it is a useful addition as a secondary treatment, or in combination with a tricyclic antidepressant. Yet other reports allege that a therapeutic dose of this group of drugs can induce depression, while a further suggestion is that it is withdrawal of the drug that induces depression.

An examination of the prescribing habits of doctors may give us some clues as to how these drugs are regarded by clinicians. Bellantuono *et al.* (1980) concluded, from market data, that in the UK some 20% of benzodiazepine prescriptions are motivated by the treatment of depressive symptoms. Some general practice studies have suggested that many family doctors appear to prescribe tricyclic antidepressant drugs and benzodiazepines as almost interchangeable drugs, with the benzodiazepines being prescribed as much for depression as anxiety (Johnson, 1973a; Tyrer, 1978). Other studies carried out at the General Practice Research Unit of the Institute of Psychiatry (Clare, 1981) reported that this was only true for women treated for depression. Approximately half the population of depressed women received tricyclic antidepressants, but in contrast almost all men diagnosed as depressed received a recognized antidepressant. In a further analysis of the family doctors' prescribing habits, Johnson (1974, 1981) reported that while most doctors started treatment for a new episode of illness with a tricyclic antidepressant, the longer the patient remained ill with depression the more likely they were to receive a non-therapeutic dose of the tricyclic drug, or have their treatment changed to a benzodiazepine. The explanation offered by general practitioners was based more upon the problems of side effects, and their influence upon patient compliance, than a positive belief that benzodiazepines were specifically antidepressant. Other authors have suggested that family doctors may be more influenced by the presenting symptoms than the use of diagnostic categories. Patients presenting with anxiety, or a mixture of anxiety and depression, irrespective of aetiology, are more likely to receive a prescription for benzodiazepines (Downing and Rickels, 1974). It is, of course, important to discover the prescribing habits and to learn the reasoning behind these habits, since both in hospital and general practice the most frequent treatment for depression is medication accompanied by a fairly brief form of reassurance (Shepherd *et al.*, 1966; Johnson, 1973a,b,c).

Any attempt to identify the differential effects of treatment upon anxiety and depression must start with an acknowledgement that the relationship between these two symptoms, or syndromes, is complex and remains an area of legitimate debate (Mendels *et al.*, 1972; Downing and Rickels, 1974; Kendell, 1975; Klerman, 1977; American Psychiatric Association, 1980). Although it is usual to divide neurotic illness into separate diagnostic categories (WHO, 1977), and some attempts to demonstrate the integrity of anxiety states and depressions have apparently been successful (Roth *et al.*, 1972; Prusoff and Klerman, 1974), the dichotomy is not by any means universally accepted (Kendell, 1975). It has also been suggested that many patients may not be able to separate and identify the symptom or experience of anxiety from depression (Leff, 1978). These factors must introduce a keen sense of caution when formulating any firm conclusions.

Two recent reviews have analysed the double-blind trials comparing benzodiazepines with more traditional antidepressant substances. Bellantuono *et al.* (1980) identified 24 studies, but these included not only tricyclic antidepressants but also phenelzine and viloxazine. Their conclusion was that 13 studies demonstrated a clear superiority for the traditional antidepressants, and 11 studies showed no difference. No study demonstrated a superiority for the benzodiazepines. Schatzberg and Cole (1981) identified 22 studies comparing the benzodiazepines specifically with the tricyclic antidepressants. They concluded that in 12 of the 22 studies the tricyclic antidepressant was clearly superior to the benzodiazepine, in nine studies the drugs were found to be equal in overall efficiency. In only one study was the benzodiazepine reported to be superior. Their comment in this latter study was that problems of methodology prevented them from agreeing that the superiority of the benzodiazepine's antidepressant properties had been clearly established.

The present review is of 25 double-blind studies comparing the relative efficiency of the benzodiazepines with tricyclic antidepressants. In 12 of these 25 studies traced by a computer search of the literature, the tricyclic antidepressant was clearly superior to the benzodiazepine (Johnstone and Claghorn, 1968; Verner, 1969; Rickels *et al.*, 1969; Kay *et al.*, 1970; Montgomery *et al.*, 1970; Butterworth and Watts, 1971; Sterlin *et al.*, 1972;

Overall *et al.*, 1973; Johnson *et al.*, 1973; Covi *et al.*, 1974; Lipman and Covi, 1976; Kleber, 1977; Feighner *et al.*, 1979). In contrast, only one study (Shammas, 1977) concluded that the benzodiazepines were superior, and this was the one identified in the Schatzberg and Cole (1981) review. However, as noted later, the high drop-out rate in the tricyclic group, a low mean dosage of amitriptyline, and the nature of the symptom reduction must lead to the conclusion that this particular result may have other explanations.

The remaining 12 studies found no difference reaching a level of statistical significance between the two drug groups (Beaubien *et al.*, 1970; Sterlin *et al.*, 1970; Rickels *et al.*, 1970, 1973; Claghorn and Kellner, 1971; Sim *et al.*, 1971; General Practitioner Clinical Trials, 1971; d'Elia *et al.*, 1974; Hare, 1974; Johnson, 1979; Feighner, 1982). Nevertheless trends can be identified and it may help clarify the issues by identifying these. In three studies (Rickels *et al.*, 1970; Feighner, 1982) a trend is claimed for the benzodiazepines, but a closer inspection reveals that in two of these studies this claim is based only upon a more rapid response to alprazolam with a similar outcome to both drugs at the completion of the study at 4 weeks (Feighner, 1982). In five studies the trend was in favour of the tricyclic antidepressant (Beaubien *et al.*, 1970; Sterlin *et al.*, 1970; General Practitioner Clinical Trials, 1971; Rickels *et al.*, 1973; d'Elia *et al.*, 1974), and in the remaining four studies no definite trend was demonstrated (Sim *et al.*, 1971; Claghorn and Kellner, 1971; Hare, 1974; Johnson, 1979).

The overall evaluation of the 24 studies identified is that the results of 17 of these studies suggest some superiority for tricyclic antidepressants, with 12 studies showing a difference reaching a level of significance. In contrast only four studies claim any superiority for the benzodiazepines, with only one study demonstrating a difference reaching a level of significance. This last study, and two of the trials claiming a trend in favour of the benzodiazepines do not justify this conclusion.

A further consideration is that on a closer inspection of the methodology of the reported studies it is clear that in the majority the tricyclic drugs were not given the opportunity to demonstrate their true antidepressant effect. In only five of the 25 studies were the patients prescribed the generally accepted full therapeutic dose for even a reasonable period (Johnstone and Claghorn, 1968; Sterlin *et al.*, 1972; Covi *et al.*, 1974; Kleber, 1977; Johnson, 1979). Four of these studies showed the benzodiazepines to be clearly inferior, and the fifth (Johnson, 1979) failed to demonstrate any difference between the drugs compared. An examination of the single study claiming a significant advantage for the benzodiazepines reveals that the mean daily dose of amitriptyline was only 94 mg. In the three trials claiming a trend in favour of the benzodiazepines the dose was substantially less than optimal in two studies, whilst in the third the dose is unclear. It is quite likely that the use of a full therapeutic dose of the tricyclic antidepressants for a 3 or 4 week period would have substantially changed the therapeutic potential in all the trials where the benzodiazepines have a possible superiority, and in the majority of trials where no difference was demonstrated.

Another consideration which has to be addressed is whether the diagnostic categories studied in the double-blind trials in fact allowed any firm conclusions about the true antidepressant effects of either drug group. Most of the patients studied had anxious, reactive, or psychoneurotic depressions. The overlap of symptoms described, coupled with the imprecision of the diagnoses used, must raise the suspicion that many patient samples could have been included in a variety of diagnostic categories. The symptoms described were certainly very frequently common to both anxiety states and depressions. This must raise the question whether in fact some of the trials offered the opportunity to demonstrate a true antidepressant effect. To overcome this objection an attempt has been made to analyse the studies to identify those which contained samples, or subsamples, of endogenous-like depressions and to delineate those symptoms which appear to be ameliorated by the benzodiazepine drugs. This was difficult because of the lack of firm operational definitions and it is acknowledged that some diagnoses may be an area for legitimate debate.

Seven studies were identified where treatment was directed at endogenous-like depressions. Three were more comprehensive in size and in the scope of the investigation into specific symptoms. Kay *et al.* (1970) compared diazepam and amitriptyline as the continuation therapy in patients treated with ECT. During a 7 month follow-up period amitriptyline was not only more effective in preventing actual relapses, but these patients had significantly lower scores on both the Hamilton Rating Scale for Depression and the Beck Depression Inventory. The Covi *et al.* (1974) study compared imipramine with diazepam in a female outpatient population and again found diazepam inferior. Feighner *et al.* (1979) compared chlordiazepoxide, amitriptyline, a combination of the two and a placebo. At the end of 4 weeks the amitriptyline-treated patients were found to be superior on a global rating and the Beck Depression Inventory, but no different to chlordiazepoxide on the Hamilton Rating Scale for Depression. Overall, three out of the seven studies of endogenous-like depressions show a clear advantage for the tricyclic antidepressant. The other four studies failed to demonstrate a difference between the two drug groups (Sim *et al.*, 1971; Hare, 1974; Feighner, 1982). However, an examination of the methodology clearly suggests reasons for these negative results. In two studies the symptomatology was particularly mild. Now Paykel (1972) has shown that this reduces the potential for demonstrating a difference between drugs since the antidepressant effect of a drug correlates with the initial severity. In addition the daily dosage of amitriptyline was only 75 mg. In a third study, although the operational definition was clear, as the Feighner Diagnostic Criteria (Feighner *et al.*, 1972) were used, it is unfortunate that the most severely depressed patients were excluded and only a mean daily dose of 124 mg of amitriptyline was used.

In the final study (Feighner, 1982) the same operational definition was used but details of dosage were either unclear or unstated. These last two studies compared alprazolam with a tricyclic and despite no overall difference between the two drug groups at final outcome, a special antidepressant effect was claimed for this new member of the benzodiazepine group.

The author's own evaluation of the trials reported is that not only is there no indication that benzodiazepines might have a superiority over amitriptyline, but there is really no clear indication that benzodiazepines have a true antidepressant effect of any degree. The claims that alprazolam may have an antidepressant effect different from, or superior to, the other benzodiazepines, also seems unfounded. However, it must be acknowledged that problems exist, and a final conclusion based on present information may be premature. For example, as already mentioned, it is not accepted by all authorities that depression and anxiety can be divided into two clear-cut diagnostic entities (Kendell, 1975). Even when their integrity has been successfully demonstrated (Roth *et al.*, 1972; Prusoff and Klerman 1974) it has not been conclusively shown that their natural courses differ (Greer and Cawley, 1966). A further consideration has been raised by a recent Medical Research Council trial (Johnstone *et al.*, 1980). In this study 240 neurotic outpatients were not allocated to a diagnostic category but were rated in terms of both depression and anxiety at weekly intervals during a 4 week trial of amitriptyline, diazepam, a combination of amitriptyline and diazepam, and placebo. The outcome tended to be good irrespective of medication, but any significant drug effects found were due to amitriptyline with both the anxiety and depressive symptoms. The overall conclusion of this study was that a distinction between anxiety and depression in neurotic outpatients is of no practical value with regard to the drug treatment prescribed, as it was found that drug treatments had a relatively small influence on patient outcome. This study, of course, tells us little about endogenous illness, but it may go some way to explain the variable results with many of the patient samples studied. In particular it may explain why a number of studies showed no difference between the drugs compared. However, despite all their reservations, Johnstone *et al.* (1980) did conclude that amitriptyline alone had a significant treatment effect upon their patients. What might have been of particular interest is the pattern of symptom response within these patients. It has already been suggested that in neurotic depression both the anxiety and depressive symptoms are relieved by a tricyclic antidepressant, even by a drug without a marked sedative effect. In their study the anxiety symptoms showed a delayed response, and only resolved after the depressive symptoms began to settle (Johnson, 1979). If this result were replicated it might contribute to the separation of anxiety and depressive states, and in drug evaluation the pattern of symptom response, particularly over the relatively short periods observed in drug trials, might be considered as relevant as the final scores.

Taking into consideration these objections it may be valuable to consider the pattern of symptom response in the main double-blind studies reported. In an analysis by Schatzberg and Cole (1981) of symptom response in the first 22 studies reported, they found that the benzodiazepines were most effective in reducing anxiety, tension, insomnia, decreased libido, and reduced interest. In contrast they exerted relatively little effect on psychomotor retardation, anergia, diurnal variation, or suicidal ideation or behaviour. The symptoms influenced appear to be those which can appear in anxiety states, depressions, and other less specific neurotic states, whilst those relatively unaffected are more specific to depression and in particular are commonly associated with endogenous depressions (Roth *et al.*, 1972). In an earlier analysis of symptoms in a different pool of patients, Cassano and colleagues (Cassano *et al.*, 1973; Cassano and Conti, 1981) also found the benzodiazepines most effective in relieving insomnia, anxiety, and agitation, but reported a lesser effect on mood and the level of general interest. They found little effect upon the traditional biological symptoms and concluded that patients with a more endogenous-like depression treated with benzodiazepines often experienced a higher level of residual symptoms.

Schatzberg and Cole (1981) further considered whether either drug group may actually exacerbate specific symptoms. Unfortunately a lack of data reported did not allow any general conclusion, but in one study (Kleber, 1977) psychomotor retardation was increased and in two other studies suicidal ideation became more prominent (McDowall *et al.*, 1966; Ryan *et al.*, 1968). Although Kay *et al.* (1970) reported three suicides in a diazepam-treated group they concluded that the absence of an antidepressant effect, rather than a positive aggravation by the benzodiazepine, was responsible.

The fact that the benzodiazepines have not been shown as efficient as the tricyclic antidepressants, or indeed that they may not have any true antidepressant effect, does not necessarily mean they have no place in the treatment of depressed patients. It is generally agreed that there is an overlap between the diagnostic categories of anxiety and depression even if the two categories can be shown to exist independently. It is also agreed that the symptom of anxiety exists in a depressive illness and vice versa. Therefore the possibility that a combination of a tricyclic and a benzodiazepine may be the most efficient treatment has to be explored. Equally it must be pointed out that there are many scientific and practical reasons why combination therapy, and in particular combination tablets with two or more drugs in a fixed ratio, should be discouraged as a general principle. Nevertheless a proper evaluation is required since combination therapy is not uncommon in both hospital and general practice.

An examination of the literature is disappointing since very little investigation under strictly controlled double-blind conditions has taken place. Hollister *et al.* (1971) suggested some benefits from combination therapy in mixed states of anxiety and depression, but in a more recent review appear to have revised these views, saying that such patients respond to non-specific treatments, and did not argue the need for benzodiazepine drugs to be prescribed (Hollister, 1981). Feighner *et al.* (1979) found a combination therapy beneficial at the beginning of a drug trial, with insomnia and anxiety selectively responding to the addition of a benzodiazepine, but by the end of the fourth week this advantage had been lost. Johnstone *et al.* (1980) found no advantage in using a mixture of amitriptyline and diazepam compared to amitriptyline alone. There are some studies where the results can be described as encouraging for combination therapy rather than conclusive, but the claims for an enhanced antidepressant effect are only noted for those patients with a high initial score for anxiety (Cassano *et al.*, 1968; Browne, 1969; Houck, 1970; Rickels *et al.*, 1970; Grainger, 1972; Smith, 1973). Even with these studies, the claims are related to an amelioration of the anxiety component rather than a true resolution of depression, and the speed of response rather than outcome after the relatively short period of 4 weeks. A factor analysis of the individual terms of the Hamilton Rating Scale for Depression and the Self-Administered Depression Scale (Cassano *et al.*, 1977) suggested that some items responded poorly to amitriptyline alone. However, the fact that some of these items coincide with symptoms identified as frequently responding to the benzodiazepines does not in itself support the claims of Cassano and Conti (1981) that a combination therapy is in the best interest of the patient. The whole subject of combination therapy with a tricyclic antidepressant drug together with a benzodiazepine has been inadequately researched, and at the present time most claims for a benefit cannot be substantiated by the results obtained.

The final question is, does the use of a benzodiazepine actually cause depression in some patients? Certainly some of our most prestigious textbooks suggest this to be the case (Hollister, 1978; Goodman and Gilman, 1980). In the analysis of symptom response to drugs it has already been mentioned that psychomotor retardation and suicidal ideation can, on occasions, be made worse by the use of a benzodiazepine drug in an already depressed patient. In addition, Weissman and Klerman (1977) have reported that the usage of benzodiazepines can be associated with a depression assuming a more chronic form. Schatzberg and Cole (1978) also reported a relatively high percentage of benzodiazepine-treated depressions as failing to respond to subsequent physical treatments. An examination of suicidal thoughts and impulses by Gundlach *et al.* (1966) found these to be associated with patients on a therapeutic dose of diazepam, but not placebo. Ryan *et al.* (1968) also reported seven patients who developed suicidal ideas after the use of diazepam. Five improved after the discontinuation of diazepam but two committed suicide. Hall and Joffe (1972) reported six patients who developed depression abruptly on a fairly high dose of diazepam, 40 mg daily, but additional symptoms were suggestive of an organic confusional state. A single case report by Zisook and De Vaul (1977) also suggests an acute diazepam-induced suicidal state.

A careful examination of these reports reveals that they are all anecdotal, and in most instances the patients either have a concomitant physical illness or are receiving additional medication (Hall and Zisook, 1981). It would be quite unsafe to make any assumptions as to the aetiology of symptoms. In the past it has been suggested that some apparently paradoxical drug responses have not in fact been unpredictable, but only a disinhibiting effect on a person of known abnormal personality (Dimascio *et al.*, 1969). In a review of the literature by Hall and Zisook (1981) it was concluded that the incidence of reported paradoxical effects of the benzodiazepines was very low overall. When they do occur they seem idiosyncratic and could not be associated with any predictable clinical indicators. Individual instances of induced depression may exist, but there seems little firm evidence that there is a constant relationship with the use of the drug, nor that it is a true consequence of the pharmacological actions of the benzodiazepines. Again a rather vague clinical impression appears to have developed into an accepted fact by some authorities without any firm foundation.

In conclusion, this review has drawn attention to the fact that it is common for the benzodiazepine drugs to be prescribed as the primary treatment for depression. However, a search of the literature has failed to support claims that the benzodiazepine drugs have any true antidepressant effect. The response of a depressive illness, particularly endogenous-like depressions with the presence of biological symptoms but also reactive or neurotic depressions, to a tricyclic antidepressant drug is superior to a benzodiazepine. This response is almost certainly due to a true antidepressant effect rather than a non-specific action. The response of depressive symptoms in patients of poorly defined diagnostic categories is also greater to the tricyclic antidepressants. There is no clear indication that the addition of a benzodiazepine, or the use of a combination therapy has any advantage except in the response of certain anxiety symptoms and insomnia during the first weeks of treatment. Equally, any claims that the benzodiazepines should be avoided because of a risk of drug-induced depression appears to be without substantial proof, and at the present time based on anecdotal comment. Unhappily this search of the literature has revealed an important area of clinical practice which requires energetic clarification based on high quality research.

## REFERENCES

American Psychiatric Association (1980). In: *Diagnostic and Statistical Manual of Mental Disorders*, 3rd edition, pp.205–224, American Psychiatric Association, Washington.

Bellantuono, C., Reggi, C., Tognoni, G. and Garattini, S. (1980). Benzodiazepines: *Clinical Pharmacology and Therapeutic Use. Drugs*, **19**, 195–219.

Beaubien, J., Ban, T. A. and Lehmann, H. E. (1970). Doxepin in the treatment of psychoneurotic patients. *Curr. Ther. Res.*, **13**, 192–194.

Browne, M. W. (1969). A comparison of two drug treatments in depressive illness. *Brit. J. Psychiat.*, **115**, 693-696.

Butterworth, A. T. and Watts, R. D. (1971). Treatment of hospitalised alcoholics with doxepin and diazepam. *Ql. J. Stud. Alc.*, **32**, 78–81.

Cassano, G. B., Castrogiovanni, P. and Conti, L. (1973). Drug responses in different anxiety states under benzodiazepine treatment. Some multivariate analyses for the evaluation of 'Rating Scale for Depression scores'. In: *The Benzodiazepines*, pp.379–390. Raven Press, New York.

Cassano, G. B., Castrogiovanni, P. and Conti, L. (1977). Automation techniques in assaying the spectrum of activity of psychoactive drugs. *Drugs exp. clin. Res.*, **1**, 61–68.

Cassano, G. B., Castrogiovanni, I., Gallevi, M. and Riccioni, R. (1968). Sperimentazione clinica controllata di una associazione farmacologica (amitriptilina—clordiazepossido) nella terapia dell'ansia delle psicosi depressive. In: *Atti Convegni Farmitalia Le Associazioni di Psicofarmaci*, pp.93–120. Edizioni Minerva Medica, Torino.

Cassano, G. B. and Conti, L. (1981). Some considerations on the role of benzodiazepines in the treatment of depression. *Brit. J. clin. Pharmac.*, **11**, 235–295.

Claghorn, J. and Kellner, R. (1971). When is tranquilliser an antidepressant? *Curr. Ther. Res.*, **13**, 575–579.

Clare, A. W. (1981). Psychotropic drug use in general practice in Britain. In: *Epidemiological Impact of Psychotropic Drugs* (Eds. Tognoni, E., Bellantuono, C. and Lader, M.), Elsevier, North-Holland Biomedical Press, Oxford.

Covi, L., Lipman, R. S. and Derogatis, L. R. (1974). Drugs and group psychotherapy in neurotic depression. *Am. J. Psychiat.*, **131**, 191–198.

Dimascio, A., Shader, R. I. and Harmatz, J. (1969). Psychotropic drugs and induced hostility. *Psychosomatics*, **10**, 46–57.

Downing, R. W. and Rickels, K. (1974). Mixed anxiety—depression. Fact or myth? *Arch. gen. Psychiat.* **30**, 312–317.

D'Elia, G., Von Knorring, L. and Marcusson, J. (1974). A double-blind comparison between doxepin and diazepam in the treatment of states of anxiety. *Acta psych. scand.*, **255**, Supplement, 35–47.

Feighner, J. P. (1982). Benzodiazepines as antidepressants. In: *Modern Problems of Pharmacopsychiatry*, pp.196–212 (Ed. Ban, T. A.), S. Karger, Basel.

Feighner, J. P., Guze, S., Robins, E., Woodruff, R., Winokur, G. and Munoz, R. (1972). Diagnostic criteria for use in psychiatric research. *Arch. Gen. Psychiat.* **26**, 57–63.

Feighner, J. P., Brauzer, B. and Gelenberg, A. J. (1979). A placebo-controlled multicentre trial of Limbitrol versus its components (amitriptyline and chlordiazepoxide) in the symptomatic treatment of depressive illness. *Psychopharmacology*, **61**, 221–225.

General Practitioner Clinical Trials (1971). Antidepressant effects of tranquillisers. *Practitioner*, **206**, 146–149.

Goodman, L. and Gilman, A. (1980). *The Pharmacological Basis of Therapeutics*, 6th Edition, pp.437–442 (Eds. Goodman, L. and Gilman, A.), Baillière Tindall, London.

Grainger, G. J. (1972). A clinical study of 'Limbitrol' in the treatment of anxiety-depression in general practice. *Practitioner*, **208**, 807–809.

Greer, H. S. and Cawley, R. H. (1966). *Some Observations on the Natural History of Neurotic Illness.* Australian Medical Association, New South Wales.

Gundlach, R., Engelhardt, D. M. and Hankoff, L. (1966). A double-blind outpatient study of diazepam (Valium) and placebo. *Psychopharmacology*, **9**, 81–92.

Hall, R. C. W. and Joffe, J. R. (1972). Aberrant response to diazepam. A new syndrome. *Am. J. Psychiat.*, **129**, 114–118.

Hall, R. C. W. and Zisook, S. (1981). Paradoxical reactions to benzodiazepines, *Brit. J. clin. Pharmac.*, **11**, 995–1045.

Hare, M. K. (1974). Treatment of anxiety and depression. A comparative trial of amitriptyline (Laroxyl) and diazepam (Valium). *Clin. Trials J.*, **11**, 39–44.

Hollister, L. E. (1978). *Clinical Pharmacology of Psychotherapeutic Drugs*, p.97. Churchill Livingstone, London.

Hollister, L. E. (1981). Benzodiazepines—an overview. *Brit. J. clin. Pharmac.*, **11**, 1175–1195.

Hollister, L. E., Overall, J. E., Pokorny, A. and Shelton, J. (1971). Acetophenazine and diazepam in anxious depressions. *Arch. gen. Psychiat.*, **24**, 273–278.

Houck, J. E. (1970). Combined therapy in anxiety-depressive syndromes. Comparative effects of Limbitrol (chlordiazepoxide-amitriptyline) and placebo. *Dis. Nerv. Syst.*, **31**, 269–273.

Johnson, D. A. W. (1973a). Treatment of depression in general practice. *Brit. med. J.*, **2**, 18–20.

Johnson, D. A. W. (1973b). An analysis of outpatient services. *Brit. J. Psychiat.*, **122**, 301–306.

Johnson, D. A. W. (1973c). A further study of psychiatric outpatient services in Manchester. An operational study of general practitioner and patient expectation. *Brit. J. Psychiat.*, **123**, 185–191.

Johnson, D. A. W. (1974). A study of the use of antidepressant medication in general practice. *Brit. J. Psychiat.*, **125**, 186–192.

Johnson, D. A. W. (1979). A double-blind comparison of flupenthixol, nortriptyline and diazepam in neurotic depression. *Acta Psych. Scand.*, **59**, 1–8.

Johnson, D. A. W. (1981). Depression: treatment compliance in general practice. *Acta Psych. Scand.*, Supplement **290**, 447–453.

Johnson, F., Sacco, F. A. and Yellowley, T. W (1973). Chlordiazepoxide and dothiepin compared in anxiety-depression in general practice. *Practitioner*, **211**, 362–364.

Johnstone, E. E. and Claghorn, J. L. (1968). Doxepin vs. chlordiazepoxide: a controlled comparison in neurotic outpatients. *Curr. Ther. Res.*, **10**, 514–519.

Johnstone, E. C., Owens, D. G. C., Firth, C. D., McPherson, K., Dowie, C., Riley, G. and Gold, A. (1980). Neurotic illness and its response to anxiolytic and antidepressant treatment. *Psychol. Med.*, **10**, 321–328.

Kay, D. W. K., Fahy, T. and Garside, R. F. (1970). A seven month double-blind trial of amitriptyline and diazepam in E.C.T. treated depressed patients. *Brit. J. Psychiat.*, **117**, 667–671.

Kendell, R. E. (1975). *The Role of Diagnosis in Psychiatry*, pp.67–68, Blackwell, Oxford.

Kleber, R. J. (1977). Depression and anxiety: a study of diagnosis and treatment. *Scientific Exhibit, American Psychiatric Association, 130th Meeting.*

Klerman, G. L. (1977). Anxiety and depression. In: *Handbook of Studies in Depression*, pp.49–68 (Ed. Burrows, G.), Excerpta Medica, New York.

Leff, J. P. (1978). Psychiatrists' versus patients' concepts of unpleasant emotions. *Brit. J. Psychiat.*, **133**, 306–313.

Lipman, R. S. and Covi, L. (1976). Outpatient treatment of neurotic depression: medication and group psychotherapy. In: *Evaluation and Psychological Therapies* (Eds Spitzer, R. G. and Klein, D. F.), Johns Hopkins University Press, Baltimore.

McDowall, A., Owens, S. and Robin, A. A. (1966). A controlled comparison of diazepam and amylobarbitone in anxiety states. *Brit. J. Psychiat.*, **112**, 629–631.

Mendels, J., Weinstein, N. and Cochrane, C. (1972). The relationship between anxiety and depression. *Arch. gen. Psychiat.*, **27**, 649–653.

Montgomery, B. A., Cullinan, T. R. and Bayley, A. J. (1970). A double-blind comparative trial of doxepin hydrochloride and chlordiazepoxide in anxiety and depression in general practice. *Brit. J. clin. Pract.*, **24**, 207–209.

Overall, J. E., Brown, D. and Williams, J. D. (1973). Drug treatment in anxiety and depression in detoxified alcoholic patients. *Arch. gen. Psychiat.*, **29**, 218–221.

Paykel, E. S. (1972). Depressive typologies and responses to amitriptyline. *Brit. J. Psychiat.*, **120**, 147–156.

Prusoff, B. and Klerman, G. (1974). Differentiating depressed from anxious neurotic outpatients. *Arch. gen. Psychiat.*, **30**, 302–308.

Rickels, K., Chung, H. R. and Feldman, H. S. (1973). Amitriptyline, diazepam and phenobarbitol sodium in depressed outpatients. *J. nerv. ment. Dis.*, **157**, 442–451.

Rickels, K., Gordon, P. E. and Jenkins, B. W. (1970). Drug treatment in depressive illness. *Dis. nerv. Syst.*, **31**, 309–42.

Rickels, K., Perloff, M. and Stepansky, W. (1969). Doxepin and diazepam in general practice and hospital clinic neurotic patients: a collaborative controlled study. *Psychopharmacologia*, **15**, 265–279.

Roth, M., Gurney, C., Garside, R. F. and Kerr, T. A. (1972). Studies in the classification of affective disorders. The relationship between anxiety and depressive illness. *Brit. J. Psychiat.* **121**, 147–161.

Ryan, H. F., Merrill, B. and Scott, G. E. (1968). Increase in suicidal thoughts and tendencies: association with diazepam therapy. *J. Am. Med. Ass.*, **203**, 1137–1139.

Schatzberg, A. F. and Cole, J. O. (1978). Benzodiazepines in depressive disorders. *Arch. gen. Psychiat.*, **35**, 1359–1365.

Schatzberg, A. F. and Cole, J. O. (1981). Benzodiazepines in the treatment of depressive, borderline personality and schizophrenic disorders. *Brit. J. clin. Pharmac.*, **11**, 175–225.

Shammas, E. (1977). Controlled comparison of bromazepam, amitriptyline and placebo in anxiety-depression. *Dis. nerv. Sys.*, **38**, 201–207.

Shepherd, M., Cooper, B., Brown, A. C. and Kalton, G. (1966). *Psychiatric Illness in General Practice*. Oxford University Press, London.

Sim, M., Bindman, E. and Conochie, B. C. (1971). The treatment of anxiety-depressive states. *Clin. Trials J.*, **8**, 22–27.

Smith, M. (1973). Clinical response to amitriptyline and chlordiazepoxide-amitriptyline (Limbitrol) in anxiety-depressive states. A double-blind study. *Psychosomatics*, **14**, 168–175.

Sterlin, C., Ban, T. A. and Jarrold, L. (1972). The place of doxepin among anxiolytic sedative drugs. *Curr. Ther. Res.*, **14**, 195–204.

Sterlin, C., Ban, T. A. and Lehmann, H. E. (1970). A comparative evaluation of doxepin and chlordiazepoxide in the treatment of psychoneurotic outpatients. *Curr. Ther. Res.*, **12**, 195–208.

Tyrer, P. (1978). Drug treatment of psychiatric patients in general practice. *Brit. Med. J.*, **2**, 1008–1010.

Verner, J. V. (1969). Comparison of imipramine and chlordiazepoxide in the treatment of the depressed and anxious patient. *J. Flanders med. Ass.* **56**, 15–21.

Weissman, M. M. and Klerman, G. L. (1977). The chronic depressive in the community. Unrecognised and poorly treated. *Comprehensive Psychiat.*, **18**, 523–531.

World Health Organization (1977). *Manual of the International Statistical Classification of Diseases, Injuries and Causes of Death*, Vol. 1, WHO, Geneva.

Zisook, S. and De Vaul, R. A. (1977). Adverse behavioural effects of benzodiazepines. *J. Fam. Pract.*, **5(6)**, 963–966.

## DISCUSSION

## CHAIRMAN: PROFESSOR A. RICHENS

DR. LINNOILA: I would like you to comment on the large-scale study by Covi and Rickels, where they compared doxepin or imipramine with diazepam which they published in 1982 in the *Psychopharmacology Bulletin*. They had almost 300 patients, and they showed that which drug came ahead depended on the time of follow-up. Initially the benzodiazepines were better, particularly in the people who complained about anxiety. This was a mixed group of anxiety and depression, a very similar study to the Johnstone study conducted here in England (Johnstone *et al.*, 1980). What was rather surprising—and I tend also to read the Johnstone study in the same way—was that if one followed up long enough (that is for about 6 weeks) the tricyclic antidepressants came ahead, even in the patients whose primary complaint was anxiety.

So it looks as though, in the maintenance treatment, tricyclics would be better in patients who complain about generalized anxiety.

DR. JOHNSON: I would agree. One of the interesting things, certainly in my own study comparing the two, was a differential response to anxiety and depression. Certainly, as you say, the time factor is crucial because the anxiety response seems to trail behind the antidepressant response. There may be some reason for looking at syndromes in the borderlands between these two in terms of drug response to help us to clarify some of the diagnostic issues.

THE CHAIRMAN: Am I getting the message, as a non-psychiatrist, that we should be using tricyclic antidepressants for all these disorders, anxiety and depression?

DR. LINNOILA: There is obviously a price to pay for the tricyclics, namely they are very toxic in overdose compared with the benzodiazepines. However, the whole field is in a great state of flux—the situation regarding what is currently available suggests that, indeed, the tricyclics might be better than the first generation of benzodiazepines in the long-term treatment of both anxious and depressed patients, if the patient is not suicidal.

DR. JOHNSON: There are really two issues here. One is whether patients who have anxiety in the absence of depression respond to tricyclic antidepressants as well as, or better than, the benzodiazepines. The other is the atypical presentation of depression. I think that the diagnosis of depression is made more often now than it was a few years ago, and people are aware that depression may present in the absence of overt mood change, at least identified by the doctor. Whether we are talking of obsessional states, phobic states, or anxiety states, a proportion of these—and I do not want to overemphasize this point—probably are atypical depressions and they respond more satisfactorily to a tricyclic antidepressant.

DR. P. TYRER: Could I just reinforce that? I think the changes in the last few years have meant that the spectrum of antidepressant treatment has been moving further into the anxiety field and replacing the benzodiazepines in groups of disorders. I think it is also fair to say there is no real evidence in the pure anxiety states, that I referred to, that tricyclic antidepressants have a definite role.

DR. M. TRIMBLE: Is there any evidence from pharmacokinetics or the biochemistry that alprazolam is in any way different from any of the other benzodiazepines? Do we have any evidence, apart from clinical evidence, that that is so?

DR. R. N. STRAW: Dr. Sultzer has some information that at least in a propanalol-altered model of beta-receptors that alprazolam appears to be somewhat different from traditional benzodiazepines. Dr. Sethy from our laboratories found similar findings in a reserpine-altered model.

DR. L. L. IVERSEN: It seems important to distinguish these new compounds—

alprazolam and the one that is looming on the horizon, ademazolam—as being atypical benzodiazepines. If they are (as they seem to be) antidepressant, it is not because they work on the benzodiazepine receptor, but because of some other secondary pharmacological property. There is a danger of semantic confusion here in that we may call these the first benzodiazepine antidepressants. They may belong to the benzodiazepine chemical class, but that particular feature probably does not belong to the standard benzodiazepine pharmacology. The question then is whether such a combination of properties is a desirable one to have clinically.

Benzodiazepines Divided
Edited by M. R. Trimble


# 19

# Benzodiazepines and Sleep

IAN OSWALD

## INTRODUCTION

I shall first consider something of what often underlies the prescribing of any hypnotic drug, I shall consider then what sleep does for us, and what it may fail to do for the insomniac, and finally turn in detail to the effects upon sleep of the benzodiazepines themselves.

## THE ACT OF PRESCRIBING

Patients often complain about their sleep, especially those who are older, female or of nervous temperament (McGhie and Russell, 1962; Karacan *et al.*, 1976). The drugs they then get are usually those that relieve anxiety and promote sleep. Insomnia, like pain, is indeed a complaint and not a diagnosis. Some people are more and some less extravagant in their use of language to convey their complaint. Some who complain of poor sleep are at times of transition in life or passing through a crisis. They may usually 'not believe in' sleeping pills and they get but a single prescription that lasts them through their temporary troubles. Others who complain reflect by their complaints a general dissatisfaction: dissatisfaction with life by day and dissatisfaction with life by night. They look to the doctor for the understanding and sympathy they feel they deserve to get elsewhere but fail to find.

The doctor likes to believe he is kindly, helpful, and always possessed of the power to relieve suffering. He feels his image would be tarnished if he said, in plain terms, that there was nothing he could do to bring relief. Most doctors are men, while most of those who complain about their sleep and succeed in getting hypnotics are women, and, over the years, some of the latter become adroit in eliciting a prescription, even if the doctor has inner doubts. There had been that nice doctor a few years before who used to understand and who helped her so much, and then after him there was that uncaring brute whose practice she soon left, now to come to you who surely are one of the nicer, kindlier, more helpful among doctors and who surely will not refuse her what she needs. Thus it may come to pass that, as a token of his caring ways the doctor pens a prescription. After an interval the patient returns for more and soon the doctor prefers to avoid seeing her and leaves the writing of prescriptions to the practice secretary (Freed, 1976). And why not, one might reply? If modern hypnotic drugs work, and people like them, then are these drugs not in the same category as modern contraceptives or telephones, to be made available to those who seek them? Certainly they are cheaper and less dangerous than alcohol (see Chapter 1). Here is the doctor's dilemma, for he may feel it wrong in principle to be a liberal prescriber but yet wants to be helpful. He may have fears about the long-term effect of what he may prescribe. He may reflect that, although hypnotics have a long history, from the days when alcohol, the mandrake root, the poppy, the barbiturates, or the thalidomide were first choice, yet medical knowledge about sleep and about hypnotics has remained sparse.

## WHAT DOES SLEEP DO FOR US?

We have to ask, what does sleep do for us? Is the sleep of insomniacs less effective in doing whatever it is? If less effective, do drugs like benzodiazepines put matters right? What benefit does sleep bring? We feel better when we have had a good night's sleep. People who sleep at irregular hours rate themselves as less happy than do regular sleepers (Taub, 1978). Severely curtailed sleep is associated with inability to sustain attention, and the most obvious benefits of sleep are associated with efficiency of the central nervous system. People feel restored by their sleep and it is indeed the case that structural renewal by mitoses and protein synthesis is facilitated in all bodily tissues during the time of sleep. The reasons for this remain the subject for future research, but the altered ratio of high energy phosphates within cells, as a consequence of the profound rest that sleep brings, seems the likely primary mechanism (Adam, 1980), with the differing hormone pictures also important. Wakefulness is a time of profligate use of energy, of highest levels of the catabolic hormones, corticosteroids, and catecholamines. Sleep is a time of maximal rest, especially for the brain, in which glucose consumption falls dramatically (Kennedy *et al.*, 1982) and is a time when the output of anabolic hormones is increased, notably growth hormone, while catabolic hormones sink to their lowest levels. Early in the night, during human sleep, there is EEG slow-wave sleep that specifically releases growth hormone (Sassin *et al.*, 1969; Schnure *et al.*, 1971), at the same time of night as corticosteroids fall to their lowest before rising in the later night to peak a couple of hours after first waking. In slow-wave sleep (SWS), rest is most extreme, with whole body oxygen consumption at its lowest (Brebbia and Altshuler, 1968; Haskell *et al.*, 1981), and responsiveness to the environment minimal (Williams *et al.*, 1966). Again, SWS has long been known to have first priority upon recovery from sleep loss (Berger and Oswald, 1962) and as sleep that is 'worth more' (Dement and Greenberg, 1966). It is this same SWS that is radically reduced in duration as a consequence of benzodiazepine intake.

## IS THE SLEEP OF INSOMNIACS LESS EFFECTIVE IN BRINGING BENEFITS?

Research into sleep has for many years now been dominated by the EEG. It is a valuable tool for telling us when someone is asleep and when awake. There are close and consistent correlations between the different depths or stages of sleep as judged, on the one hand by the EEG and, on the other behaviourally, or by other physiological means. Unfortunately, reliance on the EEG can blinker us into thinking we know more about sleep than is the case. We simply do not know if changes in the electrophysiologically recorded number of minutes of SWS or REM sleep are important, or if a minute of drugged sleep is 'worth' as much as, less than, or more than a minute of natural sleep.

If we consider first how many minutes of sleep are achieved (and this the EEG can tell us very accurately) then those who complain of poor sleep actually sleep more than they believe, but somewhat less than controls of the same age. There are plenty of people who have short and broken sleep yet have no complaints, while others of the same age sleep unbrokenly, and for longer, and are full of vivid complaints. There are patients who claim that, for example, they have not slept at all for many years, but who, upon investigation, are found to sleep (Oswald and Adam, 1980a). The degree of subjective inaccuracy on the part of even the average complainer is considerable (Carskadon *et al.*, 1976; Frankel *et al.*, 1976). As an example Frankel *et al.* (1976) studied in the laboratory a group of 18 people of mean age 45 who persistently complained of poor sleep, and compared them with 18 age-matched controls who had no complaints. The non-complainers overestimated their sleep, while the complainers took only half as long to fall asleep as they themselves believed, and slept 10% longer than they themselves believed, albeit they slept three-quarters of an hour less than the non-complainers.

Monroe (1967) had earlier studied a group of young adults who thought themselves good sleepers, and compared them with others who thought themselves poor sleepers and reported similar findings. He also made physiological measures, and it is of interest that through the night the mean rectal temperature of the poor sleepers remained significantly higher than that of the good sleepers, suggesting a higher rate of catabolism and poorer rest.

A similar study of young adults was described by Johns *et al.* (1971), with persistently higher levels of urinary corticosteroids by night and by day among the poor sleepers. In a recently completed study by my colleagues, (Dr Adam and Miss Tomeny), good sleepers and poor sleepers of mean age 52 were compared in pairs, matched for height, weight, age, and exercise. The poor sleepers were significantly hotter by day and there was some supporting evidence for higher levels of overnight urinary output of corticosteroids. The higher day temperature might be related to the higher levels of trait anxiety that were also found among the poor sleepers. Even the anxiety of first sleeping in unfamiliar surroundings is associated with a higher rate of overnight catabolism, manifested by greater whole body oxygen consumption through the night, as Webb and Hiestand (1975) reported. These latter authors, in their paper, stated that the difference did not achieve significance, but Webb (personal communication) has since reported that the statement should be amended and that, using a correlated *t*-test, the difference between a first night and a second night was indeed significant.

All these metabolic data suggest that, in the balance between continual degradation of the body's cells and their continual renewal, there are factors that, in the poor sleepers, would shift the balance in favour of degradation not only by day but also by night, with less than optimal metabolic conditions for restorative sleep at night. Consequently, even if those who complain of poor sleep do exaggerate or are inaccurate, they may have a metabolic basis for their feeling of not having been fully restored.

Poor sleepers, it may thus be hypothesized, include some who are more anxious and hotter, with a correspondingly greater need for restoration, yet with sleep of lesser duration and poorer restorative quality at night. Would benzodiazepines improve things (Adam, 1979)?

## WHAT DO BENZODIAZEPINES DO FOR SLEEP?

### Subjective ratings

In subjective terms, the benzodiazepines improve the quality of sleep and shorten the time spent awake before the onset of sleep. Figure 1 shows smoothed curves for self-rated sleep quality during 32 weeks while 25 poor sleepers took placebos nightly, another 25 took nitrazepam 5 mg for the middle 24 weeks, and 47 took lormetazepam 2 mg for the middle 24 weeks, the latter weeks being preceded and followed by placebos. Either drug caused improvement, and this improvement was to an extent sustained for 24 weeks. There was then a rebound upon withdrawal, with sleep becoming temporarily worse than would have been the case had drugs never been taken (Oswald *et al.*, 1982). There were similar findings with subjective ratings of sleep latency.

In clinical practice, if hypnotics are to be withdrawn, placebos are not customarily given and the patient is often fearful lest she will be quite unable to fall asleep without her customary capsule. This fearfulness may itself delay

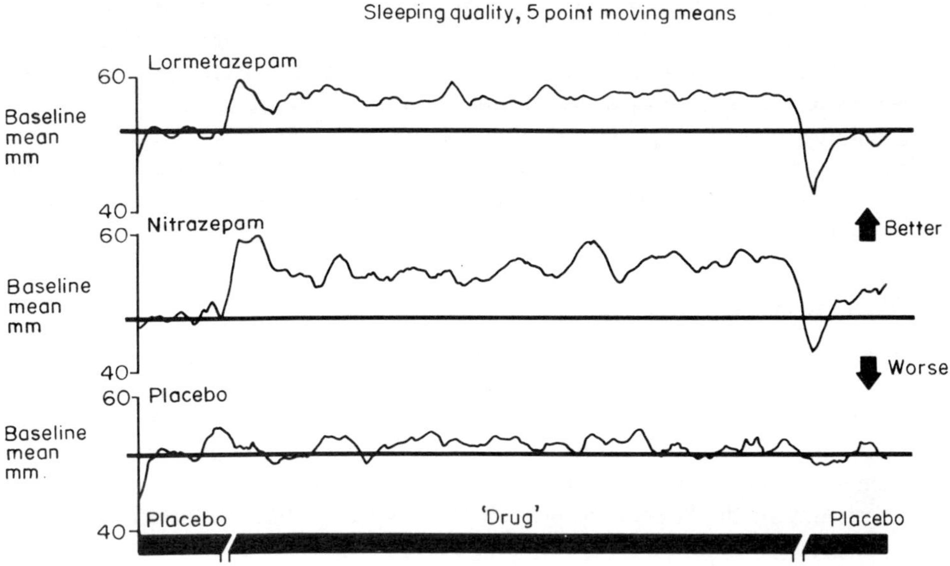


Figure 1 Daily ratings of sleep quality during 32 weeks, smoothed and shown as five-point moving means. Compared with placebo, both drugs cause sustained improvement, with rebound worsening after withdrawal (Oswald *et al.*, 1982)

the onset of sleep, and the doctor should explain to the patient that he understands her fear, and that because the nervous system has got used to the drug there really may be poor sleep for several weeks and that persistence on her part is needed in attempting to sleep without drugs. Support from the doctor through the initial withdrawal period is of great importance for such patients.

The same fearfulness plays a part while drugs are taken regularly: the patient fears that she will not get to sleep *tonight* unless she takes her pill. This very fear will itself delay sleep till, at one o'clock in the morning, she finally swallows a dose. It is not possible to divorce this fear from evening anxiety of pharmacological origin, from rebound effects. The regular intake of a short-acting hypnotic in the evening relieves anxiety and promotes sleep. Next day the tissue levels have fallen to a point where withdrawal symptoms begin to appear, notably anxiety and difficulty in falling asleep. Alcohol is the most familiar example. A bottle of gin each evening (alcohol being about 50% metabolized in 4 hours) means withdrawal anxiety and tension the next day and difficulty in falling asleep till another dose is taken. The same appears true of, for example, triazolam 0.5 mg, this benzodiazepine derivative having a similarly short persistence. Taken nightly for 3 weeks by 21 poor sleepers, triazolam 0.5 mg was found by us to be associated with mounting daytime anxiety (on visual analogue scale ratings), whereas when the same poor sleepers took the longer acting loprazolam 1 mg, their daytime anxiety fell (Morgan and Oswald, 1982). Greater anxiety is, as mentioned, associated with greater difficulty in falling asleep, and Dement *et al.* (1982) used their sleep latency test to measure how long it took subjects to fall asleep when deliberately given the opportunity every 2 hours from morning until evening. When patients or normals were given triazolam 0.5 mg nightly for a week, they had significantly greater delay in falling asleep than when they merely took placebos for a week.

### Objective measures of sleep

Benzodiazepines promote sleep, so that measured sleep may come more quickly, be less interrupted, and last longer, and as a consequence the measured duration is increased. Many studies testify to this in the case of, for example, nitrazepam (Adam *et al.*, 1976), flurazepam (Kales *et al.*, 1975), lormetazepam (Oswald *et al.*, 1979) or triazolam (Kales *et al.*, 1976). Shortening of the latency to onset of sleep is least reliably found in research investigations as the latency depends partly on absorption time and, being always a skewed measure with a large variance, drug effects have to be considerable for statistical significance to be achieved. Deliberate awakenings are more quickly followed by resumption of sleep if a benzodiazepine has been taken (Bonnet and Webb, 1979).

As a typical example of a laboratory study, Adam and Oswald (1982) used all-night electrophysiological measures to study the effects of nitrazepam 5 mg on the sleep of 12 poor sleepers of mean age 60 years. Each slept 2 nights in the laboratory for adaptation purposes in one week, and then 2 nights in the next week while baseline recordings were made, and while receiving inert capsules nightly. Genuine nitrazepam capsules were then taken nightly for 3 weeks and 2 nights were recorded in the first drug week. Then, after another adaptation night, another two nights were recorded in the third drug week before inert capsules were resumed for a further week, during which latter week another 3 nights were recorded to assess withdrawal effects. During the first week on nitrazepam the subjects on average fell asleep significantly more quickly and they also slept some 50 min longer. By the third week of intake there was no longer the significant shortening of sleep latency, but the increase in total duration of sleep above baseline was still present, yet now significantly less than in the first week of nitrazepam, demonstrating a degree of *tolerance*. The proportions of different sleep stages were altered by nitrazepam, there being a small but significant decrease in the duration of REM sleep during the earlier part of the night and, by the third week of intake, a halving in the total duration of SWS, stages 3 + 4.

The marked effect on SWS is a consistent one for benzodiazepines and has been particularly studied as a feature of flurazepam intake (Johnson *et al.*,

1979). The brief groups of EEG slow wave with faster components, known as K-complexes, are also fewer during sleep under flurazepam (Johnson *et al.*, 1979).

The cardinal EEG features of sleep are the sleep spindles, namely groups of continuous waves at 12–14 Hz of about a second or two in duration. Mere slow waves occur whenever the cortex is functioning inefficiently. All the benzodiazepines greatly enhance the prominence and duration of the sleep spindles, and this has again been specially studied with flurazepam (Johnson *et al.*, 1976). Such changes remind one that the brain is not functioning in the same way during drugged sleep as during natural sleep. Sleep is too a time normally associated with enhanced consolidation or strengthening of new memories, but clinical doses of such benzodiazepines as lorazepam, flurazepam, or triazolam alter the brain's functioning sufficiently to impair that strengthening, with reduced recall in the morning of material newly learned the previous evening (Roth *et al.*, 1980). A further reminder of the way that hypnotics have been blithely prescribed for years without a good understanding of what they are doing to patients is provided by the fact that only in 1982 has it been realized that flurazepam or triazolam, taken at bedtime, causes an increase in heart rate for several hours (Muzet *et al.*, 1982).

When hypnotics such as benzodiazepines increase total sleep and reduce REM sleep, their withdrawal leads to a rebound with short sleep and excess REM sleep, but this has not proved true for slow-wave sleep, which seems simply to return to normal values as the drug leaves the tissues and without causing rebound.

## The withdrawal rebound

Drugs that act on the CNS gradually induce changes in the CNS that become manifest partly as tolerance during intake and then by rebound upon withdrawal. The partial tolerance mentioned above for nitrazepam has also, for example, been seen with flunitrazepam (Scharf *et al.*, 1979). Consider a drug that reduces anxiety, reduces restlessness, reduces the propensity for fits, reduces REM sleep duration, reduces the vividness of dreams, but increases sleep duration. It will induce changes in the CNS such that when, after prolonged use (or after a single very large overdose), it leaves the CNS, then there will appear a rebound into fearfulness, restlessness, enhanced propensity for fits, excess REM sleep, and bizarre dreams, even with the latter breaking into wakefulness as hallucinations and paranoid fears, and all accompanied by reduced sleep duration. In severe form we thus see the picture of delirium tremens, including as it does almost total insomnia, especially after older shorter acting hypnotics, including alcohol, but rare in its full form after benzodiazepines. More commonly in present-day clinical practice, after the withdrawal of benzodiazepines there is simply a temporary enhancement of anxiety (Allen and Oswald, 1976; Petursson and Lader, 1981), with fleeting paranoid ideas, restlessness, and moderate insomnia. Fits do occur, but one encounters them much less often than in the days of barbiturates. The enhancement of REM sleep as part of the rebound makes possible precise and convenient measurement and reveals that some 5 weeks or so are needed for recovery, whatever the drug. The long duration should presumably be attributed to the slow turnover time of cerebral proteins and not to any individual features of the drug.

Figure 2 illustrates that, when 10 poor sleepers of mean age 57 years took nitrazepam 5 mg regularly, their objectively measured sleep was by the eighth week still less broken than under earlier baseline conditions, but that upon withdrawal, sleep was more broken than would have been the case had the drug never been taken. The rebound, an inevitable feature, makes it genuinely difficult for patients to stop accustomed hypnotics, so that intake of benzodiazepines tends to be self-perpetuating. Rebound insomnia has not been described with flurazepam and this may be attributed to the fact that abrupt withdrawal never occurs owing to the very long-persisting active metabolites that make withdrawal a very gradual process. The most immediate rebounds occur after the short-life drugs, such as triazolam (Kales *et al.*, 1976), indeed in a recently completed EEG study of triazolam 0.5 mg nightly

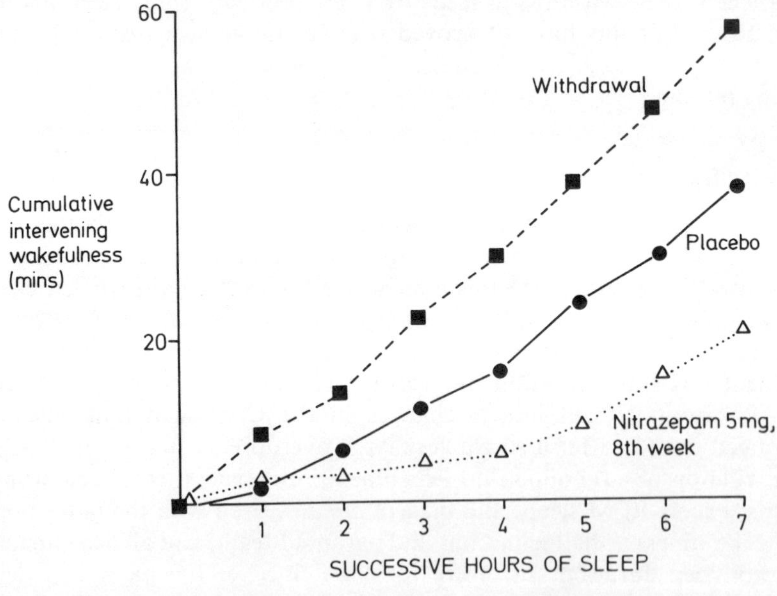


Figure 2 Mean cumulative minutes of wakefulness intervening during the sleep of 10 volunteer poor sleepers, mean age 57. All points are based upon 6 nights for each person under each condition, with the withdrawal data being drawn from the first 2 weeks after stopping nitrazepam (Adam *et al.*, 1976)

for 3 weeks, followed by withdrawal, there was the most severe and immediate rebound insomnia this author has encountered in any research study.

Recently there were proposals that rebound insomnia was 'a new clinical syndrome' in some way peculiar to the benzodiazepines (Kales *et al.*, 1978, 1979). The syndrome was not new, and the literature on the withdrawal of all other hypnotics, including alcohol, is replete with references to the insomnia so caused. Indeed, it was recognized for paraldehyde withdrawal nearly a hundred years ago, and was well described as part of the barbiturate withdrawal syndrome by Wulff (1959).

**Relation to sleep's restorative qualities**

Patients usually like their sleep better after an hypnotic, and if they *feel* restored, perhaps that should be taken as a guide. On more objective grounds, evidence is thin. Although benzodiazepines reduce SWS, as manifested by the EEG waves, and although SWS is the stimulus for the principal secretion of growth hormone during the 24 hours, the underlying CNS events governing growth hormone secretion at such times seem to be unaltered. There are several reports in which two or three subjects have been reported to have their growth hormone unchanged after benzodiazepine intake and Adam *et al.* (1976) found no effect on growth hormone among seven middle-aged subjects when nitrazepam 5 mg had been taken for 8 weeks, and despite the customary reduction of EEG slow-wave sleep.

Among catabolic hormones, it is to be expected that both catecholamines and corticosteroids would be lowered by anxiety-reducing benzodiazepines. In one Edinburgh study reported by Ogunremi *et al.* (1973), venous blood had been sampled at half-hourly intervals during sleep via an indwelling catheter and without disturbing sleep. The minor tranquillizer benzoctamine, taken nightly by eight subjects, was then associated with significantly lower plasma corticosteroids (as assessed by areas under the curve between fixed times), though with a later significant rebound above baseline upon withdrawal. Similarly, in another recent Edinburgh study of nine poor sleepers of mean age 55 years, Adam has found both triazolam 0.5 mg and loprazolam 1 mg to be associated with a tendency to lowered overnight urinary cortisol levels, but then a significant rebound above baseline levels upon withdrawal, the rebound being immediate and large with the dose of triazolam used. Since cortisol enhances amino acid degradation and inhibits protein synthesis, sleep associated with withdrawal of benzodiazepines may be inferred to be of poorer restorative value, quite apart from any reduction in sleep duration. If it can be confirmed that there are lower cortisol (and adrenaline) values during sleep after benzodiazepines then, on those grounds, sleep of better restorative potential might be presumed. The same would be inferred, of course, from the increased duration of sleep, though it should be remembered that for patients with emphysema and chronic bronchitis, benzodiazepines such as nitrazepam (Gaddie *et al.*, 1972; Rudolf *et al.*, 1978) and possibly temazepam (Pleuvry *et al.*, 1980) may cause carbon dioxide retention and so impede the benefits of sleep.

While numerous papers show enhancement of mitoses at the time of sleep, there are no reports of the effect of benzodiazepines, though Bullough (1948) reported that the pinnal mitoses of mice could be enhanced by inducing sleep with barbiturates. When we gave benzodiazepines to 75 volunteer poor sleepers and blank capsules to another 25 poor sleepers, we found a small but significant loss of body weight after 5 months of intake of benzodiazepines, with no change among those taking the blanks (Oswald and Adam, 1980b). The site of loss is unknown (we think it was *not* through atrophy of brain!), though one remembers that the benzodiazepines are muscle relaxants and that diminished tone might lead to some slight wasting in the postural muscles. A lot of middle-aged women receive diazepam or other benzodiazepines, and a lot of middle-aged women complain of backache. Phenobarbitone had earlier been held to be a possible cause of the shoulder–hand syndrome of stiffness in the shoulder and some atrophy of the hand (Van der Korst *et al.*, 1960), and one wonders if benzodiazepines might cause back trouble.

## A BENZODIAZEPINE FOR SLEEP?

If an hypnotic is to be taken at all, then the benzodiazepines are at present the most suitable. Overdosages are our modern epidemic and the barbiturates are too often lethal (Johns, 1977). In the Edinburgh Poisons Unit, having some 2000 admissions per year, the number of unconscious patients admitted has steadily declined year by year since the benzodiazepines came increasingly to be taken, and deaths as a consequence of benzodiazepines are rare. An overdose of, for example, nitrazepam is followed by excessive sleepiness and inertia, the drug is slowly eliminated over a period of 10–12 days and during this time the brokenness of sleep increases until finally this withdrawal rebound subsides by the fourth or fifth week, as Figure 3 illustrates (Haider and Oswald, 1970).

## TEN-HOUR HALF-LIFE BENZODIAZEPINES MAY BE THE BEST

The choice among benzodiazepines is large. I used to say they were all the same. They generally were, being mostly long-acting. Increasing experience of the daytime impairments (Oswald *et al.*, 1979; Johnson and Chernik, 1982), and particularly experience of daytime emotional crises and accidents released by flurazepam 30 mg nightly (Oswald *et al.*, 1979) have left me in no doubt that the really long-acting benzodiazepines should be avoided.

I used to suppose that a very short-acting hypnotic, all of it vanishing by

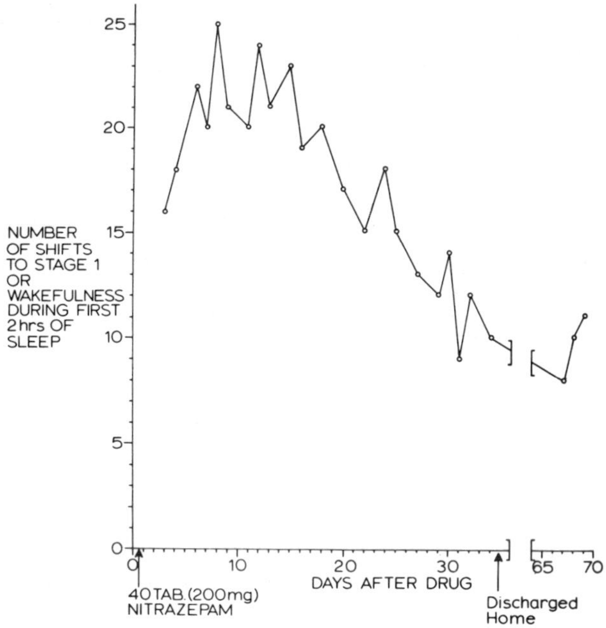


Figure 3 Brokenness of sleep, shown on the ordinate, during the early night, rises to high levels about 10 nights after an overdose of nitrazepam and declines gradually in the succeeding 3 weeks (Haider and Oswald, 1970)

breakfast time, would be ideal, but I should have remembered the alcoholic's morning shakes. Experience of an extensive research project with the very short-life triazolam and the daytime anxiety that it caused, as already mentioned, and adverse reports from the Netherlands about the same drug have disillusioned me. On the other hand, experience over several years of research with lormetazepam as a relatively trouble-free hypnotic, leads me to believe that an hypnotic with a half-life of around 10 hours, such as lormetazepam or temazepam, offers a sensible compromise. The cumulative flurazepam dopes people about as much by day as by night; the ultrashort-life triazolam causes rapid see-sawing in CNS drug concentrations. A benzodiazepine that does not see-saw as violently, is not cumulative, that acts at night, is only half gone by breakfast time, while by then too low in concentration to cause appreciable impairment, and persisting enough to prevent rebound anxiety before the next dose, would seem about the best. Even it, however, will not offer escape from the final withdrawal rebound.

## REFERENCES


Adam, K. (1979). Do drugs alter the restorative value of sleep? In: *Pharmacology of the States of Alertness*, pp.105–111 (Eds. Passouant, P. and Oswald, I.), Pergamon, Oxford.

Adam, K. (1980). Sleep as a restorative process and a theory to explain why. *Prog. Brain Res.*, **53**, 289-305.

Adam, K., Adamson, L., Brezinova, V., Hunter, W. M. and Oswald, I. (1976). Nitrazepam: lastingly effective but trouble on withdrawal. *Brit. med. J.*, **1**, 1558-1560.

Adam, K. and Oswald, I. (1982). A comparison of the effects of clormezanone and nitrazepam on sleep. *Brit. J. clin. pharmac.*, **14**, 57-65.

Allen, S. and Oswald, I. (1976). Anxiety and sleep after fosazepam, *Brit. J. clin. Pharmac.*, **3**, 165-168.

Berger, R. J. and Oswald, I. (1962). Effects of sleep deprivation on behaviour, subsequent sleep and dreaming. *J. ment. Sci.*, **108**, 457-465.

Bonnet, M. H. and Webb, W. B. (1979). The return to sleep. *Biol. Psychol.*, **8**, 225-233.

Brebbia, D. R. and Altshuler, K. Z. (1968). Stage related patterns and nightly trends of energy exchange during sleep. In: *Computers and Electronic Devices in Psychiatry*, pp.319-336 (Eds Kline, N. S. and Laska, E.), Grune and Stratton, New York.

Bullough, W. S. (1948). The effects of experimentally induced rest and exercise on the epidermal mitotic activity of the adult male mouse, Mus musculus L. *Proc. R. Soc. (Series B)*, **135**, 233-242.

Carskadon, M. A., Dement, W. C., Mitler, M. M., Gilleminault, C., Zarcone, V. P. and Spiegel, R. (1976). Self-reports versus sleep laboratory findings in 122 drug-free subjects with complaints of chronic insomnia. *Am. J. Psychiat.*, **133**, 1382-1388.

Dement, W. and Greenberg, S. (1966). Changes in total amount of stage four sleep as a function of partial sleep deprivation. *EEG and clin. Neurophysiol.*, **20**, 523-526.

Dement, W., Seidel, W. and Carskadon, M. (1982). Daytime alertness, insomnia and benzodiazepines. *Sleep*, **5**, S28-S45.

Frankel, B. L., Coursey, R. D., Buchbinder, R. and Snyder, F. (1976). Recorded and reported sleep in chronic primary insomnia. *Arch. gen. Psychiat.*, **33**, 615-623.

Freed, A. (1976). Prescribing of tranquillisers and barbiturates by general practitioners, *Brit. med. J.*, **2**, 1932-1933.

Gaddie, J., Legge, J. S., Palmer, K. N. V., Petrie, J. C. and Wood, R. A. (1972). Effect of nitrazepam in chronic obstructive bronchitis. *Br. med. J.*, **2**, 688-689.

Haider, I. and Oswald, I. (1970). Late brain recovery processes after drug overdose. *Brit. med. J.*, **2**, 318-322.

Haskell, E. H., Palca, J. W., Walker, J. M., Berger, R. J. and Heller, H. C. (1981). Metabolism and thermoregulation during stages of sleep in humans exposed to heat and cold. *J. appl. Physiol.*, **51**, 948-954.

Johns, M. W. (1977). Self-poisoning with barbiturates in England and Wales during 1959-74. *Brit. med. J.*, **1**, 1128-1130.

Johns, M. W., Gay, T. J. A., Masterton, J. P. and Bruce, D. W. (1971). Relationship between sleep habits, adrenocortical activity and personality. *Psychosom. Med.*, **33**, 499-508.

Johnson, L. C. and Chernik, D. A. (1982). Sedative-hypnotics and human performance. *Psychopharmacology*, **76**, 101-113.

Johnson, L. C., Hanson, K. and Bickford, R. G. (1976). Effect of flurazepam on sleep spindles and K-complexes. *EEG and clin. Neurophysiol.*, **40**, 67-77.

Johnson, L. C., Seales, D. M., Naitoh, P., Church, M. W. and Sinclair, M. (1979). The effects of flurazepam hydrochloride on brain electrical activity during sleep. *EEG and clin. Neurophysiol.*, **47**, 309-321.

Kales, A., Kales, J. D., Bixler, E. O. and Scharf, M. B. (1975). Effectiveness of hypnotic drugs with prolonged use: flurazepam and pentobarbital. *Clin. Pharmac. Ther.*, **18**, 356-363.

Kales, A., Kales, J. D., Bixler, E. O., Scharf, M. B. and Russek, E. (1976). Hypnotic efficacy of triazolam: sleep laboratory evaluation of intermediate-term effectiveness. *J. clin. Pharmac.*, **16**, 399–406.

Kales, A., Scharf, M. B. and Kales, J. D. (1978). Rebound insomnia: a new clinical syndrome. *Science*, **201**, 1039–1041.

Kales, A., Scharf, M. B., Kales, J. D. and Soldatos, C. R. (1979). Rebound insomnia: a potential hazard following withdrawal of certain benzodiazepines. *J. Am. med. Ass.*, **241**, 1692–1695.

Karacan, I., Thornby, J. I., Anch, M., Holzer, C. E., Warheit, G. J., Schwab, J. J. and Williams, R. L. (1976). Prevalence of sleep disturbance in a primarily urban Florida county. *Soc. Sci. Med.*, **10**, 239–244.

Kennedy, C., Gillin, J. C., Mendelson, W., Suda, S., Miyaoka, M., Ito, M., Nakamura, R. K., Storch, F. I., Pettigrew, K., Mishkin, M. and Sokoloff, L. (1982). Local cerebral glucose utilization in non-rapid eye movement sleep. *Nature (Lond.)*, **297**, 325–327.

McGhie, A. and Russell, S. M. (1962). The subjective assessment of normal sleep patterns. *J. ment. sci.*, **108**, 642–654.

Monroe, L. J. (1967). Psychological and physiological differences between good and poor sleepers. *J. abnorm. Psychol.*, **72**, 255–264.

Morgan, K. and Oswald, I. (1982). Anxiety caused by a short-life hypnotic. *Brit. med. J.*, **284**, 942.

Muzet, A., Johnson, L. C. and Spinweber, C. L. (1982). Benzodiazepine hypnotics increase heart rate during sleep. *Sleep*, **5**, 256–261.

Ogunremi, O. O., Adamson, L., Brezinova, V., Hunter, W. M., Maclean, A. W., Oswald, I. and Percy-Robb, I. W. (1973). Two anti-anxiety drugs: a psychoneuroendocrine study, *Brit. med. J.*, **2**, 202–205.

Oswald, I. and Adam, K. (1980a). The man who had not slept for 10 years. *Brit. med. J.*, **281**, 1684–1685.

Oswald, I. and Adam, K. (1980b). Benzodiazepines cause small loss of body weight. *Brit. med. J.*, **281**, 1039–1040.

Oswald, I., Adam, K., Borrow, S. and Idzikowski, C. (1979). The effects of two hypnotics on sleep, subjective feelings and skilled performance. In: *Pharmacology of the States of Alertness*, pp.51–63 (Eds Passouant, P. and Oswald, I.), Pergamon, Oxford.

Oswald, I., French, C., Adam, K. and Gilham, J. (1982). Benzodiazepine hypnotics remain effective for 24 weeks. *Brit. med. J.*, **284**, 860–863.

Petursson, H. and Lader, M. H. (1981). Withdrawal from long-term benzodiazepine treatment. *Brit. med. J.*, **283**, 643–645.

Pleuvry, B. J., Maddison, S. E., Odeh, R. B. and Dodson, M. E. (1980). Respiratory and psychological effects of oral temazepam in volunteers. *Brit. J. Anaesth.*, **52**, 901–906.

Roth, T., Hartse, K. M., Saab, P. G., Piccione, P. M. and Kramer, M. (1980). The effects of flurazepam, lorazepam and triazolam on sleep and memory. *Psychopharmacology*, **70**, 231–237.

Rudolf, M., Geddes, D. M., Turner, J. A. McM. and Saunders, K. B. (1978). Depression of central respiratory drive by nitrazepam. *Thorax*, **33**, 97–100.

Sassin, J. F., Parker, D. C., Johnson, L. C., Rossman, L. G., Mace, J. W. and Gotlin, R. W. (1969). Effects of slow wave sleep deprivation on human growth hormone release in sleep: preliminary study. *Life Sci. (Part I)*, **8**, 1299–1307.

Scharf, M. B., Bixler, E. O., Kales, A. and Soldatos, C. R. (1979). Long-term sleep laboratory evaluation of flunitrazepam. *Pharmacology*, **19**, 173–181.

Schnure, J. J., Raskin, P. and Lipman, R. L. (1971). Growth hormone secretion during sleep: impairment in glucose tolerance and non-suppressibility by hyperglycemia. *J. clin. Endrocrinol.* **33**, 234–241.

Taub, J. M. (1978). Behavioural and psychophysiological correlates of irregularity in chronic sleep routines. *Biol. Psychol.*, **7**, 37–53.

Van der Korst, J. K., Colenbrander, H. and Cats, A. (1960). Phenobarbital and the shoulder–hand syndrome. *Ann. Rheumatic Dis.*, **25**, 553–555.

Webb, P. and Hiestand, M. (1975). Sleep metabolism and age. *J. appl. Physiol.*, **38**, 257–262.

Williams, H. L., Morlock, H. C. and Morlock, J. V. (1966). Discriminative responses to auditory signals during sleep. *Psychophysiology*, **2**, 208–215.

Wulff, M. H. (1959). The barbiturate withdrawal syndrome. *EEG and clin. Neurophysiol.*, Supplement **14**, 1–161.

## DISCUSSION

## CHAIRMAN: PROFESSOR A. RICHENS

THE CHAIRMAN: Perhaps I could open up the discussion by asking Professor Oswald about rapid eye movement sleep. When nitrazepam was introduced, it was argued then that the drug suppressed rapid eye movement sleep less than the barbiturates. This was a good feature because suppression of rapid eye movement sleep was undesirable, and impaired the quality of sleep. Could you tell us what the present view is about this?

PROFESSOR OSWALD: I think I was inadvertently somewhat responsible for that. In 1965 we published a paper on the suppression of rapid eye movement sleep and a rebound on withdrawal from nitrazepam, and of course rapid eye movement sleep was very popular, everybody identified it with dreaming. My colleague Dr. Adam now has, for the second time, shown in a very large study that if you take middle-aged people of stable body weight the amount of REM sleep is proportional to gross body weight, and it is no longer seen that you have got to dream in order to stay sane. All these drugs do diminish the amount of REM sleep. They are not terribly powerful in doing so compared with, say, the tricyclic antidepressants or the monoamine oxidase inhibitors, but they do reduce it. You get a rebound on withdrawal, but we do not know any clinical significance of that, except I should say there is good evidence that people in delirium tremens have — and indeed we have seen this ourselves — paradoxical or REM sleep bursting into wakefulness, abruptly. The suppression of REM sleep by the drug leads to this rebound on withdrawal, and as anxiety is high with the rebound, so they are getting fearful dreamlike experiences. That is the only clinical significance I can attach to it.

DR. TRIMBLE: Am I right in assuming, from the data you have shown, that we are correct to prescribe benzodiazepines for our patients who complain of insomnia? Thus patients actually say they sleep better when they have benzodiazepines, and that effect continues contrary to what we are often told. It seems to me there may be justification here for my patient who says, 'Well, doctor, I sleep better on them and therefore I want them to be prescribed'.

PROFESSOR OSWALD: I think that there is tolerance. We published a paper earlier this year on nitrazepam showing a significantly reduced effect after 3 weeks compared with the first week, but there still was a significant effect though reduced at a larger time. I am sure there is a degree of tolerance but it is not complete. The same is true of barbiturates. There is tolerance to barbiturates, but it is never complete and you never get barbiturate addicts taking a hundred capsules a day in the way that amphetamine addicts will take their tablets.

If it goes on being effective, why should we not go on giving it to patients? You may think that, like telephones and the contraceptive pill, sleeping pills are part of modern life and people might as well have them, or you may have a stern attitude to prescribing and the doctor's responsibility. I do not think it is an easy matter, but my own attitude is only to prescribe these drugs where I can foresee that there is likely to be a time when they can be stopped.

DR. COBB: It seemed to me from your interesting data about the discrepancy between actual sleep and reported sleep that the right clinical advice to patients on night sedation would be, 'Do not take your tablets before you go to bed but go to bed and if after half-an-hour you are still awake then take a tablet'.

PROFESSOR OSWALD: A lot of people do say that, but of course then they are going to be a little bit more doped in the morning than they would otherwise have been. You have two factors: they are anxious lest they do not fall asleep, and they are anxious because they are going into withdrawal in some cases. Some time the drugs have got to stop and that is where the doctor comes in. He tells his patient that he is going to sleep badly, he is going to have nightmares, he is going to have several rough weeks but that if he persists and keeps it up he will sleep just as well without his drugs. It is up to the doctor to support the patient and let the patient be dependent on him instead of being dependent on the drug, and then some weeks later to wean the patient off that dependence.

DR. TYRER: I have two questions which are quite important clinically. The first is, what would you regard as the minimum length of time that a person could remain on a hypnotic without having rebound insomnia on withdrawal? Second, do you think there are important differences in the rebound effects of benzodiazepine hypnotics between 3 and 20 hours' half-life? Do you think it is a question of half-life more than anything else or are there other factors involved?

PROFESSOR OSWALD: I am quite sure, and I see no reason why it should be to the contrary, that a single dose will do what I have described. But, of course, a single dose is not going to do as much as repeated doses, and it is a matter of degree and the size of the dose.

Your second point was whether there was much difference between one of 3 hours' half-life and one of 20 hours' half-life. A 20 hour half-life one will accumulate a bit and a 3 hour one will not. I used to be one who took the view that the ideal hypnotic would be one with a half-life of about 3 hours: take it tonight and it is all gone by breakfast time. But I should have given a bit more thought to the long-standing hypnotic alcohol. The alcoholic creates his own anxiety and tension by the drug he takes and he keeps taking the drug to keep anxiety down.

DR. COHN: We repeated your studies in a different way. We gave triazolam, lorazepam, and flurazepam and we got what you call rebound anxiety, but we called it arousal. Would you say that your people who were more anxious, were also more aroused and more eager to do something?

PROFESSOR OSWALD: They were making ratings, using a visual analogue scale, each evening of how anxious they had been during the day. That is the measure. The concept of arousal is an abstract concept that was in the ordinary language and then become much modified with the discovery of the reticular formation. It is always a little uncertain what people mean by this term 'arousal', but I think most of us have a sort of vague understanding that people are more awake, and also often more anxious. I can only report what we measured.

PROFESSOR HAMILTON: Accepting your principle that hypnotics should never be prescribed except for a limited period, would it be of help if, during that time they were prescribed for only 5 nights a week and stopped during the weekend? Would that diminish dependence and all these other difficulties you have been talking about?

PROFESSOR OSWALD: I suppose patients rather like rules handed down by their doctor and so there might be some advantage in that, but I would have thought that all you would do would be to ensure that the patient got a bad night's sleep each weekend.

PROFESSOR HAMILTON: It would not diminish the tendency to have dependence and severe after-effects?

PROFESSOR OSWALD: I am sure it would, yes.

DR. ROSE: My experience is that some people have difficulty getting off to sleep at night and some people tend to wake up early in the mornings. I am well aware that early morning waking is a symptom of depression, but it seems to me that a lot of the younger patients tend to have difficulty getting off and some of the older patients seem to develop this pattern of early morning waking which really is not part of a depressive disease.

PROFESSOR OSWALD: It is a natural feature of ageing.

DR. ROSE: That was one of the questions I was going to ask you. Is it, in fact, appropriate to treat it, and, if you are going to treat it, is a benzodiazepine the right drug to use?

PROFESSOR OSWALD: I think a benzodiazepine is the right drug to use, if you are going to use one, because it is safe. Whether you are going to treat it is another question because what you treat is the patient's complaint. You are trying to please the patient and to tell yourself that you are a kindly, helpful doctor. You know perfectly well that the patient sleeps far more than she says she sleeps, but you want an easy life, you want to feel comfortable inside, and so you write a prescription.

Benzodiazepines Divided
Edited by M. R. Trimble


# 20

# Benzodiazepines in Epilepsy

MICHAEL R. TRIMBLE

## INTRODUCTION

The earlier data with regard to the anticonvulsant effects of the benzodiazepines were reviewed in 1973 by Browne and Penry, and several selective reviews of individual drugs are available (see Woodbury *et al.*, 1982). A précis of these data will therefore briefly be given, prior to the results of some recent work that has been carried out on the use of oral clobazam as adjunctive therapy in epilepsy. This will be followed by a discussion on future possibilities and an exploration of some links between psychiatric illness and epilepsy, based on the acknowledged role of the usefulness of benzodiazepines in both categories of illness.

## BENZODIAZEPINES IN EPILEPSY

Epilepsy is a term which covers a wide range of convulsive disorders. Following the international classification, as recommended by the International League Against Epilepsy (Gastaut, 1969), seizures are broadly divided into two groups, namely generalized and partial (see Table 1). In generalized seizures there is no evidence, clinical or otherwise, to imply a local onset, and the manifestations, usually loss of consciousness with motor changes, reflect bilateral disturbances of the brain. Partial seizures begin focally, the symptom pattern being highly dependent on the area of the brain from which the abnormality arises. Complex partial seizures are focal attacks that usually, but not always, originate within the temporal lobes, during which consciousness is altered, and which, in the past may have included many attacks referred to as either temporal lobe epilepsy, or as psychomotor epilepsy.

Treatment for epilepsy depends to some extent on the type of seizures patients have, and their responsiveness to anticonvulsant drugs. Some, such as

Table 1 A classification of epilepsy

| | |
|---|---|
| Partial seizures | With simple symptomatology<br>1. with motor symptoms<br>2. with sensory or somatosensory symptoms<br>3. with autonomic symptoms<br>4. compound |
| | With complex symptomatology<br>1. with impaired consciousness alone<br>2. with cognitive symptoms<br>3. with affective symptoms<br>4. with psychosensory symptoms<br>5. with psychomotor symptoms<br>6. compound |
| Generalized seizures | 1. absences (petit mal)<br>2. with myoclonus<br>3. infantile spasms<br>4. clonic seizures<br>5. tonic seizures<br>6. tonic–clonic seizures (grand mal)<br>7. atonic seizures |
| Unilateral seizures | |
| Unclassified seizures | |

After the International League against Epilepsy recommendations.

generalized absence (petit mal) seizures respond well to ethosuccimide, the latter being virtually specific for such episodes. With generalized tonic–clonic and partial seizures, the commonest forms of seizures in epilepsy, the choice of drugs is wider, and a summary of the use of anticonvulsants for some forms of seizures is given in Table 2.

In addition, the benzodiazepines have a recognized clinical niche. Diazepam is a drug of choice intravenously for status epilepticus, 63–83% of patients achieving lasting control (Browne and Penry, 1973). Absence status seems especially sensitive, infantile myoclonic status responding poorly. Orally, however, it has never found acceptance, and there are few trials of its use as a sole anticonvulsant. Chien and Keegan (1972) randomly divided 42 epileptic patients into two groups, one of which was taken off their former drugs and started on diazepam (from 10 mg thrice daily), which was given for 6 months. Although no differences in the number of patients having seizures was noted, the diazepam group had a significantly higher number of generalized tonic–clonic attacks, while the standard treatment group had more 'minor seizures'. In a double-blind study of 32 patients, diazepam or pheneturide was given as adjunctive therapy in uncontrolled epilepsy (Hershon and Parsonage, 1969). Fifty per cent of those on the benzodiazepine and 31% of the pheneturide

Table 2 A summary of some currently prescribed anticonvulsant drugs and their clinical use

| Drug | Recommendations |
|---|---|
| Phenytoin (Epanutin) | P, G |
| Phenobarbitone | P, G |
| Primidone (Mysoline) | P, G |
| Ethosuccimide (Zarontin) | GA |
| Methsuccimide (Celontin) | P |
| Troxidone (Tridione) | GA |
| Carbamazepine (Tegretol) | P, G |
| Sodium valproate (Epilim) | G, GA |

P, partial seizures; G, generalized seizures; GA, generalized absence seizures. Note: list excludes benzodiazepines

group had a satisfactory improvement after 6 months, which was best in those with 'subcortical' seizures, or those whose seizures clustered, but neither drug was of value in night-time seizures. One reviewer of this subject reported that the findings suggest there is some limited effectiveness of diazepam in the treatment of psychomotor epilepsy (Mattson, 1972).

Table 3 Benzodiazepines that have been investigated in clinical studies (alphabetical order)

| | |
|---|---|
| Chlordiazepoxide | (Librium) |
| Clorazepate | (Tranxene) |
| Clobazam | (Frisium) |
| Diazepam | (Valium) |
| Lorazepam | (Ativan) |
| Nitrazepam | (Mogadon) |
| Oxazepam | (Serenid-D) |

Table 3 lists other benzodiazepines that have been examined in clinical studies. Few have been controlled, or used double-blind techniques. Lon (1968) gave oxazepam (15 mg thrice daily) or a placebo to 11 cases with predominantly complex partial seizures in a crossover design, in which the active drug was given in addition to existing anticonvulsant drugs for a period of 2 months. Three became seizure-free, and nine had a reduction of seizures greater than 50%. Evaluation of the electroencephalograms revealed six to be 'less paroxysmal' at the end of the active period.

Nitrazepam has been used orally in epilepsy since 1964 (Baruzzi *et al.*, 1982). It is found to be effective in a variety of seizure types, but its use is mainly in the treatment of infantile spasms with hypsarrhythmia, and in myoclonic epilepsies of childhood. Reviewing the literature, Baruzzi *et al.* also commented on case studies suggesting that nitrazepam was of value in the Lennox Gastaut syndrome in doses of up to 75 mg daily. However tolerance to its effects occurred in some 50% of patients within 3 months, and side effects were common but mild. Open studies of its value in primary generalized epilepsy suggests it is of less benefit, although several authors note improvement in some intractable cases of partial seizures, sometimes lasting many months.

The literature on clonazepam in epilepsy has been well reviewed (Browne, 1976, 1978), and of all the benzodiazepines in current use it has found the most acceptance as oral adjunctive therapy in epilepsy. It has been shown in double-blind trials to be as effective as ethosuccimide, and significantly superior than placebo or diazepam for the management of generalized absence seizures (Chandra, 1973; Mikkelsen *et al.*, 1976; Sato *et al.*, 1977). Doses of 3–6 mg a day are typical, and seizures seem controlled with serum concentrations of up to 70 ng/ml. Double-blind studies have also confirmed its value in myoclonic seizures (Nanda *et al.*, 1977). Its potential for the management of generalized tonic–clonic seizures, however, is less clear. While one controlled study against placebo showed it to be effective (Nanda *et al.*, 1977), in another (Feldman *et al.*, 1981) no difference was noted.

There have been several double-blind studies of its use in partial seizures. Mikkelsen *et al.* (1981) compared it with carbamazepine in 36 newly diagnosed patients with previously untreated psychomotor epilepsy. No significant differences between the drugs emerged at 6 months. In a smaller study, Bensch *et al.* (1977) gave clonazepam (maximum 10 mg daily) or placebo to 14 children with a variety of seizures, adding the therapy to the existing drug regimen. The design was a crossover study, with each therapy given for 3 months. Clonazepam was statistically superior to placebo, five patients becoming seizure-free. Shakir *et al.* (1979) carried out a crossover comparative study of clonazepam and sodium valproate in 15 adults already receiving anticonvulsant drugs. Both drugs reduced 'minor' seizure frequency, but valproate had the more significant result. In this study, pharmacokinetic data was also given. Serum concentrations of other anticonvulsants were unchanged by the addition of clonazepam, but patients receiving higher doses of other anticonvulsants had lower serum clonazepam levels. Similar data have been collected by Nanda *et al.* (1977), who, in an open study of clonazepam, found a significant negative correlation between clonazepam and phenobarbitone serum levels.

Lance and Anthony (1977), in a less well designed study than that of Shakir *et al.*, also compared clonazepam to sodium valproate in intractable epilepsy. Both were effective for the control of petit mal absences and myoclonic jerks, but clonazepam was superior in the management of partial seizures, and sodium valproate for the control of generalized tonic–clonic and atonic attacks.

In a more recent study, Wilensky *et al.* (1981) have evaluated the value of clorazepate against phenobarbitone in a double-blind study. Forty-three patients were on phenytoin throughout the investigation and both treatments were given for 4 months. Thirty-one preferred clorazepate and 12 phenobarbitone. The former was favoured especially by patients with complex partial seizures. No significant differences on seizures were noted, although subjects with many seizures during a baseline period of assessment had significantly better control with the clorazepate. Toxicity was significantly more frequent with phenobarbitone, and tolerance to the anticonvulsant effect of clorazepate was not seen. Serum level monitoring did not reveal any interaction between the clorazepate and phenytoin, and a serum level of desmethyldiazepam of around 1 mg/litre was thought to be therapeutic.

Other 1,4-benzodiazepines have not been the subject of much controlled investigative data so far. A summary of the value of these drugs would thus suggest that they are valuable across a wide spectrum of epileptic seizures, and often produce quite dramatic changes in EEG patterns. They seem to have more value against focal seizures than generalized attacks, and the tendency has been towards their acceptance as adjunctive, rather than first-line, therapy. Several of the studies discussed record patients whose control actually deteriorates following treatment (Browne and Penry, 1973), usually with exacerbation of generalized tonic–clonic seizures. In view of the paucity of studies, it is hardly surprising that little pharmacokinetic data are available, regarding both effective serum levels for seizure control and interaction with other anticonvulsant drugs. Most data are available for clonazepam for which it has been shown that steady-state plasma levels rise in direct proportion to the drug dose, and that phenytoin levels may fall in patients on combined therapy (Eadie and Tyrer, 1980), although generally interaction with other anticonvulsants is minimal.

Most authors that have used these benzodiazepines in epilepsy have commented on the relatively high frequency of side effects, especially behaviour problems (see Browne, 1978). Drowsiness and ataxia are recorded in 6–80% of cases, and interaction with barbiturates can be particularly severe. These problems tend to occur early in treatment, and to subside with chronic administration. Other problems include nausea, headache, double vision, speech disturbance, loss of appetite, listlessness, and hypotonia.

Behavioural disorders are frequent. While they are especially noted in children, they also occur in adults and include irritability, restlessness, aggression, outbursts of violence and disinhibition, and — more rarely — frank psychiatric illness. Psychotic episodes have been reported (see Browne and Penry, 1973), although their precise phenomenology is unclear. Nearly all reference to behaviour changes is anecdotal, but the findings bear a resemblance to the similar statements that were made about phenobarbitone and behaviour disorder following its use in epilepsy. Although there is some suggestion that it is patients, especially children, with pre-existing problems, that have these exacerbated by the anticonvulsant, who are prone, this is probably not the whole story. In particular, several authors have commented on the role of 'forced normalization' in the precipitation of behaviour problems (Livingston and Paull, 1977). Thus, in the epilepsy literature, there has been discussed for many years the so-called antagonism theory of the link between psychiatry and epilepsy (for review see Trimble, 1981). At the turn of this century it was thought that seizures and psychosis were somehow mutually exclusive, a concept that led to the introduction of convulsive therapies in psychiatry. Landolt (1958) recorded the electroencephalograms (EEG) of patients with epilepsy who had psychotic episodes that lasted several days, or sometimes longer, and noted an improvement in their previously abnormal records during the psychosis. On resolution of the psychosis, sometimes initiated by a seizure, the EEGs returned to abnormality, leading Landolt to refer to 'forced normalization' of the EEG as a mechanism for the development of the psychosis. Such observations have been confirmed by others, albeit in far fewer cases than Landolt collected.

Clinically, while such phenomena are probably quite rare, their existence raises to question the effects of normalizing the EEG in epileptic patients by anticonvulsant drugs. The investigations with benzodiazepines, where EEG monitoring has been carried out, show a reduction of abnormal background activity, and suppression of abnormal discharges, often with rapid and dramatic effects (Browne and Penry, 1973). While this seems more frequent with generalized discharges, focal abnormalities may be equally responsive. The extent to which these changes interlink with the initiation or exacerbation of behaviour problems in epileptic patients has not been examined, but clearly requires investigation.

## 1,5-BENZODIAZEPINES IN EPILEPSY

The 1,5 configuration of the benzodiazepines may permit a superior therapeutic ratio in epilepsy, although the only drug studied so far in this group is clobazam. In animal models, this is shown to be effective against pentylenetetrazol and audiogenic seizures in rodents, and photosensitive seizures in the baboon *Papio papio* (Chapman *et al.*, 1978). In the latter model, there is relative absence of toxic side effects, even after three times the effective anticonvulsant dose, which is in contrast to the actions of some other anticonvulsants such as phenytoin. In man, Gastaut and Low (1979) have reported on their clinical experience with 103 patients suffering from a variety of forms of epilepsy. Antiepileptic effects were observed in 72% of cases, 'a percentage [we] never observed before with any antiepileptic medication'. Responses were better in partial seizures (63–68%), than in primary or secondary generalized attacks (50–55%); however, tolerance occurred in one-third, usually before the third month. Interestingly, the authors reported a decrease in behaviour problems, especially anxiety and hyperkinesia, in 32% of cases and referred to 'a psychomotor arousal with increased attention, energy and participation in everyday activities'.

Critchley *et al.* (1982) have carried out a double-blind trial of 10–20 mg clobazam in 28 patients with resilient seizures, comparing it as adjunctive therapy with placebo. Treatment periods were for 6 weeks, and clobazam led to a significant fall in seizure frequency. No changes in the serum levels of phenobarbitone, phenytoin, or carbamazepine were noted.

We have recently evaluated further the role of clobazam in the management of intractable seizures in a double-blind crossover trial against placebo (Allen *et al.*, 1983). The patients were 26 residents from the Chalfont Centre for Epilepsy with uncontrolled seizures at a rate of four or more per month. The frequency of attacks was monitored by experienced staff at the Centre, and clobazam or identically matched placebo capsules were given to patients for 9 weeks, using a crossover design with an 8-week washout period between treatments. Half received the placebo first, and half clobazam. The clobazam (30 mg at night) was given in addition to the patients' existing anticonvulsant therapy, and the patients were assessed at weekly intervals for side effects and dose adjustment. If side effects were noted, the dose was lowered, one tablet being withdrawn until side effects ceased or the patient withdrew from the trial.

For analysis of the results, seizures were classified following the ILAE guidelines and divided into two broad groups, namely partial with or without secondary generalization, and generalized. Response to treatment was graded according to the percentage fall in seizures on the active treatment, a 50% or greater drop in frequency in those patients completing the trial being taken as a good therapeutic result. Tolerance to the effect of the drug was examined by comparing the seizure frequency in the first and second half of the active treatment epoch for those responding to the drug, who had no change in the clobazam dose. Withdrawal seizures were assessed by noting the number of attacks in a 10 day period following withdrawal of clobazam, in comparison with a similar phase after placebo.

The results of this trial are summarized in Figure 1. Six patients dropped from the study, one during the placebo period. Two patients had the dose of clobazam lowered, but completed the trial. Figure 1 shows the significant fall in seizure frequency during the active period, the most significant results being with partial seizures. If drop-outs are considered as non-responders there is still a significant result in favour of the active drug, 12 patients showing a 50% or greater fall, three patients having no seizures during the clobazam period (Figure 2).

No tolerance to the effect of the drug was noted in the responders for the 9 weeks of the trial, but significantly more seizures were seen in the clobazam withdrawal period, compared with placebo ($P<0.01$).

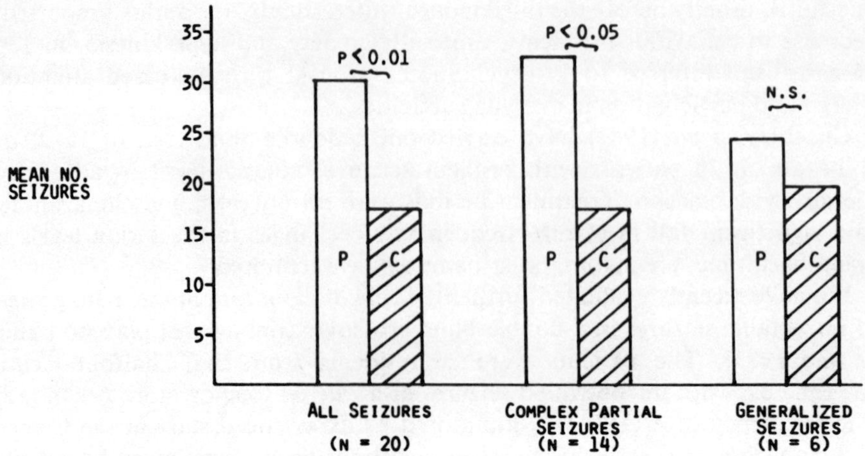


Figure 1 Change in seizure frequency P = placebo C = clobazam

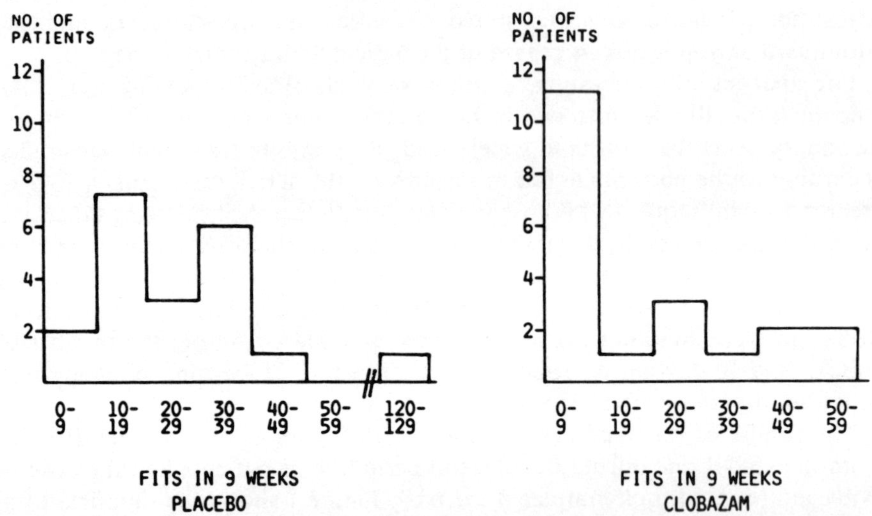


Figure 2 Total seizure frequency over 9 weeks in 20 patients on clobazam or placebo

Feely *et al.* (1982) have used clobazam for the management of catamenial epilepsy. They compared 20–30 mg to placebo, patients taking their medication for a 10 day period, when exacerbation of seizures was expected. Patients significantly preferred the active drug, although some actually responded to placebo.

These data suggest that the 1,5-benzodiazepines may be effective in the management of epilepsy, and that they probably lead to fewer side effects than the 1,4 compounds. Some evidence for clobazam having less sedative and cognitive effects than other benzodiazepines is discussed elsewhere (see chapter 22), and, if compared with phenytoin, in a double-blind placebo controlled investigation using volunteers (Thompson and Trimble, 1981) it had less influence on several psychological tests, including those of memory function. In epilepsy, the effects of tolerance are still noted, although some patients seem to achieve lasting benefit. Withdrawal seizures occur, and may be a problem, especially if they are not anticipated. Once initiated, such therapies in epileptic patients should be only slowly withdrawn.

This review of the use of benzodiazepines in epilepsy suggests that further encouragement should be given to the development of benzodiazepines that are anticonvulsant and can be used clinically in the management of epilepsy, and more work needs to be carried out on existing compounds specifically to disentangle some important questions. Paramount among these would be:

1. the profile of the antiepileptic effect;
2. the mechanism of tolerance;
3. the relationship between the anxiolytic and antiepileptic effects;
4. the role of metabolites in the anticonvulsant effects;
5. the influence of benzodiazepines on the pharmacokinetics of other anticonvulsant drugs, and vice versa;
6. the nature and mechanism of behaviour changes that occur with treatment, both adverse and psychotropic.

## PSYCHIATRY, EPILEPSY, AND THE BENZODIAZEPINES

Questions (3) and (6) above have a direct bearing on the fascinating, but clearly established, link between psychiatry and epilepsy (for review see Trimble, 1981). While most work has concentrated on personality disorder or schizophreniform psychoses and the links with temporal lobe epilepsy, there are hints that the associations go much further. Depression and the ECT experience have been mentioned above in relation to antagonism. Dysphoria, with inclusion of anxiety symptoms, panic, and fear, are often recorded as aura of epileptic attacks, and the latter are noted in particular in patients with anterior temporal lesions (Williams, 1956). In addition, neurotocism, as assessed by rating scales (Eysenck, 1950), or neurosis, as documented clinically (Shukla *et al.*, 1979), are seen with higher frequency in epileptic, more especially temporal lobe epileptic populations. While there are several possible reasons for this, not the least being the unpleasant, unpredictable nature of epilepsy, and the associated social stigmatization, biological links may well exist and deserve consideration. The role of the hippocampus and medial temporal structures in anxiety has been discussed elsewhere by Gray (see chapter 9), and it is therefore difficult to fail to notice the persistent reference to temporal lobe epilepsy, with lesions also in medial temporal structures, in the epilepsy and psychiatry literature. Hermann *et al.* (1982) have recently explored these links using the Minnesota Multophasic Personality Inventory (MMPI). Patients with either temporal lobe or generalized epilepsy were given the scale, and the former were divided into those with and without an aura of ictal fear. The temporal lobe group with this symptomatology scored higher on all but two scales, significantly so on several including the Pt—which measures anxiety and tension symptoms.

The growing knowledge of the biochemical aspects of the benzodiazepines, especially the discovery of benzodiazepine receptors, takes the links between psychiatry and epilepsy even further. Thus:

1. epilepsy, psychophathology, and the temporal lobes have some biological relationship;
2. benzodiazepines are both anxiolytic and anticonvulsant, especially for partial seizures;
3. benzodiazepine withdrawal leads to overt psychopathology, sometimes even a psychosis, but in addition also to seizures;
4. the benzodiazepine receptor is intimately linked to the GABA receptor, benzodiazepines facilitating GABA-ergic transmission;
5. GABA is anticonvulsant, and GABA-ergic drugs are anxiolytic (see Gray, chapter 9).

Not only clinically therefore are associations apparent, but now experimentally the same neurotransmitter and neuroreceptor systems, namely those of the benzodiazepines and GABA, may turn out to be implicated in different expressions of neuronal dysfunction, namely anxiety and epilepsy, in man. Similar parallels are seen with monoamine systems, the involvement of dopamine in both movement disorders such as Parkinson's disease or Huntington's chorea, and in psychiatric illnesses such as schizophrenia being an example. Clearly the biology of the benzodiazepines, and their future development, has much to teach us regarding fundamental mechanisms in neurobiology, especially with regard to the neuroses, but also may provide substantial therapeutic advances.

## REFERENCES

Allen, J. W., Oxley, J., Robertson, M. M., Trimble, M. R., Richens, A. and Jawad, S. S. M. (1983). Clobazam as adjunctive treatment in refractory epilepsy. *Brit. Med. J.*, **286**, 1246–1247.

Baruzzi, A., Michelucci, R. and Tassinari, C. A. (1982). Nitrazepam. In: *Antileptic Drugs*, pp.753–769 (Eds. Woodbury, D. M., Penry, J. K. and Pippenger, C. E.), Raven Press, New York.

Bensch, J., Blennow, G., Ferngren, H. *et al.* (1977). A double-blind study of clonazepam in the treatment of therapy resistant epilepsy. *Dev. Med. Child Neurol.*, **19**, 335–342.

Browne, T. R. (1976). Clonazepam: a review of a new anticonvulsant drug. *Arch. Neurol.*, **33**, 326–332.

Browne, T. R. (1978). Clonazepam. *New Engl. J. Med.*, **299**, 812–815.

Browne, T. R. and Penry, J. K. (1973). Benzodiazepines in the treatment of epilepsy. *Epilepsia*, **14**, 277–310.

Chandra, B. (1973). Clonazepam in the treatment of petit mal. *Asian J. Med.*, **9**, 433–438.

Chapman, A. G., Horton, R. W. and Meldrum, B. S. (1978). Anticonvulsant action of a 1,5 benzodiazepine, clobazam, in reflex epilepsy. *Epilepsia*, **19**, 293–299.

Chien, C. and Keegan, D. (1972). Diazepam as an oral long-term anticonvulsant for epileptic mental patients. *Dis. nerv. Syst.*, **33**, 100–104.

Critchley, E. M. R., Vakil, S. D., Hayward, H. W. *et al.* (1982). Double-blind clinical trial of clobazam in refractory epilepsy. In: *Clobazam: RSM International Congress and Symposium Series No. 43*, RSM and Academic Press, London.

Eadie, M. J. and Tyrer, J. H. (1980). *Anticonvulsant Therapy*, Churchill Livingstone, Edinburgh.

Eysenck, M. D. (1950). Neurotic tendencies in epilepsy. *J. Neurol.,Neurosurg. Psychiat.*, **13**, 237–240.

Feely, M., Calvert, R. and Gibson, J. (1982). Clobazam in catamenial epilepsy. *Lancet*, **ii**, 71–72.

Feldman, R. G., Hayes, M. K. and Browne, T. R. (1981). A double-blind comparison of clonazepam with placebo for refractory tonic-clonic seizures. *Neurology*, **31**, 159.

Gastaut, H. (1969). Clinical and electroencephalographic classification of epileptic seizures. *International League against Epilepsy Suppl., Epilepsia*, **10**, S.2–13.

Gastaut, H. and Low, M. D. (1979). Antiepileptic properties of clobazam, a 1,5 benzodiazepine in man. *Epilepsia*, **20**, 437–446.

Herman, B. P., Dikmen, S., Schwartz, M. S. and Karnes, W. E. (1982). Interictal psychopathology in patients with ictal fear. A quantitative investigation. *Neurology*, **32**, 7–11.

Hershon, H. I. and Parsonage, M. (1969). Comparative trial of diazepam and pheneturide in treatment of epilepsy, *Lancet*, **ii**, 859–862.

Lance, J. W. and Anthony, M. (1977). Sodium valproate and clonazepam in the treatment of intractable epilepsy, *Arch. neurol.*, **34**, 14–17.

Landolt, H. (1958). Serial EEG investigations during psychotic episodes in epileptic patients and during schizophrenic attacks. In: *Lectures on Epilepsy*, pp.91–133 (Ed. Lorentz de Hans, A. M.), Flsevier, London.

Livingston, S. and Paull, L. L. (1977). Clorazepate in epilepsy. *J. Am. med. Ass.*, **237**, 1561.

Lon, H. O. C. (1968). Oxazepam in the treatment of psychomotor epilepsy. *Neurology*, **18**, 986–990.

Mattson, R. H. (1972). The benzodiazepines. In: *Antiepileptic Drugs*, pp.497–516. (Eds. Woodbury, D. M., Penry, J. K. and Schmidt, R. P.), Raven Press, New York.

Mikkelsen, B., Berggreen, P., Joensen, P. *et al.* (1981). Clonazepam and carbamazepine in psychomotor epilepsy: a randomised multicentre trial. *Epilepsia*, **22**, 415–420.

Mikkelsen, B., Birket-Smith, E., Brandt, S. *et al.* (1976). Clonazepam in the treatment of epilepsy. *Arch. Neurol.*, **33**, 322–325.

Nanda, R. N., Johnson, R. H., Keogh, H. J. *et al.* (1977). Treatment of epilepsy with clonazepam and its effect on other anticonvulsants. *J. Neurol. Neurosurg. Psychiat.*, **40**, 538–543.

Sato, S., Penry, J. K., Dreiuss, F. *et al.* (1977). Clonazepam in the treatment of absence seizures. A double-blind clinical trial. *Neurology*, **27**, 371.

Shakir, R. A., Nanda, R. N., Lambie, D. G. and Johnson, R. H. (1979). Comparative trial of sodium valproate and clonazepam in chronic epilepsy. *Arch. Neurol.*, **36**, 301–304.

Shukla, G. D., Srivastava, O. N., Katiyar, B. C. *et al.* (1979). Psychiatric manifestations of temporal lobe epilepsy: a controlled study. *Brit. J. Psychiat.*, **135**, 411–417.

Thompson, P. J. and Trimble, M. R. (1981). Clobazam and cognitive functions. In: *RSM International Congress and Symposium Series*, pp.33–38, Academic Press, London.

Trimble, M. R. (1981). *Neuropsychiatry*, John Wiley, Chichester.

Wilensky, A. J., Ojemann, L. M., Temkin, N. R., Troupin, A. S. and Dodrill, C. B. (1981). Clorazepate and phenobarbital as antiepileptic drugs. A double-blind study. *Neurology*, **31**, 1271–1276.

Williams, D. (1956). The structure of emotions reflected in epileptic experiences. *Brain*, **79**, 29–67.

Woodbury, D. M., Penry, J. K. and Pippenger, C. E. (Eds) (1982). *Antiepileptic Drugs*, Raven Press, New York.

## DISCUSSION

## CHAIRMAN: PROFESSOR RICHENS

DR. TYRER: There has been no mention in the conference so far about the place of benzodiazepines in the treatment of tardive dyskinesia. It is perhaps fair to say that clonazepam has been shown to be effective as a treatment of this condition, presumably, it is felt, through its GABA mimetic effects.

DR. TRIMBLE: Measuring tardive dyskinesia is extraordinarily difficult and a lot of other compounds such as sodium valproate are said to be effective.

THE CHAIRMAN: There is very little controlled evidence that anything works in tardive dyskinesia.

DR. TYRER: I am quoting a paper by Mackay and Sheppard which did have a control group and produced fairly convincing results.

THE CHAIRMAN: I think paediatricians find the benzodiazepines of great value in myoclonic epilepsy, particularly nitrazepam. The reason for that I have not really understood. In your review of the literature does nitrazepam stick out as being a drug of choice in the myoclonic epilepsies?

DR. TRIMBLE: It is effective in myoclonic epilepsies in childhood, yes.

THE CHAIRMAN: It appears as if the effect is more persistent in the myoclonic epilepsies. Tolerance does not seem to occur very readily. What about clonazepam?

DR. TRIMBLE: I think that clonazepam is not a good drug in epilepsy because of the associated behaviour problems. It is highly sedative and it can interact very badly with both sodium valproate and phenobarbitone.

DR. SCHMUTZ: Indeed, it is true that there is much evidence for a link between benzodiazepines, GABA-benzodiazepine receptors, and epilepsy. On the other hand, we also have drugs that are active in especially complex partial seizures, such as carbamazepine that do not seem to bind to benzodiazepine receptors. This drug also has been shown to have psychotropic effects. I only want to say that there are different modes of action leading to similar clinical pictures.

DR. TRIMBLE: The interesting thing about carbamazepine is that in some patients it makes the electroencephalogram worse, whereas with the benzodiazepines — and indeed we see this with clobazam—you tend to get normalization of the EEG. There is a marked difference between those two compounds.

DR. HERBERT: I am trying to put together the fact that people with temporal lobe epilepsy tended to have a fear aura, with your earlier information that the benzodiazepine you used, clobazam, was particularly effective against complex partial seizures. How do you think that those two bits of information fit together?

DR. TRIMBLE: One speculates what the differences are between a structural lesion which is placed in the brain at one time in life and a functional lesion which develops at some other time during life. The clinical consequences of those two may look entirely different, but they may both lead us back into the temporal lobe. If you put a probe into such a structure and stimulate it in patients, what will you see? You get fear auras. If you stimulate enough, you get a complex partial seizure. Clinically, psychiatry and neurology are united very closely. It may not even be so much a qualitative thing, it may be a quantitative thing, that distinguishes between the clinical expression of temporal lobe lesions. This brings us back to the benzodiazepine receptor. I think for the field of neurosis, these developments are going to be extremely important. There is a biology to the neurosis as much as there is a biology to the psychosis, and indeed there are treatments for the two.

Benzodiazepines Divided
Edited by M. R. Trimble


# 21

# Benzodiazepines and Alcoholism

MARKKU LINNOILA*

Drugs with effects on the central nervous system are used for several different indications in alcoholic patients:

1. to treat symptoms of alcohol withdrawal;
2. to reduce drinking in chronic alcoholics; and
3. to alleviate symptoms of mental disorders in abstaining or moderately drinking alcoholics.

Recent studies concerning the *heritability of alcoholism* have delineated different familial patterns of inheritance of the illness. Specifically, a form of father-to-son transmission of alcoholism associated with criminality, asociality, and early onset of drinking has been contrasted with a form often inherited from the mothers and characterized by relatively late onset of heavy drinking, no excess of criminality, and significant environmental impact on the severity of alcohol abuse (Bohman *et al.*, 1981; Cloninger *et al.*, 1981) (see Table 1). These two forms of alcoholism described with the Swedish-American team of investigators may cover the concept of 'primary' and 'secondary' alcoholism which has been suggested by Tarter *et al.* (1977). His 'primary' alcoholics were mainly men who had a history of behavioural disorders such as hyperactivity, and who started heavy alcohol abuse at an early age. Moreover, the prevalence of 'secondary' alcoholism was postulated by Tarter to be relatively high in women; the illness started at a later age and often after a period of symptoms of mental distress.

Several other authors have described an excess of alcoholism in the families of patients with agoraphobia and social phobia (Munjada and Moss, 1981), with a type of primary, major depression, unipolar, 'the depression spectrum disease' (Schlesser *et al.*, 1981), drug abuse (Quitkin *et al.*, 1972),

*In conjunction with P. R. Martin.

Table 1 Two types of alcoholism

| | Type 1 (milieu-limited) | Type 2 (male-limited) |
|---|---|---|
| Prevalence in adopted men | 13% | 4% |
| Relative risk in predisposed sons | 2 with and 1 without provocation | 9 regardless of provocation |
| Prevalence in adopted women | 7% | |
| Relative risk in predisposed daughters | 3 with or without provocation | |

Bohman *et al.*, 1981; Cloninger *et al.*, 1981.
Prevalence of alcoholism in the general population: men, 5%; women, 1% (Martin, 1981)

'hyperactivity' (Cantwell, 1972), and anorexia nervosa (Eckert *et al.*, 1979). The implication of these observations is that alcoholism is probably a biologically heterogeneous disorder. To further complicate the matter, alcohol abuse may produce secondary symptoms of depression (Schuckit, 1982).

A useful approach to understanding mental disorders has involved the study of *biogenic amines*. The biochemistry of biogenic monoamines in alcoholism, however, has not been thoroughly studied, and the available animal models have yielded some diametrically opposite findings and are likely to have only limited relevance to the disorder in man. We will focus, therefore, primarily on findings from human studies. Attention has been drawn to the effects of alcohol on serotonin (Ballenger *et al.*, 1979) and to whether abnormalities in this neurotransmitter system reflect trait changes in the nervous system of alcoholics. Reserpine-like effects of alcohol have been speculated to alleviate acutely an alleged serotonergic deficiency in alcoholics but to aggravate it during chronic abuse of alcohol (Ballenger *et al.*, 1979). It is important to emphasize in this context that quite a few of the alcoholics in the study of Ballenger *et al.* had exhibited aggressive and violent behaviour prior to hospitalization. Depressed patients with alcoholic relatives also have been reported to have lower lumbar cerebrospinal fluid (CSF) 5-hydroxyindoleacetic acid (5HIAA) concentrations than depressed patients without alcoholic relatives (Rosenthal *et al.*, 1980).

Recently, we studied 25 incarcerated murderers undergoing extensive evaluation in a forensic psychiatry ward. Murderers with antisocial personality, past history of alcohol abuse and impulsive behaviour had a low CSF 5HIAA concentration in samples obtained a minimum of 90 days after their last drinking episode compared to normal controls and murderers with paranoid personality (Linnoila *et al.*, unpublished). This finding is consistent with studies concerning coexistence of alcohol abuse and criminality (see above), and it may be pertinent to an alleged poor therapeutic response to benzodiazepines in this group of patients (see below).

No consistent differences have been demonstrated in indices of norepinephrine and dopamine functioning between alcoholics and healthy volunteers. However, changes in CNS norepinephrinergic functioning during acute intoxication with ethanol have been postulated based on an increase in the 3-methoxy-4-hydroxyphenylglycol (MHPG) concentration in the lumbar CSF after drinking a high dose of ethanol (Borg *et al.*, 1981). However, the MHPG concentration in the CSF is strongly influenced by plasma MHPG concentration (Kopin *et al.*, in press), which could be affected by circulatory changes produced by alcohol. Furthermore, aldehyde reductase is essential for the formation of MHPG (Rutledge and Jonason, 1967); this enzyme could be affected by acetaldehyde produced from ethanol and the MHPG concentration in the CSF could be secondarily altered without concomitant changes in the central release of norepinephrine. Therefore, an alternate explanation for the elevation of CSF MHPG concentration after drinking is plausible. Moreover, alcohol withdrawal (a state supposed to be characterized by certain neurochemical changes opposite to those observed during intoxication) is associated with clinical signs of norepinephrinergic hyperactivity (see below). Thus, the present information concerning norepinephrinergic activity during alcohol intoxication in man is inadequate, and there is a clear need for additional experiments.

## ROLE OF ACETALDEHYDE

Intraventricularly administered acetaldehyde, unlike alcohol, maintains self-administration in the rat (Brown *et al.*, 1979). In addition, alcoholics (Korsten *et al.*, 1975) as well as the college-age offspring of alcoholics have been reported to have higher blood acetaldehyde concentrations after a given dose of alcohol than non-alcoholics and their offspring (Schuckit and Rayses, 1979). Moreover, alcoholics without cirrhosis of the liver have been reported to have low aldehyde dehydrogenase activity compared to non-alcoholic controls (Jenkins and Peters, 1980). If a high production rate of acetaldehyde would be typical of alcoholics and their offspring even prior to the manifestation of alcohol abuse, then there would be a biochemical marker for individuals at risk and a theoretical basis for constructs concerning the psychobiology of alcoholism. However, in a pilot study we could not find any differences in blood and breath acetaldehyde concentrations between children of alcoholics and non-alcoholics after an alcohol challenge (Behar *et al.*, submitted). Hence, it seems that elevated acetaldehyde levels after alcohol ingestion may be a result rather than a cause of alcoholism. Even if alcoholics and individuals at risk of developing alcoholism do not have higher blood acetaldehyde levels after a given dose of alcohol than non-alcoholics, acetaldehyde could still influence the course of alcoholism. This is because those genetically at risk to develop alcoholism might have to drink more alcohol to obtain the same degree of intoxication as those not at risk and consequently produce more acetaldehyde per drinking session as suggested by Schuckit (1980).

Tetrahydroisoquinolines, the condensation products of acetaldehyde and catecholamines, have opiate-like potency, and their concentration may be elevated in the urine of alcoholics who have recently consumed alcohol (Collins *et al.*, 1979). On the other hand, the condensation products of acetaldehyde and indoleamines, beta-carbolines, are capable of producing symptoms of anxiety and a state of catecholaminergic hyperactivity when administered to monkeys. This can be specifically blocked by benzodiazepines (Ninan *et al.*, 1983). However, the presence of increased amounts of either tetrahydroisoquinolines or beta-carbolines during alcohol abuse and withdrawal is currently controversial (Bloom and Barchas, 1982). None the less, Bhattacharaya *et al.* (1982) have speculated that an endogenous monoamine oxidase inhibitor they find to be elevated in the urines of alcoholics after withdrawal could be a beta-carboline.

## EFFECTS OF BENZODIAZEPINES

Benzodiazepines bind to specific, high affinity binding sites in the central nervous system, which are coupled to a recognition site for gamma-aminobutyric acid (GABA) and chloride the ionophore. They have a potency to increase the affinity of the GABA recognition site for its ligand (Tallman *et al.*, 1980). Among a host of events that result from the binding of benzodiazepines to their receptors are an acute inhibition of norepinephrine turnover and a chronic reduction of serotonin turnover (Stein *et al.*, 1974). These biochemical effects may be of particular importance in the treatment of alcoholism and alcohol withdrawal. Administration of alcohol to the rat alters benzodiazepine (Ticku and Davis, 1981) and probably GABA binding (Linnoila *et al.*, 1981). Thus, there is an overlap between the multitude of biochemical and membrane effects of alcohol and those that result from benzodiazepine binding to their receptors. Physiologically, the benzodiazepines reduce sympathetic nervous system activity in man (Hossmann *et al.*, 1980). Clinically, their anxiolytic, hypnotic, and anticonvulsant properties are most pertinent to their therapeutic usefulness in alcoholism withdrawal.

## ALCOHOL TOLERANCE, DEPENDENCE, AND WITHDRAWAL

There is considerable controversy, mostly theoretical, concerning the definitions of alcohol tolerance, dependence, and withdrawal (Kalant *et al.*, 1971; WHO, 1981). *Tolerance* is produced by most central nervous system CNS depressants. Briefly, after repeated exposure to a given agent, a greater dose is required to produce intoxication of the same magnitude; alternatively, a smaller degree of intoxication results from the same dose. This is due to adaptation of the CNS (functional tolerance) and increased drug clearance (dispositional tolerance). Tolerance to one CNS depressant usually results in some tolerance to many chemically unrelated depressants (cross-tolerance) which, in turn, may have both functional and dispositional components. The clinician evaluating a patient's level of tolerance is best guided by relating his behavioural state to blood ethanol concentration and to the results of an adequate drug screen for other psychoactive agents in blood or urine.

Alcohol *dependence* is also produced by repeated exposure and usually, but not always (Ritzmann and Tabakoff, 1976), develops in concert with tolerance. In man, at present, it can only be quantitated indirectly in terms of tolerance to ethanol, the severity of the abstinence syndrome and craving for alcohol observed during and after alcohol withdrawal. Attempts have been made in experimental animals to characterize the biochemical changes that occur concomitantly with the development of tolerance and dependence, as well as to modify these processes by behavioural, pharmacological, or physiological manipulations (Kissin, 1979). Significant alterations in all major neurotransmitter systems have been described. Of particular interest are observations concerning, for example, a low seizure threshold for electroshock or pentylenetetrazol, and audiogenic stimuli in alcohol-tolerant animals (Kalant *et al.*, 1971), because these functions are affected by benzodiazepines.

The issue of causality of the changes is far from resolved as there are many conflicting findings, and most of the observed changes might simply be epiphenomena in a more fundamental process. Less transitory phenomena that require structural changes within the neuron as a result of altered nucleic acid metabolism, membrane composition, or protein synthesis need also to be considered (Tewari and Noble, 1975; Chin and Goldstein, 1977). Therefore, though it is agreed that the functional state of the CNS is modified by continued alcohol consumption, and this presents to the clinician as tolerance, dependence, and the presence of signs of non-specific, long-term CNS depression, what this means in terms of the pharmacotherapy of such patients must await further understanding of fundamental processes.

Qualitatively similar *withdrawal* syndromes pertain for alcohol, barbiturates, non-barbiturate hypnosedatives, and benzodiazepines, all of which exhibit cross-tolerance and cross-dependence (Kalant *et al.*, 1971). This forms a partial rationale for drug treatment of alcohol withdrawal. When alcohol consumption is abruptly stopped or rapidly decreased, often as a result of related or concurrent disease, such as gastritis, trauma, or pneumonia, the CNS, non-specifically depressed by alcohol, undergoes 're-equilibration' manifested by emergent signs and symptoms of alcohol withdrawal. Alcohol withdrawal syndromes (see Table 2) lie on a continuum of increasing severity, from the acute hangover to delirium tremens, determined by both the intensity and duration of preceding alcohol exposure as modified by the presence of cross-tolerant medications and concurrent medical and psychiatric diseases (Kalant, 1977; Majchrowicz, 1981). Within 8–12 hours after the last drink, at blood ethanol concentrations of 200–100 mg/dl, the early, so-called 'minor'

Table 2 Signs and symptoms of alcohol withdrawal

| | |
|---|---|
| 'Minor' withdrawal | |
| | Anxiety/Apprehension/Restlessness |
| | Insomnia |
| | Tremor |
| | Hyperreflexia/Irritability |
| | Muscle fasciculations/Weakness |
| | Paroxysmal EEG discharges |
| | Anorexia/Nausea/Vomiting/Dehydration |
| | Diaphoresis/Hyperthermia |
| | Tachycardia/Arrhythmia |
| 'Major' withdrawal | |
| | 12–24 hours: generalized tonic–clonic seizure |
| | 48–72 hours: Delirium tremens (agitation, disorientation, fluctuating level of consciousness, visual and auditory hallucinations, intense autonomic hyperactivity) |

withdrawal symptoms develop. They generally include signs of CNS hyperexcitability (anxiety, apprehension, restlessness, insomnia, tremor, muscle twitches, weakness, hyperreflexia, and paroxysmal discharges on the electroencephalogram), gastrointestinal disturbances (anorexia, nausea, vomiting, and weight loss), and excessive central sympathetic nervous system activity (profuse diaphoresis, elevated body temperature, tachycardia, and cardiac arrhythmias). In more severe cases, the CNS hyperexcitability may progress to one or two generalized tonic–clonic seizures. Almost 70% of convulsions occur within 24 hours and less than 10% after 48 hours of the last drink. The most severe withdrawal reaction, commonly referred to as delirium tremens, occurs in less than 5% of hospitalized patients, usually starting 48–72 hours following the end of alcohol ingestion (Victor and Brausch, 1967). It is characterized by agitation, disorientation, fluctuating level of consciousness, vivid visual and auditory hallucinations, and intense autonomic hyperactivity. But mortality at present is less than 2%, a substantial improvement over reports of 15% in the older literature (Kalant, 1977). Whether a protracted withdrawal syndrome exists beyond 4–7 days after alcohol ingestion is discontinued is somewhat controversial (Goldstein, 1979; Kissin, 1979). Unless longitudinal studies are conducted, there is no way to settle the issue of why alcoholics are often abnormal in several respects for months or even years after alcohol withdrawal. These abnormalities might predate drinking altogether or may be degenerative consequences of prolonged alcohol consumption. In the following discussion of drug treatment of alcohol withdrawal, we are referring to the first 4–7 days after alcohol ingestion is discontinued.

## TREATMENT OF ALCOHOL WITHDRAWAL

The key first step in management of the alcoholic patient is effective symptomatic treatment of the alcohol withdrawal syndrome. Clinical evaluation must begin with a careful quantitation of the severity and progression of the alcohol withdrawal syndrome, as well as a search for medical complications of alcoholism, such as trauma, malnutrition, fluid and electrolyte disturbances, infections, gastritis, pancreatitis, hypoglycaemia, liver disease, cardiac or pulmonary disease, and past history of seizures, as well as abuse of drugs other than alcohol.

Thereafter, the clinician must decide whether pharmacological intervention is necessary at all, and if so, which drug from among the more than 100 that have been used for the treatment of alcohol withdrawal in the past offers the best therapeutic profile for the task at hand. In this discussion, we focus on the benzodiazepines, which are currently considered the drugs of choice for the treatment of alcohol withdrawal. The goals of drug treatment of the alcohol withdrawal syndrome are:

1. symptom relief;
2. prevention or treatment of serious complications of withdrawal, such as seizures, hallucinations or cardiac arrhythmias;
3. allowing a smooth transition to treatment programmes and ultimately to long-term rehabilitation.

Most patients with mild withdrawal symptoms and adequate social support do not require hospitalization. Adequate provisions must be made for patient follow-up so as to assure participation in a long-range rehabilitation programme. All patients with severe withdrawal reactions or with complicating medical, surgical, or psychiatric conditions which may augment the risk of progression to major withdrawal signs (Tavel *et al.*, 1972) should be admitted to the hospital. Good general medical management at this stage is essential and is probably the reason for improved clinical outcome in the alcohol withdrawal syndrome in recent years (see above). Since sympathetic hyperactivity often dominates the clinical picture, any treatment that reduces this hyperadrenergic state is likely of some benefit. On the basis of pharmacodynamic considerations, alcohol-related compounds may best approximate the pharmacological effects of ethanol (Majchrowicz *et al.*, 1976) and in fact, under some circumstances, an ethanol treatment regimen may prove more beneficial to the healthy alcoholic patient than current regimens which employ other psychoactive medication (Funderburk *et al.*, 1978). This approach is, however, inappropriate in the management of the severely ill alcoholic (Sellers and Kalant, 1976). Alcohol withdrawal responds to non-pharmacological interventions in 98% of patients in a detoxification centre (Whitfield *et al.*, 1978) and in approximately 80% of patients without medical complications treated in an emergency room or admitted to hospital (Shaw *et al.*, 1981; Naranjo *et al.*, 1982). Supportive care, however, has been demonstrated ineffective against hallucinations, seizures, and arrhythmias (Sellers *et al.*, personal communication). Consequently, the efficacy of time-honoured remedies for alcohol withdrawal, e.g. barbiturates, paraldehyde, and chloral hydrate and those of more recent addition to the clinician's armamentarium such as phenothiazines and butyrophenones, various anticonvulsants, sympatholytic agents as well as benzodiazepines, need to be re-evaluated in the light of these high success rates for supportive care and the low current prevalence of major withdrawal signs. If pharmacotherapy may offer only limited advantage over supportive care in many patients, treatment with any but a minimally toxic drug seems unjustified. Benzodiazepines have wider therapeutic indices than other psychoactive drugs which have been used in the treatment of alcohol withdrawal (see Table 3). Therefore, they are the current drugs of choice for this indication. It is questionable whether the choice of one benzodiazepine over another really affects treatment outcome (Greenblatt and Shader, 1974).

Table 3 Drugs used in treatment of alcohol withdrawal

| Drug class | Relative safety | Cross-tolerance with alcohol | Anxiolysis/ sedation | Anticonvulsant |
|---|---|---|---|---|
| Benzodiazepines | +++ | +++ | +++ | ++ |
| Thiazoles | ++ | ++ | ++ | ++ |
| Barbiturates | + | ++ | ++ | +++ |
| Chloral derivatives | + | ++ | + | ++ |
| Phenothiazines | ++ | + | + | — |
| Butyrophenones | ++ | + | ++ | 0 |
| Antihistamines | ++ | + | 0 | — |
| Anticonvulsants | + | ++ | — | +++ |
| Cations | 0 | + | 0 | 0 |
| $\beta$-Antagonists | ++ | 0 | ++ | 0 |
| $\alpha_2$-Agonists | + | 0 | ++ | 0 |
| Dopamine agonists | + | 0 | ++ | 0 |

Nevertheless, certain pharmacokinetic characteristics of the benzodiazepines may dictate the selection of one drug over another (see Table 4). Benzodiazepines, except perhaps lorazepam (Hosein *et al.*, 1979), should not be given by intramuscular injection due to their erratic absorption by this route (Greenblatt *et al.*, 1974). All benzodiazepines are extensively bound to serum albumin, and hence patients with hypoalbuminaemia due to liver disease have higher free drug concentrations, greater volumes of distribution, and lower total body clearances than alcoholics without liver disease (Thiessen *et al.*, 1976; Morgan *et al.*, 1981). Although the side effect of drowsiness is reported to be more common in such patients, it is not clear that this is due to an

Table 4 Advantages and disadvantages of benzodiazepines in alcohol withdrawal*

| Drug | Clinical experience | Half-life (h) | Active metabolite | Reduced clearance with liver disease | Intramuscular bioavailability | Comments |
|---|---|---|---|---|---|---|
| Chlordiazepoxide | + + + | 10 (4–16) | Desmethylchlordiazepoxide,† demoxepam, oxazepam, desmethyldiazepam | Yes | Poor | Inexpensive; parenteral formulation inconvenient |
| Clorazepate | + | Very short | Desmethyldiazepam,† oxazepam | Yes | — | Expensive; no advantage over diazepam |
| ( = Desmethyldiazepam) | | 51 (44–55) | Oxazepam | Yes | — | |
| Diazepam | + + + | 31 (50–170) | Desmethyldiazepam,† temazepam, oxazepam | Yes | Poor | Inexpensive; easy parenteral formulation |
| Lorazepam | + + | 14 (10–17) | Inactive glucuronide | No | Good | Expensive; intravenous formulation; most potent |
| Oxazepam | + + | 12 (4–17) | Inactive glucuronide | No | — | Expensive; no parenteral formulation |

* Adapted from Sellers, 1978.
†Major active metabolite in blood; prolongs biological half-life and causes cumulation.

increased free fraction, but may also reflect organic CNS dysfunction due to hepatic disease (Greenblatt and Koch-Weser, 1974). The biotransformation of chlordiazepoxide, diazepam, and desmethyldiazepam is impaired in patients with liver disease and the half-lives may increase up to sixfold (Klotz *et al.*, 1977). These drugs have long half-lives and they are transformed to active metabolites resulting in accumulation and prolonged pharmacological activity and possible toxicity. Oxazepam and lorazepam are inactivated by glucuronidation and hence may be preferable in patients with hepatic disease (Shull *et al.*, 1976).

Disposition of benzodiazepines may be altered during the course of alcohol withdrawal, due to the initial presence of alcohol (Whiting *et al.*, 1979) and more rapid distribution to tissues (Pond *et al.*, 1979). Upon alcohol elimination, chlordiazepoxide clearance can double, perhaps due to unmasking of induction of ethanol of drug-metabolizing enzymes (Sellers *et al.*, 1978). The high lipid solubility of diazepam allows rapid penetration of the blood–brain barrier (Paulson *et al.*, 1982). This accounts for this benzodiazepine's efficacy in management of status epilepticus, but also explains its greater subjective effect compared to the less lipid-soluble benzodiazepines which presumably increases its relative abuse liability (Bliding, 1974). The benzodiazepines, except clonazepam, have only modest long-term anticonvulsant activity, and prophylactic treatment with phenytoin is recommended for patients with a well-documented history of withdrawal seizures (Sellers and Kalant, 1976). Rebound insomnia is less problematic after discontinuation of those benzodiazepines with active metabolites and longer elimination half-lives (Kales *et al.*, 1978). This is a relevant consideration upon withdrawal of the benzodiazepine. Clinicians tend to use haloperidol for the treatment of hallucinations resulting from the organic brain syndrome associated with alcohol withdrawal (Sellers and Kalant, 1976), but this may not be desirable if dopaminergic neurotransmission is indeed decreased during alcohol withdrawal (Tabakoff and Hoffman, 1979). Cardiac tachyarrhythmias may be treated with propranolol (Sellers, 1977); when there is a history of asthma or diabetes or clinical signs of cardiac failure, the $\alpha_2$-agonist clonidine may be preferable (Walinder *et al.*, 1981).

## PHARMACOLOGICAL TREATMENTS TO REDUCE DRINKING IN ALCOHOLICS

The maintenance treatment of an alcoholic may be approached from different conceptual frameworks. The common goal is obviously to keep the patient socially functional. One school regards this problem as primarily non-psychiatric and another as psychiatric.

In the non-psychiatric mode it is relatively common to advocate the use of disulfiram as the pharmacological treatment of choice, and, if the patient is so inclined, to get him involved in Alcoholics Anonymous or some other self-help group. These interventions may help some alcoholics, but there are few good controlled studies to document their efficacy (Fuller and Roth, 1979). Disulfiram as such is relatively toxic, and it reduces the clearance of benzodiazepines such as diazepam and chlordiazepoxide, which require dealkylation and hydroxylation in their biotransformation. Thus, conservative dosing of these drugs is recommended in patients receiving disulfiram (MacLeod *et al.*, 1978).

In the psychiatric mode, a careful psychiatric and family history is elicited in an attempt to classify alcoholism as 'primary' or 'secondary'. In the latter case, it may be important to understand the patient's psychopathology prior to the onset of alcoholism and to take a careful history concerning psychopathology in the blood relatives. Then the pharmacological intervention can be 'tailored' to match this psychopathology.

Benzodiazepine treatment may be relatively contraindicated in 'primary' alcoholics with criminality in the family, particularly so if this is associated with impulsive and violent acts. It has been suggested that the benzodiazepines increase impulsive violence in prisoners, even though controlled studies are unavailable (Lion *et al.*, 1975; Brown, 1978). This would be theoretically consistent with a primary deficiency in serotonergic neurotransmission which predisposes them to impulsive violence and is aggravated by further benzodiazepine-induced reductions in serotonin turnover. These patients may benefit from treatment with new serotonin reuptake inhibiting antidepressants, such as zimelidine or citalopram, or with lithium (Marini and Sheard, 1977).

Patients with alcoholism secondary to affective disorders or from a pedigree with 'depression spectrum disease' may benefit from treatments with antidepressants or lithium. However, controlled studies addressing this issue are still in their initial stages (Reynolds *et al.*, 1979). In a controlled study imipramine significantly reduced the attrition rate of all alcoholic patients in a long-term treatment programme compared to placebo (Kissin, 1975).

Patients with a personal or family history of anxiety disorders suffering from alcoholism should probably receive an adequate trial of an appropriate psychotropic medication. Agoraphobics with or without panic attacks may benefit from antidepressants and possibly from norepinephrinergic beta-receptor blocking agents; obsessive-compulsives from behavioural interventions and serotonin reuptake inhibitors; and social phobics or patients with generalized anxiety disorder from antidepressants or benzodiazepines (for review see Linnoila, (1983). In a controlled study, effective anxiolytic doses of chlordiazepoxide were claimed to reduce attrition rate in a long-term treatment programme of alcoholics (Kissin, 1975). The price for this was suggested in another uncontrolled study to be a 5% incidence of addiction to the benzodiazepines (Rothstein *et al.*, 1976). However, the potency of benzodiazepines to maintain self-administration in man is probably less than that of barbiturates

(Griffiths *et al.*, 1980). Consequently, they should be less addictive than the barbiturates, which were used to treat alcoholics prior to the availability of the benzodiazepines. If the benzodiazepines are used in a long-term treatment programme some special circumstances may arise when the choice of a particular benzodiazepine may make a difference (see Table 5). Should a patient be drinking while in the programme, then a benzodiazepine with relatively mild additive interaction with alcohol, such as chlordiazepoxide, clorazepate, or oxazepam (Palva and Linnoila, 1978), might be preferred over diazepam or lorazepam, which have a relatively strong additive interaction with alcohol (Linnoila and Mattila, 1973; Seppala *et al.*, 1982). Should a patient's gastritis or ulcer be treated with cimetidine or tuberculosis with isoniazid, which inhibit dealkylation and hydroxylation (Klotz and Reimann, 1980a,b; Ochs *et al.*, 1981), then a benzodiazepine, such as oxazepam or lorazepam, which is eliminated via glucuronidation, should be used. The same pertains to cirrhosis of the liver. Finally, should the patient show hostile behaviour, oxazepam might be preferable over chlordiazepoxide (Kochansky *et al.*, 1975).

Table 5 Special problems in long-term treatment of alcoholism with benzodiazepines

| | | |
|---|---|---|
| Interacton with alcohol | Strong: lorazepam, diazepam | Mild: clorazepate, chlordiazepoxide, oxazepam |
| Cimetidine, isoniazid, disulfiram, cirrhosis | Inhibit biotransformation of diazepam, clorazepate, chlordiazepoxide, prazepam | Do not inhibit biotransformation of lorazepam, oxazepam |
| Hostility | Aggravated by chlordiazepoxide | Not aggravated by oxazepam |

In conclusion, there is a dire need for large-scale controlled studies concerning the efficacy of psychotropic medications in the long-term treatment of alcoholics. At the present time, we do not know whether clinical outcome is favourably affected by pharmacotherapy or whether choice of the psychiatric or non-psychiatric approaches alters the likelihood of treatment success. The benzodiazepines are the drugs of choice in patients undergoing alcohol withdrawal, but their value in the maintenance treatment of alcoholism has not been established. Furthermore, they may have a potential to cause insidious long-term side effects and should not be used on a chronic basis or for too liberal indications (Lader and Petursson, 1981).

## REFERENCES

Ballenger, J. C., Goodwin, F. K., Major, L. F. and Brown, G. L. (1979). Alcohol and central serotonin metabolism in man. *Arch. gen. Psychiat.*, **36**, 224–227.

Behar, D., Berg, C. J., Rapoport, J. L., Nelson, W., Linnoila, M., Cohen, M., Bozevich, C. and Kopin, I. J. (1983). Behavioral and physiological effects of ethanol in high risk and control children. Submitted for publication.

Bhattacharaya, S. K., Glover, V., Sandler, M., Clow, A., Topham, A., Bernadt, M. and Murray R. (1982). Raised endogenous monoamine oxidase inhibitor output in postwithdrawal alcoholics: Effects of L-dopa and ethanol. *Biol. Psychiat.*, **17**, 829–836.

Bliding, A. (1974). Effects of different rates of absorption of two benzodiazepines on subjective and objective parameters. *Eur. J. clin. pharmac.*, **7**, 201–211.

Bloom, F. E. and Barchas, J. D. (1982). Occurrence and significance of beta-carbolines and tetrahydroisoquinolines—cellular actions and localization of beta-carbolines and tetrahydroisoquinolines. *Psychopharmac. Bull*, **18(3)**, 198–203.

Bohman, M., Sigvarsson, S. and Cloninger, C. R. (1981). Maternal inheritance of alcohol abuse. *Arch. gen. Psychiat.*, **38**, 965–969.

Borg, S., Kvande, H. and Sedvall, G. (1981). Central norepinephrine metabolism during alcohol intoxication in addicts and healthy volunteers. *Science*, **213**, 1135–1137.

Brown, C. R. (1978). The use of benzodiazepines in prison populations. *J. clin. Psychiat.*, **38**, 219–222.

Brown, G. L., Goodwin, F. K., Ballenger, J. C., Goyer, P. F. and Major, L. F. (1979). Aggression in humans correlates with cerebrospinal fluid amine metabolites. *Psychiat. Res.*, **1**, 130–140.

Cantwell, D. P. (1972). Psychiatric illness in the families of hyperactive children. *Arch. gen. Psychiat.*, **27**, 414–417.

Chin, J. H. and Goldstein, D. B. (1977). Drug tolerance in biomembranes: a spin label study of the effects of ethanol. *Science*, **196**, 684–685.

Cloninger, C. R., Bohman, M. and Sigvardsson, S. (1981). Inheritance of alcohol abuse. *Arch. gen. Psychiat.*, **38**, 861–868.

Collins, M. A., Nijin, W. P., Bonge, G. F., Teas, G. and Goldfarb, C. (1979). Dopamine-related tetrahydroisoquinolines: significant urinary excretion by alcoholics after alcohol consumption. *Science*, **206**, 1184–1186.

Eckert, E. D., Goldberg, S. C., Halmi, K. A., Casper, R. C. and Davis, J. M. (1979). Alcoholism in anorexia nervosa. In: *Psychiatric Factors in Drug Abuse*, pp.267–283 (Eds. Pickens, R. W. and Hestan, L. L.), Grune and Stratton, New York.

Fuller, R. K. and Roth, H. P. (1979). Disulfiram for the treatment of alcoholism: an evaluation of 128 men. *Ann. intern. Med.*, **90**, 901–904.

Funderbunk, F. R., Allen, R. P. and Wagman, A. M. I. (1978). Residual effects of ethanol and chlordiazepoxide treatment for alcohol withdrawal. *J. Nerv. Ment. Dis.*, **166**, 195–203.

Goldstein, D. B. (1979). Some promising fields of inquiry in biomedical alcohol research. *J. Stud. Alcohol*, **8**, 204–215.

Greenblatt, D. J. and Koch-Weser, J. (1974). Clinical toxicity of chlordiazepoxide and diazepam in relation to serum albumin concentrations: a report of the Boston Collaborative Drug Surveillance Program. *Eur. J. clin. Pharmac.*, **7**, 259–263.

Greenblatt, D. J. and Shader, R. I. (1974). *Benzodiazepines in Clinical Practice*, Raven Press, New York.

Greenblatt, D. J., Shader, R. I. and Koch-Weser, J. (1974). Slow absorption of intramuscular chlordiazepoxide. *New Engl. J. Med.*, **291**, 1116–1118.

Griffits, R. R., Bigelow, G. E., Liebson, I. and Kaliszak, J. E. (1980). Drug preference in humans: double blind choice comparison of pentobarbital, diazepam and placebo. *J. Pharmac. exp. Ther.*, **215**, 649–661.

Hosein, I. N., de Freitas, R. and Beaubrun, M. H. (1979). Intramuscular/oral lorazepam in acute alcohol withdrawal and incipient delerium tremens. *W. I. med. J.*, **28**, 45–48.

Hossman, V., Maling, T. J. B., Hamilton, C. A., Reid, J. L. and Dollery, C. T. (1980). Sedative and cardiovascular effects of clonidine and intrazepam, *Clin. Pharmac. Ther.*, **28**, 167–176.

Jenkins, W. J. and Peters, T. J. (1980). Selectively reduced acetaldehyde dehydrogenase in alcoholics. *Lancet* **i**, 628–629.

Kalant, H. (1977). Alcohol withdrawal syndromes in the human: comparison with animal models. In: *Alcohol Intoxication and Withdrawal*, Vol. 3B, pp.57–64 (Ed. Gross, M. M.), Plenum Press, New York.

Kalant, H., LeBlanc, A. E. and Gibbins, R. J. (1971). Tolerance to and dependence on some non-opiate psychotropic drugs. *Pharmac. Rev.*, **23**, 135–191.

Kales, A., Scharf, M. B. and Kales, J. D. (1978). Rebound insomnia: a new clinical syndrome. *Science*, **201**, 1039–1041.

Kissin, B. (1975). The use of psychoactive drugs in the long term treatment of chronic alcoholics. *Ann. N. Y. Acad. Sci.*, **252**, 385–395.

Kissin, B. (1979). Biological investigations in alcohol research. *J. Stud. Alcohol*, **8**, 146–161.

Klotz, U., Antonin, K. H., Brugel, H. and Bieck, P. R. (1977). Disposition of diazepam and its major metabolite desmethyldiazepam in patients with liver disease. *Clin. Pharmac. Ther.*, **21**, 430–436.

Klotz, U. and Reimann, I. (1980a). Influence of cimetidine on the pharmacokinetics of desmethyldiazepam and oxazepam. *Eur. J. clin. Pharmac.*, **18**, 517–520.

Klotz, U. and Reimann, I. (1980b). Delayed clearance of diazepam due to cimetidine. *New Engl. J. Med.*, **302**, 1012–1014.

Kochansky, G. E., Salzman, C., Shader, R. L., Harmaz, J. S. and Ogeltree, A. M. (1975). The differential effects of chlordiazepoxide and oxazepam on hostility in a small group setting. *Am. J. Psychiat.*, **132**, 861–863.

Kopin, I. J., Blomberg, P., Ebert, M. H., Gordon, E. K., Jimerson, D. C., Markey, S. P. and Polinsky, R. J. (1983). Disposition and metabolism of MHPG-$CD_3$ in humans: Plasma MHPG as the principal pathway of norepinephrine metabolism and as an important determinant of CSF levels of MHPG. *Proceedings of the Nobel Conference 'Frontiers in Biochemical and Pharmacological Research in Depression'*, Raven Press, New York, in press.

Korsten, M. A., Matsuzaki, S., Feinman, L. and Lieber, C. S. (1975). High blood acetaldehyde levels after ethanol administration. Difference between alcoholic and nonalcoholic subjects. *New Engl. J. Med.*, **292**, 386–389.

Lader, M. H. and Petursson, H. (1981). Benzodiazepine derivatives-side effects and dangers. *Biol. Psychiat.*, **16**, 1195–1201.

Linnoila, M. (1983). Pharmacotherapy of anxiety disorders. *Proceedings of the Meeting, Pharmacotherapy in Psychiatry*, Clarke Institute of Psychiatry, Toronto, in press.

Linnoila, M. and Mattila, M. J. (1973). Drug interaction on psychomotor skills related to driving: diazepam and alcohol. *Eur. J. clin. Pharmac.*, **5**, 186–194.

Linnoila, M., Stowell, L., Marangos, P. J. and Thurman, R. G. (1981). Effect of ethanol and ethanol withdrawal on $^3$H-muscimol binding and behaviour in the rat: a pilot study. *Acta pharmac. toxicol.*, **49**, 407–411.

Lion, J. R., Azcavate, C. L. and Koepke, H. H. (1975). 'Paradoxical rage reaction' during psychotropic medication. *Dis. nerv. Syst.*, **36**, 557–558.

MacLeod, S. M., Sellers, E. M., Giles, H. G., Billings, B. J. and Martin, P. R. (1978). Interaction of disulfiram with benzodiazepines. *Clin. Pharmac. Ther.*, **24**, 583–589.

Majchrowicz, E. (1981). Reversal in central nervous system function during ethanol withdrawal in humans and experimental animals. *Fed. Proc.*, **40**, 2065–2072.

Majchrowicz, E., Hunt, W. A. and Piantadosi, C. (1976). Suppression by 1,3-butanediol of the ethanol withdrawal syndrome in rats. *Science*, **194**, 1181–1182.

Marini, J. L. and Sheard, M. H. (1977). Antiaggressive effect of lithium ion in man. *Acta psychiat. scand.*, **55**, 269–286.

Martin, P. R. (1981). The human genetics of alcoholism. *Substance and Alcohol Actions/Misuse*, **2**, 389–406.

Morgan, D. D., Robinson, J. D. and Mendenhall, C. L. (1981). Clinical pharmacokinetics of chlordiazepoxide in patients with alcoholic hepatitis. *Eur. J. clin. Pharmac.*, **19**, 279–285.

Munjada, D. J. and Moss, H. B. (1981). Affective disorder and alcoholism in families of agoraphobics. *Arch. gen. Psychiat.*, **38**, 869–871.

Naranjo, C. A., Sellers, E. M., Chater, K., Iversen, P., Roach, C. and Sykora, K. (1982). Importance of non-pharmacologic interventions in the treatment of acute alcohol withdrawal. *Clin. Pharmac. Ther.*, **31**, 254–255.

Ninan, P. T., Insel, T. R., Cohen, R. M., Cook, J. M., Skolnick, P. and Paul, S. M. (1983). Benzodiazepine receptor mediated experimental 'anxiety' in primates. *Science*, in press.

Ochs, H. R., Greenblatt, D. J., Roberts, G.-M. and Dengler, H. J. (1981). Diazepam interaction with antituberculosis drugs. *Clin. Pharmac. Ther.*, **29**, 671–678.

Palva, E. and Linnoila, M. (1978). Effect of active metabolites of chlordiazepoxide and diazepam, alone or in combination with alcohol, on psychomotor skills related to driving. *Eur. J. clin. Pharmac.*, **13**, 345–350.

Paulson, O. B., Gyory, A. and Hertz, M. M. (1982). Blood-brain barrier transfer and cerebral uptake of antiepileptic drugs. *Clin. Pharmac. Ther.*, **32**, 466–477.

Pond, S. M., Phillips, M., Benowitz, N. L., Galinsky, R. E., Tong, T. G. and Becker, C. E. (1979). Diazepam kinetics in acute withdrawal. *Clin. Pharmac. Ther.*, **25**, 832–836.

Quitkin, F. M., Rifkin, A., Kaplan, J. and Klein, D. F. (1972). Phobic anxiety syndrome complicated by drug dependence and addiction. *Arch. gen. Psychiat.*, **27**, 159–162.

Reynolds, C. M., Merry, J. and Coppen, A. (1979). Prophylactic treatment of alcoholism by lithium carbonate: an initial report. In: *Affective Dsorders*, pp.31–37 (Eds. Goodwin, D. W. and Erickson, C. K.), SP Medical and Scientific Books, New York.

Ritzmann, R. F. and Tabakoff, B. (1976). Dissociation of alcohol tolerance and dependence. *Nature*, **263**, 418–420.

Rosenthal, N. E., Davenport, Y., Cowdry, R. W., Webster, M. H. and Goodwin, F. K. (1980). Monoamine metabolites in cerebrospinal fluid of depressive subgroups. *Psychiat. Res.*, **2**, 113–119.

Rothstein, E., Cobble, J. C. and Sampson, N. (1976). Chlordiazepoxide: long-term use in alcoholism. *Ann. N. Y. Acad. Sci.*, **273**, 381–384.

Rutledge, C. O. and Jonason, J. (1967). Metabolic pathways of dopamine and norepinephrine in rabbit brain *in vitro*. *J. Pharmac. exp. Ther.*, **157**, 493–502.

Schlesser, M. A., Winokur, G. and Sherman, B. M. (1981). Hypothalamic-pituitary-adrenal axis activity in depressive illness. *Arch. gen. Psychiat.*, **37**, 737–743.

Schuckit, M. A. (1980). Self-rating of alcohol intoxication by young men with and without family histories of alcoholism. *J. Stud. Alcohol*, **41**, 242–249.

Schuckit, M. A. (1982). Prevalence of affective disorder in a sample of young men. *Am. J. Psychiat.*, **139**, 1431–1436.

Schuckit, M. A. (1982). Prevalence of affective disorder in a sample of young men. *Am. J. Psychiat.*, **139**, 1431–1436.

Schuckit, M. A. and Rayses, V. (1979). Ethanol ingestion: differences in blood acetaldehyde concentrations in relatives of alcoholics and controls. *Science*, **203**, 54–55.

Sellers, E. M. (1977). Comparative efficacy of propranolol and chlordiazepoxide in alcohol withdrawal. *J. Stud. Alcohol*, **38**, 2096–2108.

Sellers, E. M. (1978). Clinical pharmacology and therapeutics of benzodiazepines. *Can. Med. Ass. J.*, **118**, 1533–1538.

Sellers, E. M., Greenblatt, D. J., Zilm, D. H. and Degani, N. (1978). Decline in chlordiazepoxide plasma levels during fixed dose therapy of alcohol withdrawal. *Brit. J. clin. Pharmac.*, **6**, 370–371.

Sellers, E. M. and Kalant, H. (1976). Alcohol intoxication and withdrawal. *New Engl. J. Med.*, **294**, 757–762.

Seppala, T., Aranko, K., Mattila, M. J. and Shrotiya, R. (1982). Effects of alcohol and buspirone and lorazepam actions. *Clin. Pharmac. Ther.*, **32**, 201–207.

Shaw, J. M., Kolesar, G. S., Sellers, E. M., Kaplan, H. L. and Sandoz, P. (1981). Development of optimal tactics for alcohol withdrawal. I. Assessment and effectiveness of supportive care. *J. clin. Psychopharmac.*, **1**, 382–387.

Shull, H. J., Wilkinson, G. R., Johnson, R. and Schenker, S. (1976). Normal disposition of oxazepam in acute viral hepatitis and cirrhosis. *Ann. intern. Med.*, **84**, 420–425.

Stein, L., Wise, C. D. and Beluzzi, J. D. (1974). Effects of benzodiazepines on central serotonergic mechanisms. *Adv. Biochem. Psychopharmac.*, **14**, 29–44.

Tabakoff, B. and Hoffman, P. L. (1979). Development of functional dependence on ethanol in dopaminergic systems. *J. Pharmac. exp. Ther.*, **208**, 216–222.

Tallman, J. F., Paul, S. M., Skolnick, P. and Gallagher, D. (1980). Receptors for the age of anxiety: pharmacology of the benzodiazepines. *Science*, **207**, 274–281.

Tarter, R. E., McBride, H., Buonpane, N. and Schneider, D. U. (1977). Differentiation of alcoholics. *Arch. gen. Psychiatry*, **34**, 761–768.

Tavel, M. E., Davidson, W. and Batterton, I. D. (1972). A critical analysis of mortality associated with delirium tremens: a review of 39 fatalities in a 9 year period. *Am. J. Med. Sci.*, **242**, 429–431.

Tewari, S. and Noble, E. P. (1975). Alterations in cerebral polynucleotide metabolism following chronic ethanol ingestion. In: *Alcohol Intoxication and Withdrawal, Experimental Studies—II*, pp.37–53 (Ed. Gross, M. M.), Plenum Press, New York.

Thiessen, J. J., Sellers, E. M., Denbeigh, P. and Dolman, L. (1976). Plasma protein binding of diazepam and tolbutamide in chronic alcoholics. *J. clin. Pharmac.*, **16**, 345–351.

Ticku, M. K. and Davis, W. C. (1981). Evidence that ethanol and pentobarbital enhance [3H] diazepam binding at the benzodiazepine–GABA receptor–ionophore complex indirectly. *Eur. J. Pharmac.*, **71**, 521–522.

Victor, M. and Brausch, C. (1967). The role of abstinence in the genesis of alcoholic epilepsy. *Epilepsia*, **8**, 1–20.

Walinder, J., Balldin, J., Bokstrom, K., Karlsson, I., Lundstrom, B. and Svensson, T. H. (1981). Clonidine suppression of the alcohol withdrawal syndrome. *Drug and Alcohol Depend.*, **8**, 345–348.

Whitfield, C. L., Thompson, G., Lamb, A., Spencer, V., Pfeifer, M. and Browning-Ferrande, M. (1978). Detoxification of 1,024 alcoholic patients without psychoactive drugs. *J. Am. med. Ass.*, **239**, 1409–1410.

Whiting, B., Lawrence, J. R. and Skellern, G. G. (1979). Effects of acute alcohol

intoxication on the metabolism and plasma kinetics of chlordiazepoxide. *Brit. J. clin. Pharmac.*, **7**, 95–100.
WHO (1981). Memorandum nomenclature and classification of drug- and alcohol-related problems. *WHO Bull.*, **59**, 225–242.

## DISCUSSION

## CHAIRMAN: PROFESSOR RICHENS

THE CHAIRMAN: One drug that you have not mentioned, which surprised me, was chlormethiazole. I thought there was an important role for this drug in the management of alcoholism.

DR. LINNOILA: In my opinion it is lethal and, therefore, I do not want to mention it in the treatment of alcoholism. I purposely left it out.

PROFESSOR SANDLER: Could I just ask you about interaction between amphetamine and alcohol, and whether you agree that some of these psychopaths may actually be a manifestation of minimal brain dysfunction children grown old, and one may control it with amphetamine-like drugs? Would you be able to suppress hostility and aggression?

DR. LINNOILA: That is not known.

DR. L. L. IVERSEN: You mentioned the phenomenon of cross-tolerance between ethanol and benzodiazepines. I wonder what you meant by that because tolerance is not a very notable phenomenon for the benzodiazepines. Patients on these drugs do not tend to escalate dose, or at least it is quite rare.

DR. LINNOILA: What I mean by cross-tolerance is the issue that there are well-documented phenomena of alcoholics requiring very high doses of benzodiazepines. There is both pharmacodynamic and pharmacokinetic cross-tolerance. There is a very clear pharmacodynamic cross-tolerance in the sense that alcoholics can take large doses of benzodiazepines without sedation, some surprisingly large.

DR. TRIMBLE: I am very interested that you come down so heavily in favour of benzodiazepines for alcohol abuse, because there is an alternative school that would feel that you were in danger of replacing one drug of addiction by another. There is a growing literature, mainly from Scandinavia, on the use of carbamazepine in the acute withdrawal phase. This is advocated really on two grounds, first because it is anticonvulsant and, second, it is non-sedative. A third ground is that it may itself have some psychotropic properties.

DR. LINNOILA: Benzodiazepines are significantly less toxic than carbamazepine when used parenterally. So they are easy to use. They are the first choice drugs in this situation, and I think then, when the acute withdrawal is over, one has to start wondering about the long-term treatment and there the benzodiazepines are not indicated, based on present knowledge. The carbamazepine issue relates to a kindling model of alcohol withdrawal. I am not convinced at this point that we can unequivocally use this model. Carbamazepine does not show cross-tolerance with alcohol which may have some value.

THE CHAIRMAN: Is not the frequent occurrence of fits during withdrawal an argument for using a good anticonvulsant routinely for prophylaxis?

DR. LINNOILA: How frequent is it? The data suggests it is less than 5% of patients who come in with incipient withdrawal, and we are talking now of severe alcoholics. This is a matter of resources. If you can watch the patient and if you can treat the patient very well with all supportive means, you need fewer drugs. If you cannot watch the patient and you do not have nursing staff, then you may have to resort to drugs which you would not use under more optimal circumstances.

DR. D. A. W. JOHNSON: I would just like to re-emphasize that point. In Manchester we have the only hospital based detoxification unit in the country and we had 5% or fewer withdrawal seizures in chronic alcoholic patients.

Benzodiazepines Divided
Edited by M. R. Trimble


# 22

# Benzodiazepines, Psychological Functioning, and Dementia

MALCOLM LADER

## INTRODUCTION

The benzodiazepines have supplanted the barbiturates as tranquillizers, hypnotics, preoperative medication, muscle relaxants, and anticonvulsants. Many patients take these drugs sporadically or in short courses but a disconcerting trend can be detected towards long-term use. Thus, Marks (1983) presented a table showing that in 1967/8, 27% of patients on psychotropic drugs were given long-term repeat prescriptions whereas in 1977/8, the corresponding figure was 64%. Undoubtedly, patients with severe anxiety function poorly without some sedation and the advantages of taking benzodiazepines outweigh possible drawbacks. Many patients, however, are less severely ill or have largely recovered from their initial symptoms and yet still continue their medication.

A major difficulty is that little is known of either the benefits or the problems associated with long-term benzodiazepine use. Many studies have examined the therapeutic efficacy of the benzodiazepines in the various indications mentioned above. And many studies have quantified the psychological effects of these drugs given in single doses or in short courses of treatment. But the methodological problems of studying the long-term use of benzodiazepines has precluded any definitive assessment of either long-term efficacy or long-term unwanted effects. Prospective studies have concentrated on efficacy, or more recently on withdrawal, with few attempts at measuring psychological effects.

A further problem relates to possible morphological changes in the brain. The advent of computerized brain tomography led to the confirmation that alcohol abusers may develop anatomical changes in the brain such as ventricular dilation (Ron, 1977). The possibility that benzodiazepines given for years on end might also lead to morphological brain changes, reversible or irreversible, cannot be dismissed without further consideration.

The purpose of this presentation is to review the psychological effects of benzodiazepines. Where possible, long-term studies will be emphasized. Some data from our studies on benzodiazepine users will be outlined.

## PROBLEMS OF METHOD

Anxious patients can be defined operationally as those people whose anxiety levels have led them to seek medical advice. Accordingly, normal subjects are those not under medical care: yet they may still have high anxiety levels, as high as those of patients. Some screening procedure is therefore needed to separate out appropriate groups. This can be informal as a brief psychiatric interview or formal using a standardized rating scale.

Anxiety, itself, affects psychological functioning, quite marked impairments being found on some measures. We compared 30 drug-free patients suffering from chronic anxiety states with 30 normal controls matched for age, sex, and social class (Bond *et al.*, 1974a). Card-sorting into categories and simple piles, digit symbol substitution test, symbol copying, simple arithmetic, and tachistoscopic recognition were all significantly impaired in the patients. Auditory reaction time, simple tapping, Gibson spiral maze, and cancellation tests were not affected. We concluded that as task complexity increased, patient performance was more impaired.

The corollary of this finding is, of course, that treatments which lower anxiety will tend to improve performance indirectly which nullifies any direct depressant effect of the medication. Those direct effects are consequently better studied in normal subjects, at least initially in the programme of research. Armed with this knowledge, the researcher can better interpret his data from patients. Empirically, it is important to establish whether patients are psychologically impaired while on benzodiazepines. Dosage is crucial: a high dose will produce impairment in patients. What is more important is to see whether impairment supervenes at clinically effective doses.

Motivational factors can affect the results of performance studies. The expectations of experimenter and subjects, the level of payment, and the context in which the study is conducted can modify test results. Double-blind procedures, careful screening of volunteers, well-trained experimenters, and strict adherence to a carefully constructed protocol are essential.

Practice effects are particularly important with tests involving the coordination of sensory and motor system functions. One approach is to test every subject repeatedly until they reach a plateau of performance, but this can be very tedious as improvement in performance can continue over many repetitions of the test. Other tests may need the use of parallel versions to prevent the subject becoming familiar with the test content.

A further complication concerns tolerance. Clinical reports suggest that patients with initial complaints of sedation on benzodiazepines often find these symptoms waning over the course of the first week or two. This tolerance is quite substantial as it supervenes despite cumulation of the longer acting benzodiazepines such as diazepam and clorazepate.

## IMMEDIATE EFFECTS

Two major uses of the benzodiazepines are as tranquillizers and hypnotics. In the former use, interest centres on the immediate effects of the drugs on psychological functioning, whereas in the latter use there is more concern with residual or 'hangover' effects, detectable when the patient awakes the next morning.

Many studies have evaluated the acute effects of benzodiazepines on various psychometric functions. Considerations of space preclude a detailed review of the literature, which have been compiled by McNair (1973), Wittenborn (1978, 1979) and Hindmarch (1980).

The number of tests used is legion. Hindmarch (1980) lists the following: proof reading ability, spiral after effect duration, low speed car handling tasks, card sorting ability, car driving simulator, pursuit rotor, symbol copying, absolute auditory threshold, short- and long-term memory, verbal learning, discrimination conditioning of the eyelid response, kinaesthetic figural after effect, muscular grip strength, adaptive tracking, beam balancing task, digit symbol substitution task, delayed auditory feedback, ocular convergence, the speed of putting caps on ballpoint pens, tapping speed, hidden word task, auditory reaction time, Gibson spiral maze, critical flicker fusion frequency, time estimation procedure, digit span test, response time, body sway, duration of after images, serial subtraction of numbers, Purdue pegboard, stabilometer, concentration, concept identification task, group vigilance task, cancellation of numbers, category clustering, saccadic eye movements, rudder control test, choice reaction time task, car driving ability, spontaneous reversals of the Necker cube, two handed coordination, Whipple's tracing board and a trigram recognition task. This list is by no means exhaustive.

These tests can be roughly subsumed under the following headings: sensory function and sensory processing ability; CNS function and central processing ability including memory and learning; motor function and behavioural coordination; sensorimotor performance. Psychomotor performance is the outcome of coordinated sensory and motor systems through the integrative and organizational activities of the brain. Personality, memory, and motivation influence the processing of sensory information. The level of arousal of the central nervous system governs the degree of integration of these functions. The coordinated behavioural responses are themselves modified by adaptive and feedback mechanisms.

The most commonly used tests are reaction time, digit symbol substitution, cancellation, tapping, card sorting, pursuit rotor, and critical flicker fusion. The most sensitive, i.e. those which have discriminated most significantly between a benzodiazepine and a placebo, are critical flicker fusion, learning and memory, digit symbol substitution, cancellation, and card sorting (Hindmarch, 1980). Functions that seem to be relatively insensitive are complex visual motor coordination, visual spatial performance, and auditory perception. Simulated driving seems less impaired than actual driving.

Before interpreting such data the caveat must be entered that some tests may be inherently less reliable than others even before drugs are administered. None the less, it seems that the benzodiazepines have little effect on such established functions as visual–spatial, perceptual, and verbal tasks whereas the acquisition of new material as sampled by memory functions and digit symbol substitutions were sensitive to these drugs. Speed of repetitive movements such as tapping, cancellation, and card sorting are relatively sensitive to drug effects. Thus, in summary, learning, memory, and simple repetitive tasks are affected by benzodiazepines, well established higher mental faculties are less or not affected.

## RESIDUAL EFFECTS

Studies on the residual effects of benzodiazepines, like those on the immediate effects, have concentrated on normal subjects. Of 52 studies reviewed by Johnson and Chernik (1982), only eight used insomniac patients. A wide range of benzodiazepines has been evaluated and in general the time course of any impairments can be predicted from the pharmacokinetic properties of each drug. However, the pharmacokinetic parameters of a benzodiazepine must be known in detail in order to make accurate predictions. For example, the short alpha half-life (redistribution phase) of diazepam means that its short-term effects wear off rapidly, and only on repeated administration does accumulation occur because of the metabolite, desmethyldiazepam, with a very long beta (elimination) half-life. Hypnotic drugs can be roughly divided into long-acting and short-acting, the dividing point being whether cumulation would be expected in normal dosage. We have recently reviewed all these studies on residual effects and concluded that the long-acting compounds such as nitrazepam and flurazepam are generally associated with residual effects the next day, whereas short-acting compounds such as temazepam and triazolam do not result in residual effects unless the dose is high or the subject is an untypically slow metabolizer of the drug (Bond and Lader, 1981).

Johnson and Chernik (1982) have listed the tests used and the proportion of investigations in which each test was sensitive to benzodiazepine effects. Card sorting was most useful in discriminating between hypnotic/sedative and placebo with 11 out of 18 test comparisons (61%) being positive. Symbol copying, tapping rate, digit symbol substitution, memory, arithmetic, and vigilance tasks were all discriminatory in a third or more of studies. Coordination tasks, critical flicker fusion, pursuit rotor, Purdue pegboard, and sample of choice reaction times were least useful. The main discrepancy between these lists and those for tests for the immediate effects of benzodiazepines is the failure of critical flicker fusion in residual studies. However, all these negative results emanated from one laboratory. Otherwise, the same sort of conclusion is warranted: the speed at which simple acts of a repetitive nature are performed are most likely to be impaired by benzodiazepines, especially where the motor component is linked to a learning or memory component.

This finding raises the possibility that performance decrements are due, at least in part, to the muscle relaxant effects of benzodiazepines rather than their central effects on arousal or learning. If so, then many of the apparent psychological impairments produced by these drugs could be minimized or even obviated by developing benzodiazepines devoid of muscle relaxant actions. Clobazam has a minor action on muscle tone and several studies have indicated that moderate doses have little if any effect on psychomotor functioning (Steiner-Chaskel and Lader, 1981).

## EFFECTS IN PATIENTS

Our study published several years ago demonstrated the difficulty of detecting any effects of benzodiazepines given for a few weeks on psychological functioning in anxious patients (Bond *et al.*, 1974b). Tranquillization improves performance because it counteracts the disruptive effects of the anxiety state. Similar conclusions were obtained in a study of the residual effects of hypnotics in a sample of 60 severely anxious inpatients (Tansella *et al.*, 1974). Card sorting and Gibson spiral maze time were marginally affected after a week of treatment with *N*-desmethyldiazepam, 20 mg at night.

Over the short term, then, the symptomatic relief afforded by the benzodiazepines also tends to improve psychological functioning, provided the dose level is judiciously chosen. Underdosage will be associated with failure to improve and too high a dose will push the patient over the top of the classical inverted U-shaped curve resulting in definite impairment.

Over the longer term, the situation becomes even more complex. Cumulation of longer acting benzodiazepines is inevitable and, unless counteracted by tissue tolerance, would lead to gross impairment. But remission of the anxiety state will also complicate the issue. If the anxiety lessens, then anxiety-related performance decrements will also lessen and the benzodiazepine is much more likely to result in psychological impairments. Of course, patients in remission would be expected to relinquish their benzodiazepine taking although some patients may develop normal dose dependence and continue their medication indefinitely.

## PSYCHOMETRIC STUDIES

Under these circumstances of long-term use, some psychological impairments might occur in these patients. We took the opportunity to evaluate the chronic effects of benzodiazepines as part of our work on benzodiazepine withdrawal and tolerance. The main aim was to assess psychological performance in patients during long-term benzodiazepine treatment and withdrawal, and in particular whether tolerance and rebound could be demonstrated.

Twenty-two patients (13 males, 9 females) who had been on normal-dose, long-term benzodiazepine treatment were withdrawn from their drugs. Thirteen of the patients were studied as outpatients, and nine were inpatients. Their mean (±s.d.) age was 40.2 ± 11.5 years, range 22–70. All the patients had received benzodiazepines in therapeutic doses for at least one year. Thirteen were on diazepam (mean daily dose 15.2 mg, range 6–30 mg); five had received lorazepam (mean daily dose 4.6 mg, range 1.0–7.5 mg); two were on clobazam, 30 mg daily; one was on oxazepam, 90 mg daily; and one had received lorazepam 2.5 mg plus triazolam 0.25 mg daily.

Most patients were referred by their general practitioners for the purpose of withdrawal from their long-term (7.6 ± 4.6 years) benzodiazepine therapy. The withdrawal was gradual, double-blind, and placebo controlled: patients were randomly allocated to two groups (A and B). Both groups continued with their drugs, full dose, for the first 2 weeks; group A was then reduced to half dose for a further 2 weeks, before the medication was discontinued. Group B received the full dose of their medication for the first 4 weeks, but were then withdrawn in the same manner as group A, i.e. 2 weeks later. During these phases placebo was substituted for the active drugs, and after withdrawal of the drugs both groups continued on placebo only for 4 and 2 weeks respectively, followed by 2 weeks without any tablets or capsules. In the course of the study period which comprised 14 occasions over 64 days, patients were assessed at regular intervals of 3, 4, or 7 days, on a battery of clinical, physiological, and psychological tests.

Two control groups were studied. The main control group consisted of 16 (8 females, 8 males) healthy, drug-free individuals recruited from the community. They were matched as closely as possible with the patients in terms of age, sex, and social class. Their mean age (± s.d.) was 39.3 ± 12.2 years, range 21–60. These individuals served as controls for the paper-and-pencil psychological assessments (DSST, SCT, CT), and were tested 14 times.

The second abbreviated control group comprised 14 (7 females, 7 males) drug-free, healthy individuals, most of whom were members of research or technical staff of the Institute of Psychiatry. Their mean age (± s.d.) was 35.3 ± 8.7, range 21–55. These individuals served as part-controls for the laboratory assessments (RT, KTR), but were only assessed on three occasions.

## Digit-Symbol Substitution Test (DSST)

This task is a measure of cognitive skills involving coding. It entails the subject coding symbols for numbers and is a subtest of the Wechsler Adult Intelligence Schedule. The score was the mean time (in seconds) taken by the patient to complete each correct item during the 90-second test period (i.e. 90/no. of items completed). Coding performance improved over time significantly in both patients and controls ($F(13,23) = 17.92$; $P < 0.0001$). The overall improvement reflected a substantial practice effect with the attainment of an asymptote on the later occasions. The overall performance of the two patient groups differed significantly ($F(1,35) = 5.86$; $P < 0.02$), and their performance was also consistently lower than control ($F(1,25) = 13.98$; $P < 0.0007$).

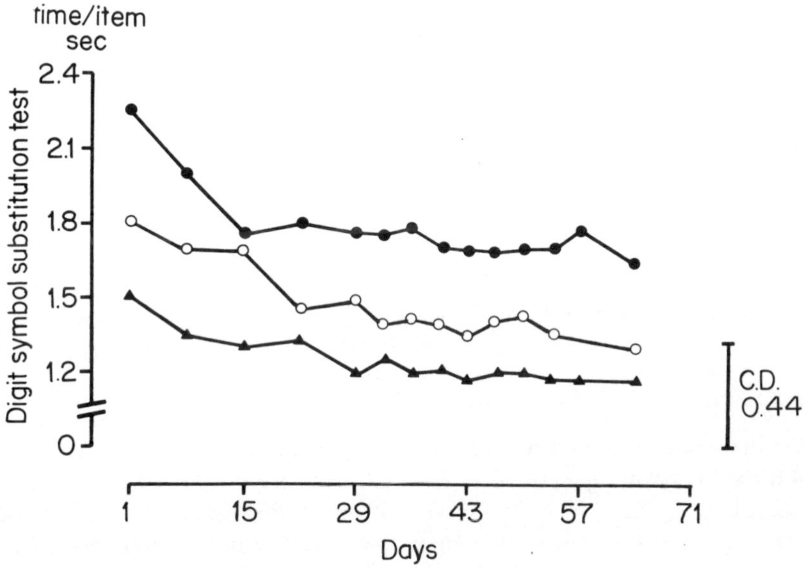


Figure 1 Mean time/item of the Digit Symbol Substitution Test in controls (▲——▲) and in patients, group A (●——●) and group B (○——○) during withdrawal of benzodiazepines (group A full dosage first 2 weeks, half dosage next 2 weeks, drug withdrawn; group B full dosage first 4 weeks, half dosage next 2 weeks, drug withdrawn); Within each group critical differences further apart than shown are significant at 5% level or more

**Symbol Copying Test**

The same symbols are used as in the DSST, but the subject has only to copy and not code them. This gives a measure of writing skills and is the motor component of the DSST. Again the score was the mean time (in seconds) the patient took to complete each correct item during the 90-second test period. A substantial practice effect was detected on the SCT ($F(13,23) = 5.13$; $P < 0.0004$). Again, the patients performed significantly worse than the controls throughout the study ($F(1,35) = 17.54$; $P < 0.0002$).

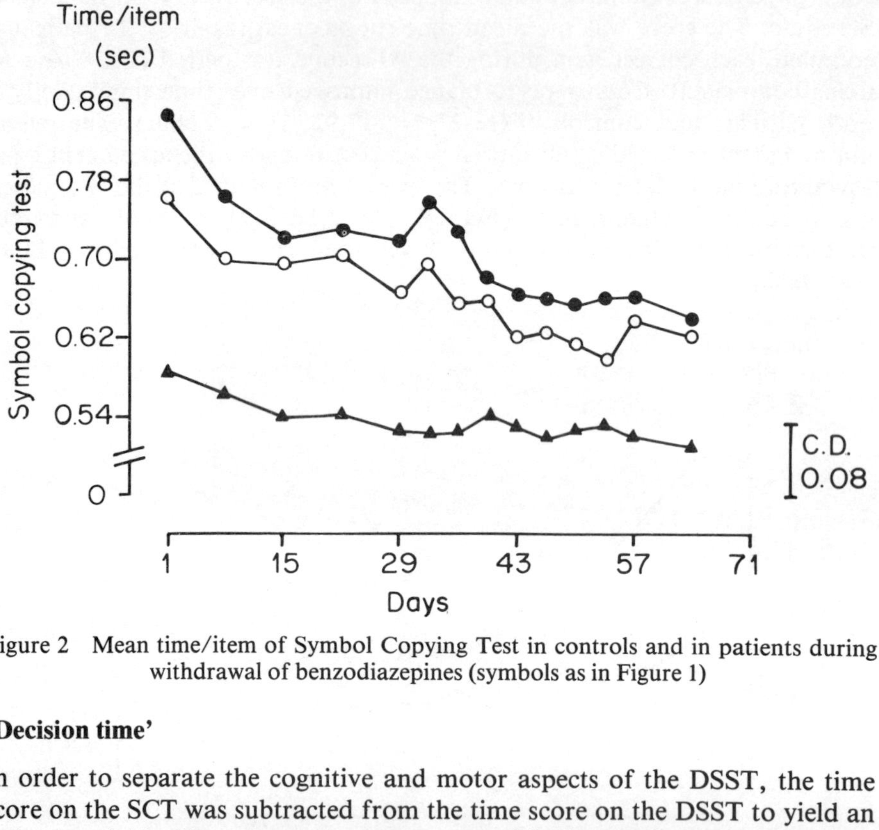


Figure 2 Mean time/item of Symbol Copying Test in controls and in patients during withdrawal of benzodiazepines (symbols as in Figure 1)

**'Decision time'**

In order to separate the cognitive and motor aspects of the DSST, the time score on the SCT was subtracted from the time score on the DSST to yield an estimate of 'decision time'. In agreement with the results on DSST both patients and controls showed change over time thus reflecting an initial practice effect. The mean results for the patients were significantly lower than those of the controls ($F(1,35) = 7.47$; $P < 0.01$).

**Cancellation test (CT)**

This is a measure of attention to close detail at speed and accurate scanning. The task involved the cancellation of 4s in a table of numbers where the frequency of 4s was 40 in 400 random digits. The time to complete the task and number of errors incurred were recorded. Improvement over time was the only significant effect on this test ($F(13,23) = 6.28$; $P < 0.0001$). The groups did not differ.

**Reaction time (RT)**

The simple auditory reaction time to 32 clicks of about 70 db was measured and a reciprocal transformation was applied to normalize the distribution and the mean calculated. This test provides a measure of sensory and motor speed. The patients did not differ significantly from controls on the first three occasions, nor was there a significant difference in the overall performance of the two patient groups ($F(1,20) = 2.43$; NS).

**Tapping test (KTR)**

Using the first two fingers of the preferred hand, the subject was asked to tap a key as quickly as possible. The computer recorded the number of key depressions made during 60 seconds, and the intertap interval (ITI) was computed in milliseconds. This task is a measure of pure motor speed. This test showed little practice effect and there was no significant difference in the performance of patients and normals.

This study demonstrates two main features. First, the DSST, SCT, and CT are all subject to substantial and prolonged practice effects. Second, patients on long-term benzodiazepines appear to be tolerant to the performance decrement on the CT, RT, and KTR, customarily associated with reduced arousal during the initial phases of benzodiazepine therapy. However, this was not demonstrated in respect of the DSST and the SCT, the patients showing a continuing deficit on these variables.

The apparently permanent deficits on the DSST, and in particular the SCT are more difficult to explain. As was to be expected this is also reflected in the results on the 'decision time' variable. Furthermore, patients performed rather worse than normals on the RT, although the difference was not statistically significant. On the whole, most cognitive skills, attention, vigilance, and pure motor speed are not adversely affected by prolonged benzodiazepine treatment. However, the patients demonstrated impaired performance on tasks requiring the combined use of sensory and finer motor skills. This was particularly evident in respect of the SCT, involving motor speed and fine coordination, i.e. handwriting.

Thus, although several years of chronic sedative use *may* result in selective but chronic psychological deficits, other explanations must be considered. This difference may be due to inadequate selection and matching of controls and patients although this is unlikely in view of the similar performance of patients and controls on the other tests. Second, reduced performance of this nature may be a trait of anxious patients although I am unaware of any evidence of such selective performance deficits. Third, the results could imply that these particular residual effects are excessively prolonged and that the patients may catch up with the controls several weeks or months after the withdrawal. The shape of the respective graphs, however, makes this unlikely.

## NEURORADIOLOGICAL STUDY

Structural brain abnormalities have been described in conjunction with cognitive impairment in subjects who have abused alcohol for prolonged periods (Ron *et al.*, 1982). It was possible that such abnormalities were present in benzodiazepine users in some of whom psychometric impairment was detectable during withdrawal. The advent of computerized tomography (CT scan) allowed us to study a group of such subjects and to compare them to normal controls and to chronic alcoholics.

Twenty patients on or recently withdrawn from long-term benzodiazepine treatment were studied. Doses were within the therapeutic range, i.e., up to 30 mg/day of diazepam or equivalent. Nine were scanned at an average of 3 months following withdrawal of the drugs. Eleven patients were investigated while still receiving their treatment. They comprised seven women and 13 men, mean age 43.3 years (±12.7). Diagnoses included anxiety, personality disorder with anxiety, insomnia, and depression, and none abused alcohol or took other drugs. The mean duration of their benzodiazepine treatment was 10.6 years (±4.8). Two groups were used for comparison, normal controls and alcoholics. Their records were available from a series of subjects already reported (Ron *et al.*, 1982). Subjects were selected by age and sex to match the benzodiazepine users. Where choices of controls or alcoholics were available, selection was random.

Patients and controls were scanned using an EMI CT1010 Head Scanner. Five or six contiguous pairs of slices were taken parallel to the orbitomeatal line. The scans were first reported on routinely by the neuroradiologists. Later, all the scans, including those of the comparison groups, were analysed 'blind' by a senior radiologist. CT scan measurements were made using the photographic negative and CT scan indices were made using the procedure described by Ron *et al.* (1982) and provided the following estimates.

1. *Sulcal widening* was rated on a 4-point scale (0–3), 0 representing normality and 3 gross widening.
2. *Sylvian fissure widening* was rated on a 3-point scale (0–2).
3. *Interhemispheric fissure widening* was rated as absent or present. A composite 'cortical score' was obtained by adding these three scores.
4. *Ventricular area* was expressed as a percentage of the total area within the

Table 1 Mean ratio of ventricle/brain area expressed as percentage, number of individuals with abnormal scans, and 'cortical score' in normal controls, long-term benzodiazepine users, and alcoholics

| Group | No. with definitely abnormal scan (sex:age) | Ventricle/brain areas (%) (mean ± s.e.m.) | 'Cortical score' (mean ± s.e.m.) |
|---|---|---|---|
| Normals ($n$ = 19) | 1 (M52) | 5.57 ± 0.43 | 1.4 ± 0.1 |
| BZ users ($n$ = 20) | 3 (M34;M32;F39) | 7.01 ± 0.49* | 1.8 ± 0.2‡ |
| Alcoholics ($n$ = 19) | 3 (M58;M40;F40) | 9.19 ± 0.65† | 2.8 ± 0.3† |

Difference from normals: *$P < 0.05$; †$P < 0.001$.
Difference of BZ users from alcoholics: ‡$P < 0.05$.

inner table of the skull. The measurements were made with a Stanley Allbrit planimeter in two contiguous slices showing the maximum ventricular area. The ventricle/brain ratio (V/B) was the mean of these two ratios.

Definite abnormalities were reported by the radiologist in three benzodiazepine users, as compared with one control and three alcoholics (Table 1). The abnormalities comprised ventricular enlargement, widening of sulci, Sylvian, and interhemispheric fissures.

The table shows the V/B ratio of the alcoholics to be significantly different from those of the normals ($P < 0.001$). The results for the benzodiazepine group are, on average, intermediate between but significantly different from those of control subjects ($P < 0.05$), and those of the alcoholics ($P < 0.02$). Among the benzodiazepine users the ventricle/brain ratios were significantly larger in males than females ($P < 0.05$), but there was no correlation with age ($r = 0.05$, NS), nor duration of previous benzodiazepine usage ($r = 0.03$, NS). Furthermore, there was no significant difference between those patients on or off their medication.

The table presents the mean cortical scores for the groups. The score for the alcoholics was significantly higher than those for the controls and for the benzodiazepine users. One-quarter of the controls, 45% of the drug users, and just over half the alcoholics had positive cortical scores.

The mean age of those benzodiazepine users who had positive cortical scores was 51.6 years ($\pm 13.2$), compared to 36.5 ($\pm 6.7$) for those with no demonstrable abnormalities ($P < 0.01$). Cortical score was positively correlated with age ($r = +0.47$; $P < 0.05$). However, similar to the planimetric data, there was no correlation between duration of previous benzodiazepine usage and cortical score ($r = 0.23$, NS). Again, for the benzodiazepine group, scores were primarily evident among the men, eight out of 13 (61.5%), compared to only one case among the seven women.

Scan appearances for the benzodiazepine patients are intermediate between those of control subjects and those of the alcoholics. One possibility is that benzodiazepines, taken long-term, result in radiological changes. Another is that individuals with radiological changes due to other causes are prone to develop anxiety states which only respond to sedatives, and consequently drug therapy becomes prolonged. The abnormalities seen in alcoholics tend to improve during abstention. The benzodiazepine withdrawal syndrome is usually associated with a loss of body weight (Petursson and Lader, 1981) due to loss of fluid. However, the present study did not reveal any significant differences between those patients still on benzodiazepine treatment, and those who had been withdrawn.

Although age correlated significantly with the cortical score, there was none between the planimetric data and age. This is consistent with results of some other studies (Jacoby *et al.*, 1980). Although our detailed evaluation of the benzodiazepine users excluded long-term alcohol abuse, it is possible that some resorted to alcohol sporadically. The reverse might apply to our alcoholic group although persistent drug use was an exclusion criterion in the original study. In view of the known potentiation of alcohol and benzodiazepines in other areas, this possibility needs further investigation.

The finding of no association between radiological changes and duration of previous benzodiazepine therapy leaves the clinical significance of these findings unclear. In view of the very extensive and often prolonged use of the benzodiazepines in therapeutic practice, with or without alcohol, it is important to establish the nature, extent, and reversibility of functional and structural brain changes by relating them to clinical factors and to detailed neuropsychological testing.

## CONCLUSIONS

The evaluation of the effects of benzodiazepines on psychological functioning is beset by problems of method such as the confounding effects of anxiety itself. Short-term impairments associated with benzodiazepines in normal subjects mainly involve learning, memory, and simple repetitive tasks; well-established higher mental faculties are not usually affected at normal dosage. Residual effects, e.g. the morning after an hypnotic dose, follow a similar pattern. In anxious patients, impairments are not apparent on short-term use; indeed, improvements may occur, associated with symptomatic relief. However, on long-term use, our personal work indicates that some psychological functions may be continuously impaired. Also, some neuroradiological changes may be associated with long-term use. The clinical implications of these last findings are unclear.

## REFERENCES

Bond, A. J., James, D. C. and Lader, M. H. (1974a). Physiological and psychological measures in anxious patients. *Psychol. Med.*, **4**, 364–373.

Bond, A. J., James, D. C. and Lader, M. H. (1974b). Sedative effects on physiological and psychological measures in anxious patients. *Psychol. Med.*, **4**, 374–380.

Bond, A. J. and Lader, M. (1981). Aftereffects of sleeping drugs. In: *Psychopharmacology of Sleep*, pp.177–197 (Ed. Wheatley, D.), Raven Press, New York.

Hindmarch, I. (1980). Psychomotor function and psychoactive drugs. *Brit. J. clin. Pharmac.*, **10**, 189–210.

Jacoby, R. J., Levy, R. and Dawson, J. M. (1980). Computed tomography in the elderly. 1. The normal population. *Brit. J. Psychiat.*, **136**, 249–255.

Johnson, L. C. and Chernik, D. A. (1982). Sedative-hypnotics and human performance. *Psychopharmacology*, **76**, 101–113.

Marks, J. (1983). The benzodiazepines for good or evil. *Int. Pharmac. psych.*, (in press).

McNair, D. M. (1973). Antianxiety drugs and human performance, *Arch. gen. Psychiat.*, **29**, 609–617.

Petursson, H. and Lader, M. H. (1981). Withdrawal from long-term benzodiazepine treatment. *Brit. med. J.*, **283**, 643–645.

Ron, M. (1977). Brain damage in chronic alcoholism: a neuropathological, neuro-radiological and psychological review. *Psychol. Med.*, **7**, 103–112.

Ron, M. A., Acker, W., Lishman, W. A. and Shaw, G. K. (1982). Computerized tomography scan changes in chronic alcoholics: A survey and follow-up study. *Brain* **105**, 497–514.

Steiner-Chaskel, N. and Lader, M. H. (1981). Effects of single doses of clobazam and diazepam on psychological functions in normal subjects. *Royal Society of Medicine International Congress and Symposium Series No. 43*, pp.23–32.

Tansella, M., Zimmermann-Tansella, C. and Lader, M. (1974). The residual effects of *N*-desmethyldiazepam in patients. *Psychopharmacologia*, **38**, 81–90.

Wittenborn, J. R. (1978). Effects of benzodiazepines on psychomotor performance. *Brit. J. clin. Pharmac.*, **5**, 61S–68S.

Wittenborn, J. R. (1979). Benzodiazepines and psychomotor performance, *Brit. J. clin. Pharmac.*, **7**, 61S–67S.

## DISCUSSION

## CHAIRMAN: DR M. TRIMBLE

DR. J. A. GRAY: Are there any data on long-term barbiturate users where one might expect the same picture?

PROFESSOR LADER: One of the controls we wanted to put in was long-term antidepressant users because this would be in a different group. It is known that barbiturates long-term can produce cerebral atrophy and the cerebellum is particularly at risk. But those are high dose users; these are all normal dose users.

DR. GRAY: Presumably you could see whether the better predictor of enlarged ventricles is number of years on benzodiazepines or chronological age.

PROFESSOR LADER: We have looked at both those, and neither correlates with the ventricular changes. But the numbers are rather small, and there may be many confounding factors which attenuate any relationship.

THE CHAIRMAN: We have some parallel evidence in epilepsy with some observations that a small number of people who take phenytoin for a long time develop a dementia. This was partially reversible when the phenytoin was stopped, and the Americans coined the term 'Dilantin dementia' to describe this subgroup of patients.

Over a number of years we have been looking at the effects of anticonvulsant drugs on cognitive function and data suggest that they impair cognitive abilities. I would go a little further, and say that removing patients from anticonvulsant drugs, or lessening their number of drugs, improves the mental state in some patients. I am very interested that you see changes after at least 2 months. In our anticonvulsant work we detect improvements at 3 months and 6 months.

We also have, in volunteer studies, shown that anticonvulsant drugs can impair cognitive function after 14 days' treatment. So I do not think I would entirely agree that after 8–15 days you would not expect to see effects.

PROFESSOR I. OSWALD: I would like to press Dr. Lader a little on one matter, and that is this idea that anxious patients will be improved in skilled performance by these drugs?

PROFESSOR LADER: I think you are very right to take me to task over it, because it is a crucial point as to whether there is a change with medication. After all, if one is saying that one is picking up these effects at the end of 5 years it is going to be very unusual if there is a 2 week, a 2 month or even longer window through which they go and are not impaired.

Certainly the problem is that often you are looking at a moving baseline, the placebo effect. In one study, these drugs were given at night to inpatients who were severely anxious, and it was found that they improved with placebo but showed no improvement with the other drugs, which we could interpret as saying there was an impairment going on. Even there, however, the effects were more at 4 days than at 8 days, as I remember.

In another study where we actually took groups of anxious patients, tested them with a group of age, sex, and social class matched normal individuals, we found very clear impairments of various psychological functioning. When we put them on to various drugs in a sort of crossover, there was actually an improvement of the performance towards the normal level. What we did not know then, of course, was what was happening if we were to retest the normals repeatedly. We did that later, and the curves do tend to go somewhat together; they come together very slightly, which suggests that there is an improvement over and above the practice effect in the anxious patients. I think what happens after that is that the performance then plateaus, and you then start to see these impairments coming in later.

I agree that it is something one has to be very careful about, because one's conclusions are based on a very small number of trials. There have been relatively few studies which have taken a full battery of these tests and looked at them over a time in both anxious patients and normal subjects.

PROFESSOR OSWALD: Is it true to say that, in the human, the beneficial effect of these drugs on such tasks is not really well established?

PROFESSOR LADER: I think that is true, and it is also true to say that it varies from task to task. I certainly think that the tasks which require a fine motor movement are probably the ones which are the least benefited. There are others, such as distraction, which comes into it, where there probably is some improvement; because one of the problems with a lot of these tasks is trying to keep motivation and distractability down. Anxious patients are terribly distractable when you are testing them in a laboratory situation.

DR. SANDRA FILE: I would like to add to something that Professor Oswald said. We were able to divide volunteers into high and low anxious groups, and the high anxious students had scores within the clinical range. On several learning and cognitive tasks, with no fine motor movement at all, they were all significantly impaired with an acute dose of benzodiazepines, and there was no interaction between the level of either state or trait anxiety and the impairment. So on non-clinically ill subjects, but certainly very anxious undergraduates, we still see impairment with the benzodiazepines. I agree with you, I do not know of any evidence of improved learning or performance on cognitive tasks with the benzodiazepines, even in anxious patients.

DR. GRAY: But there is improvement in animals in certain tasks.

DR. SANDRA FILE: Not in learning.

DR. GRAY: In performance.

DR. SANDRA FILE: Could I ask you about some of your results using 1 mg of nitrazepam, where they got significantly better on digit symbol substitution? Were those normal volunteers?

PROFESSOR LADER: They were normal volunteers. I think this is another problem, with the single dose studies—especially with the hypnotic and residual effects—if you give enough, you can usually get a fairly good correlation between the pharmacokinetics and the impairments. When you start repeating it though, you start to get into complications—that is repeating the dose night after night.

DR. SANDRA FILE: Yet on your very first dose you got significant improvement with nitrazepam on digit symbols.

PROFESSOR LADER: Yes, on occasion you can even get that.

DR. SANDRA FILE: But you have shown a much bigger improvement with 1 mg, and yet you were talking about the impairment. It was significantly above the placebos.

PROFESSOR LADER: I think it was 0.5 mg which improved performance. With 1 mg it detracted from performance. Occasionally you get this. Again, we know we have these clinical anecdotal accounts of the disinhibitory effect of low doses, whatever that might mean, and it may be that the dose effect curve is not monotonic but is, in fact, a biphasic dose effect curve.

DR. SANDRA FILE: It was interesting that your symbol copying, your control for motor impairment was reduced at just the dose that was improving the cognitive task.

PROFESSOR LADER: That is right. The decision time was very, very rapid. Instead of doing a number of items in 90 seconds, if you do the reciprocal and take the time to code and then the time to write, which is what the symbol copying is, and take one from the other, you get a thing which we call—probably wrongly—decision time. That is often made very, very fast by low doses of benzodiazepines. This may be an intentional effect, it may be that they have a narrowed attention. This, has, however, been seen in other studies as well, and it does lead to problems in interpreting what dose might clinically be useful.

THE CHAIRMAN: We found very similar things with anticonvulsants too in our volunteer studies. With some of the tests we saw impairment at higher dose levels, but at the lowest serum levels the volunteers are actually doing better on drugs than on placebo. I think this explains, in the anticonvulsant field, why most of them are at one time marketed as psychotropic drugs: in low doses they may well have some anxiolytic properties which help in performance.

DR. SCHMUTZ: I want to come to the point that fine motor movements are affected by benzodiazepines. This may well be due to the fact that benzodiazepines enhance GABA-mediated presynaptic inhibition at the level of the spinal cord. I had the idea that to detect such fine muscle relaxant effects bicycling might be a good thing for, on the one hand, various groups of muscles are activated and deactivated in a rather complex manner and, on the other hand, these are highly regular and repetitive movements that easily could be monitored by electromyography.

PROFESSOR LADER: I am not sure about bicycles. A very sensitive test is the one Professor Richens is using (see chapter 14). We are gradually looking at the effects of benzodiazepines on spinal cord function using the H reflex, but the parameters of setting up the physiology of it is rather complex and it has taken us about 3 years to work out what we should be using. There again, with some pilot studies using diazepam, you can show tremendous disruption of simple monosynaptic reflexes in the spinal cord, and this must be, I think, on a supraspinal influence coming down, but it is very marked.

DR:. COBB: I was wondering whether, in your series, Professor Lader, you found that the patients who had brain atrophy were those you could not get off the tablets.

PROFESSOR LADER: No, half of them had already come off up to 3 months or more, in fact, because we did half of the study prospectively and half of it retrospectively in the sense that we took patients who had come off, and they in a way provided their own two groups. Both groups were about equal for the number of people who were affected. With alcohol brain atrophy there is some evidence that it is slowly reversible but it is very preliminary evidence.

DR. TYRER: May I make a couple of points about the CAT scan work which I think has caused a great deal of concern and worry to clinical psychiatrists? In addition to the two points you make about dementia and organic anxiety being possible explanations of this, one other obvious one is that the benzodiazepine users are also dependent on alcohol.

Second, with the 50 or so patients I have followed up over 3 months after coming off chronic benzodiazepines there is certainly no clinical evidence, though I have to admit they have had no formal testing, that the patients in any way have any cognitive deficit. On the contrary, most of them repeatedly comment on how much more alert they are, and emphasize the point that has been made frequently, that when people are on chronic benzodiazepines they are in fact slightly under par, as far as many aspects of cognitive function are concerned.

PROFESSOR LADER: There are several points there. As far as we know clinically from interviewing the patients, they were not abusing alcohol at the same time. It does not mean to say they had not abused it previously but we think not. We have to rely here on their history. I think it is fair to say that we are not dealing with the sort of alcoholic population where you really cannot believe a word they tell you. These people are typically rather nice, somewhat bewildered middle-aged housewives. So I do not think the alcohol is a point, but I certainly am aware that what we may be looking at is a potentiation of alcohol by the benzodiazepines and as there is potentiation in other systems I do not see why there should not be one here.

As far as the withdrawal is concerned, certainly you can show quite marked CAT scan changes when you get withdrawal from steroids. This is known. We have in our benzodiazepine withdrawn patients looked at cortisol levels as a matter of routine and there were no systematic changes there, although certainly there were weight changes and perhaps fluid loss, but again, half of our patients were more than 3 months after the withdrawal and usually by then there is very little in the way of any metabolic changes.

As far as looking at them clinically is concerned, yes, clinically they seemed to be functioning better after their withdrawal than they were previously, but some of them do describe, even then, that they are 'not the person they used to be'. Again, this is not evidence, but it is sufficient for me to really want to use as objective a battery of tests as possible before I conclude there is not any danger.

# Index